Diffe
Diagnosis of Body Fluids in Small Animal Cytology

Differential Diagnosis of Body Fluids in Small Animal Cytology

Francesco Cian
and
Paola Monti

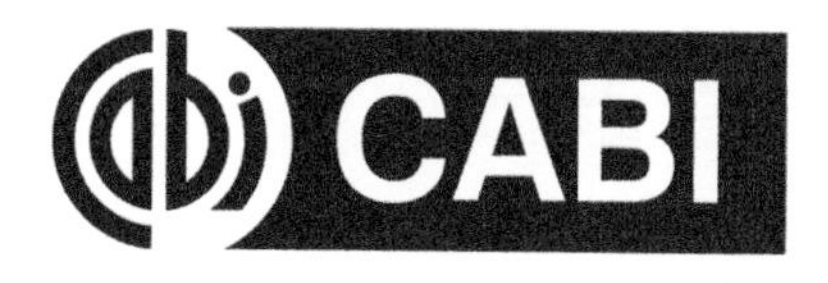

CABI is a trading name of CAB International

CABI
Nosworthy Way
Wallingford
Oxfordshire OX10 8DE
UK

Tel: +44 (0)1491 832111
E-mail: info@cabi.org
Website: www.cabi.org

CABI
200 Portland Street
Boston
MA 02114
USA

Tel: +1 (617)682-9015
E-mail: cabi-nao@cabi.org

A catalogue record for this book is available from the British Library, London, UK.

ISBN-13: 9781789247763 (paperback)
9781789247770 (ePDF)
9781789247787 (ePub)

DOI: 10.1079/9781789247787.0000

Commissioning Editor: Alexandra Lainsbury
Editorial Assistant: Emma McCann
Production Editor: James Bishop

Typeset by Straive, Pondicherry, India
Printed and bound by CPI Group (UK) Ltd, Croydon, CR0 4YY

E' meglio avere dubbi che false certezze (Luigi Pirandello)
Doubt is better than false certainties (Luigi Pirandello)

Preface

It has been four years since we published for CABI a book on small animal cytology of the skin and subcutis. From its conception, it was designed to be a practical resource for diagnostic and as a revision aid. The positive feedback we received from colleagues all over the world was so powerful that it led us to consider expanding it by covering other subjects.

In the extraordinary circumstances that have characterized the past few years we believed it was an opportune moment to embark on a new project, this time focused on body cavities fluids. These, together with the skin/subcutis and the lymph nodes, are the types of samples that are most frequently collected and analysed in general practices.

This book is not only aimed at clinical pathologists and residents, but also at all veterinarians and students who share our passion for cytology and recognize its power as a diagnostic tool. As one of our former supervisors, Dr. Kathleen Freeman, always likes to say *"Clinical pathologists (and clinicians in general), are storytellers"*. And this is our story about fluid cytology.

Francesco Cian
Paola Monti

Contents

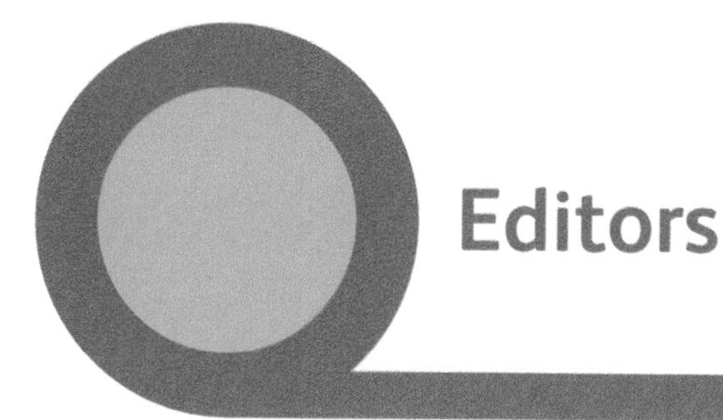

Editors

Francesco Cian, DVM, DipECVCP, FRCPath, MRCVS—Francesco graduated from the University of Padua (Italy) with a DVM in 2006. He spent the next 4 years in small animal practice. In 2010, he started a residency programme in Clinical Pathology at the University of Cambridge (UK), which he finished in 2013, attaining both the ECVCP and FRCPath diplomas. In 2015, he also received the RCVS Specialist Status in Veterinary Clinical Pathology.

Francesco joined the Animal Health Trust (AHT) in 2013 as Head of Clinical Pathology, and since September 2015, he has been working for BattLab (LABOKLIN). Francesco is the current secretary of the European College of Veterinary Clinical Pathology (ECVCP) and is a member of the cytology exam committee for the same college. He is author of several publications on peer-reviewed journals and editor of three cytology books. He also co-edited with Paola Monti the cytology chapter of the 3rd edition of the *BSAVA Manual of Veterinary Clinical Pathology.*

Francesco is a passionate educator and provides postgraduate education in cytology to veterinarians. He is the founder of the online group Veterinary Cytology.

Paola Monti, DVM, MSc, FRCPath, DipACVP (Clinical Pathology) MRCVS—Paola qualified from the University of Bologna (Italy) with a DVM in 2022. In 2005, she moved to the UK, where she spent the first years in general practice. In 2008, she started a Royal College Veterinary Surgeons (RCVS) Trust founded residency programme in Veterinary Clinical Pathology at the University of Cambridge. After her training, she obtained both the ACVP and FRCPath diplomas in Clinical Pathology, and in 2015, she received the RCVS Specialist Status in Veterinary Clinical Pathology.

In 2012, Paola joined Dick White Referrals, an internationally renowned specialist veterinary hospital, where she remained as a Senior Clinical Pathologist for 9 years. In 2021, Paola moved to Switzerland, where she co-founded the VCO-lab. Here she mostly focuses on cytology and haematology.

In these years, Paola participated in several publications and was co-author of the cytology chapter of the 3rd edition of the *BSAVA Manual of Veterinary Clinical Pathology* and co-editor of the cytology book *Differential Diagnosis in Small Animal Cytology: The Skin and Subcutis.*

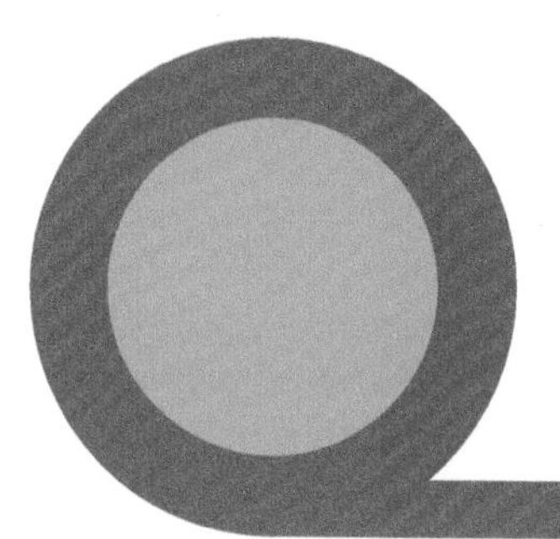

Differential Diagnosis in Small Animal Cytology: Body Fluids

Chapter 1 – Sample Collection, Preparation, General Assessment and Microbiology Testing of Fluids

This chapter covers the general recommendations for collection and analysis of fluid samples. It describes the processing and handling of the samples and slide preparation and staining. A large section is dedicated to further diagnostic techniques applied to body cavity fluids and in particular microbiology testing.

Chapter 2 – Respiratory Tract Fluids

This chapter explores the cytology of respiratory tract fluids, in particular nasal flushes, tracheal washes (TWs) and bronchoalveolar lavages (BALs). Topics covered include sampling techniques, specimens handling, analysis and slide preparation. Cytology findings of unremarkable and pathological respiratory secretions are covered in detail, exploring a wide variety of inflammatory, infectious, and neoplastic processes affecting both upper and lower respiratory airways. The chapter is enriched with numerous photomicrographs, which will represent a valid diagnostic aid for the readers.

Chapter 3 – Body Cavity Effusions

This chapter is subdivided into pleural, pericardial and abdominal effusions. The first general part is dedicated to the anatomy and physiology of these three cavities and to sample collection, handling and analysis. For each type of effusion, the pathophysiology of fluid accumulation is described, and the most common and less frequent cytological abnormalities are described in detail. The chapter is enriched with numerous photomicrographs, which represents a valid diagnostic aid for the readers.

Chapter 4 – Synovial Fluid

This chapter covers the synovial fluid cytology from the unremarkable findings to the most common pathologic conditions. Various inflammatory, infectious, degenerative and neoplastic processes are described in detail. Sampling techniques, slide preparation and staining are also included. The chapter features numerous photomicrographs that provide a visual representation of the most common cytological abnormalities encountered in this district.

Chapter 5 – Cerebrospinal Fluid (CSF)

This chapter describes the most common cytological findings encountered in CSF analysis. It includes a general part on the anatomy and physiology of the cerebrospinal fluid and a dedicated section in which the most common cytological alterations observed in inflammatory, reactive and neoplastic conditions affecting the CNS are described in detail. The chapter is enriched with plentiful photomicrographs.

Chapter 6 – Aqueous and Vitreous Humour

This chapter examines the not so widely used cytology of the aqueous and vitreous humours. Sampling techniques, handling and fluid analysis are covered and culminate in a detailed description of the most common pathological conditions that may be diagnosed via cytological examination of these fluids. This is accompanied by photomicrographs.

Chapter 7 – Bile Fluid

This short chapter covers the principles of bile cytology, from sample collection to analysis. The most common inflammatory and non-inflammatory conditions that may be diagnosed via cytology are covered and are accompanied by photomicrographs.

Chapter 8 – Urogenital Fluids

This chapter represents a guide to the cytological examination of both unstained and stained urine sediment and prostatic wash. It covers the most common inflammatory, infectious and neoplastic conditions involving the urogenital tract and is accompanied by photomicrographs for reference.

Chapter 9 – Additional Techniques to Refine the Cytologic Diagnosis in Fluid Samples

This chapter represents a practical guide to the choice of the most suitable additional techniques to complement the cytologic exam of fluids, in order to reach the most specific and accurate diagnosis. Tests covered include cytochemistry, immunocytochemistry, cell pellet immunohisto-chemistry, flow cytometry, clonality testing (PARR) and BRAF mutation.

Sample Collection, Preparation, General Assessment and Microbiology Testing of Fluids

Marta Costa

Fluid samples are often collected in veterinary clinical practice to either establish the cause for fluid accumulation (e.g. body cavity effusions) or assess underlying pathologies associated with the organs or systems where the fluid is present (e.g. bile, cerebrospinal fluid [CSF], etc.).

In some instances, fluids can be instilled and collected from lavages to help evaluating the target organs (e.g. bronchoalveolar lavage [BAL], prostatic washes).

1.1 General Recommendations for Collection of Fluid Samples

Specific collection details for each fluid type are discussed in the dedicated chapters.

Site preparation

- Sterile collection of the sample is always recommended.
- The area should be clipped and cleaned with alcohol.
- For ultrasound-guided samples, contamination with ultrasound gel should be avoided by cleaning the area and using alcohol or sterile water as a coupling medium.

Materials

- Clippers.
- Disinfectant.
- Needles (21–25 G) and butterfly needles.
- Syringes (2–10 ml).
- Three-way stopcock: this can be used to facilitate collection of large amounts of fluid. Collection into a urine collection bag may help prevent environmental contamination.
- EDTA and sterile, leak-proof plain tubes.
- Glass slides.

1.2 General Sample Processing

Macroscopic appearance

- The macroscopic characteristics of the fluid are recorded, as these can provide useful information on its composition.
- They include the following:
  - Colour: colourless, pink (blood tinged), yellow (e.g. icteric sample), green (bile), etc. The sudden appearance of blood during aspiration is a reliable indicator of a traumatic tap.
  - Turbidity: it can be assessed by the ability to read the label through a filled tube, as shown in Fig. 1.1.

DOI: 10.1079/9781789247787.0001

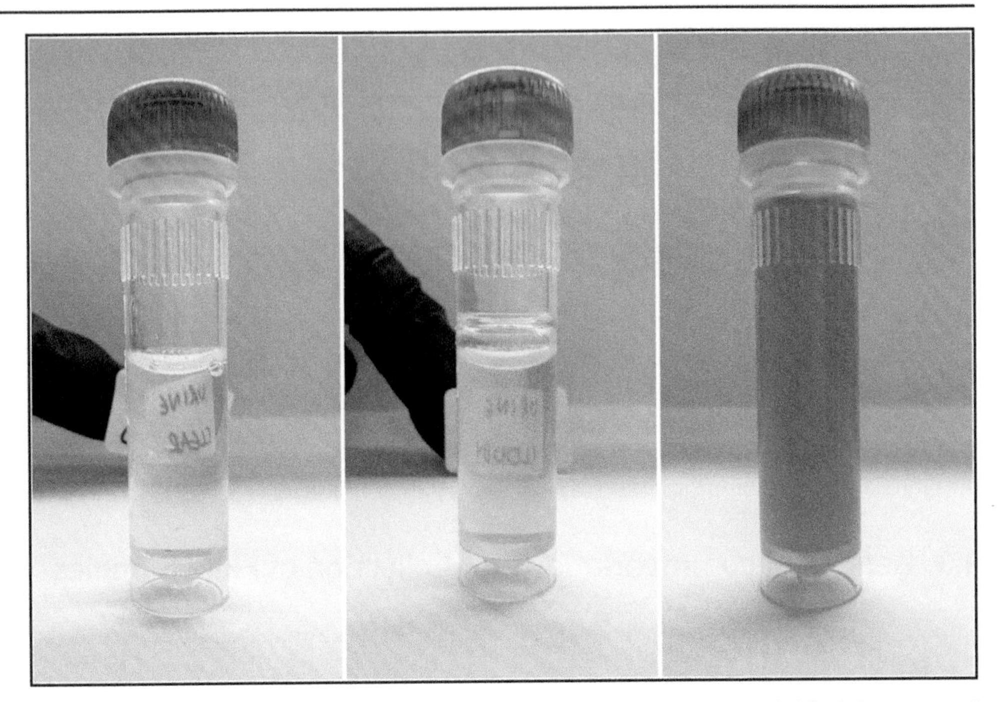

Fig. 1.1. Fluid turbidity assessment. From left to right: clear, moderately turbid and turbid fluid. Assessment of turbidity can be achieved by looking through the fluid across a label. In a clear fluid (left), a label can be read through the filled tube. In a moderately turbid fluid (centre), this becomes more difficult, and it is not possible any more in a turbid fluid (right).

Container selection and sample handling

- EDTA tube: used for preparation of cytology samples and to measure total cell count (when required). It can also be used for ancillary tests, such as polymerase chain reactions (PCRs) and flow cytometry.
- Plain sterile tubes: used for biochemistry analysis and culture testing.

Pearls and Pitfalls

- Some reference laboratories recommend to collect an aliquot of fluid into a separate EDTA tube and add a drop of formalin to improve cell preservation. However, this is discouraged if only one tube is available because formalin interferes with the staining quality of the cells and would make the sample unsuitable for any further testing.
- If sample handling and processing are delayed, specimens should be stored refrigerated until they reach the external laboratory, in order to slow down degeneration of cellular elements and decrease bacterial overgrowth.
- Refrigeration may result in some spurious changes (e.g. *in vitro* formation of urine crystals).
- Samples should not be frozen, as this will cause cell rupture.
- Samples for culture placed in transport medium should not be refrigerated.
- Sample recommendations for urine samples will depend on the collection method.
- When using serum clot activator tubes to collect fluid samples, amorphous (contaminant) structures may be found at times. These may vary in shape but often appears as rectangular, square, ladder-type, or round unstained structures.

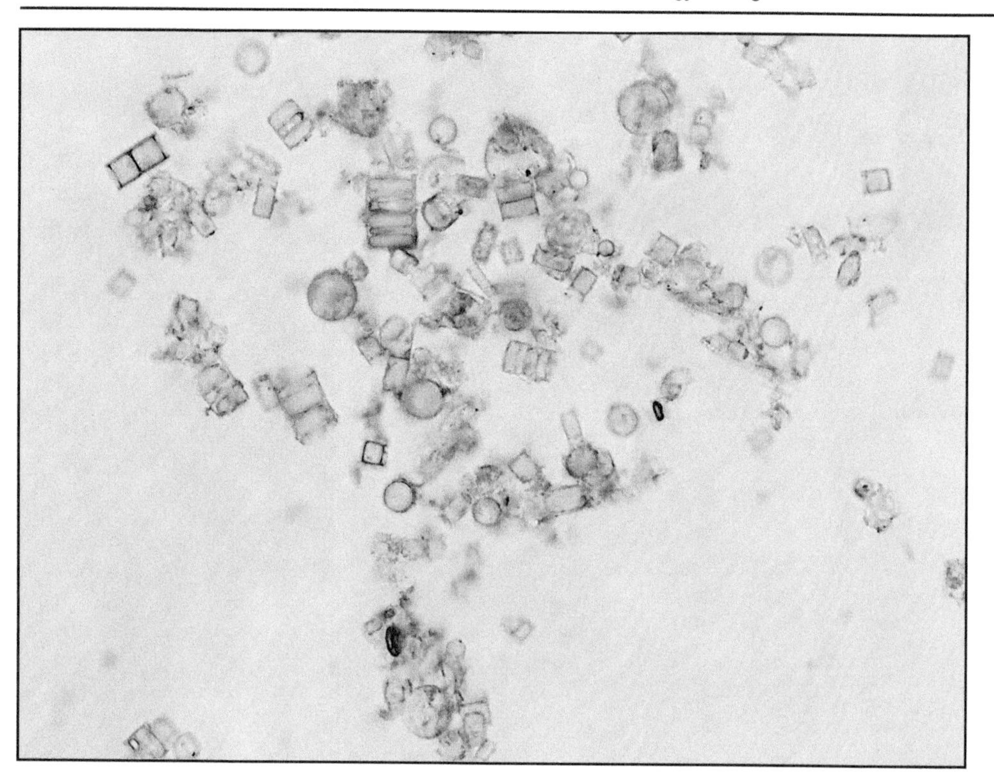

Fig. 1.2. Unstained ladder-like and round structures (contaminants) from a fluid sample collected in a serum clot activator tube. Wright-Giemsa. (Courtesy of William Gow.)

1.3 Slides Preparation

Fresh direct smears should be prepared for all fluids that are collected for cytological examination, particularly if samples are not processed immediately.

1.3.1 Smear preparation techniques

Depending on the characteristics and cellularity of the fluids, different techniques can be used to prepare fresh smears.

Squash preparation

Use

- Recommended for highly viscous fluids or when flocculent material is recovered.
- It can also be used to spread the cell pellet obtained from a fluid concentration (sediment).

Technique

- A drop of fluid is placed on one slide (Fig 1.3. A). A spreader slide is laid across the sample slide at right angle and the sample allowed to spread. With no downward pressure, the two slides are pulled apart (Fig. 1.3. B), creating two smears.
- Both smears should be retained for examination.
- Excessive downward pressure applied during the procedure may result in cell rupture.
- Slides obtained with this technique should have a *flame* shape (Fig. 1.3. C), ending before the edge of the slide. Most of the material will lie in the centre of the slide with all margins being examinable. Cells should be intact and distributed in a monolayer.

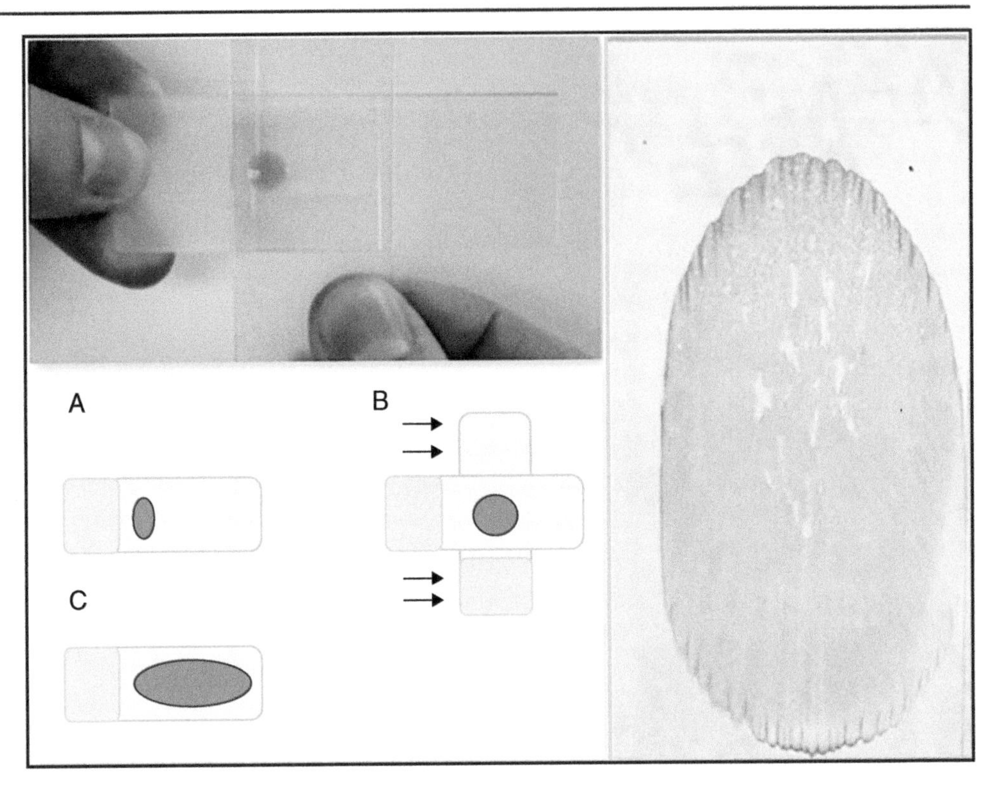

Fig. 1.3. Squash preparation technique.

Blood smear technique

Use

- Recommended for fluid samples that appear turbid or with a blood-like appearance.

Technique

- Slide can be prepared using the blood smear technique.
- A drop of specimen is placed at the end of a slide. The end of a second slide is placed in front of the drop at approximately a 30°–45° angle and slide backwards until it comes into contact with the sample drop. The sample will spread out along the width of the spreader slide. The spreader slide is advanced forwards, creating a smear with a feathered edge.
- To avoid creating excessively long smears, a greater angle of the spreader slide can be used, especially when the fluid is poorly cellular.

Line smear preparation

Use

- Used to concentrate poorly cellular fluids, when further instrumentation is not available.

Technique

- The procedure is similar to the blood smear technique, but instead of completing the smear, the spreader slide is lifted vertically prior to formation of a feathered edge. This results in concentration of cells along the 'line' where the smear is interrupted.
- This thick concentrated area (where the excess fluid has dried) allows to assess more cells in a smaller section of the slide. However, cellular morphology may be compromised by cells being poorly spread and condensed.

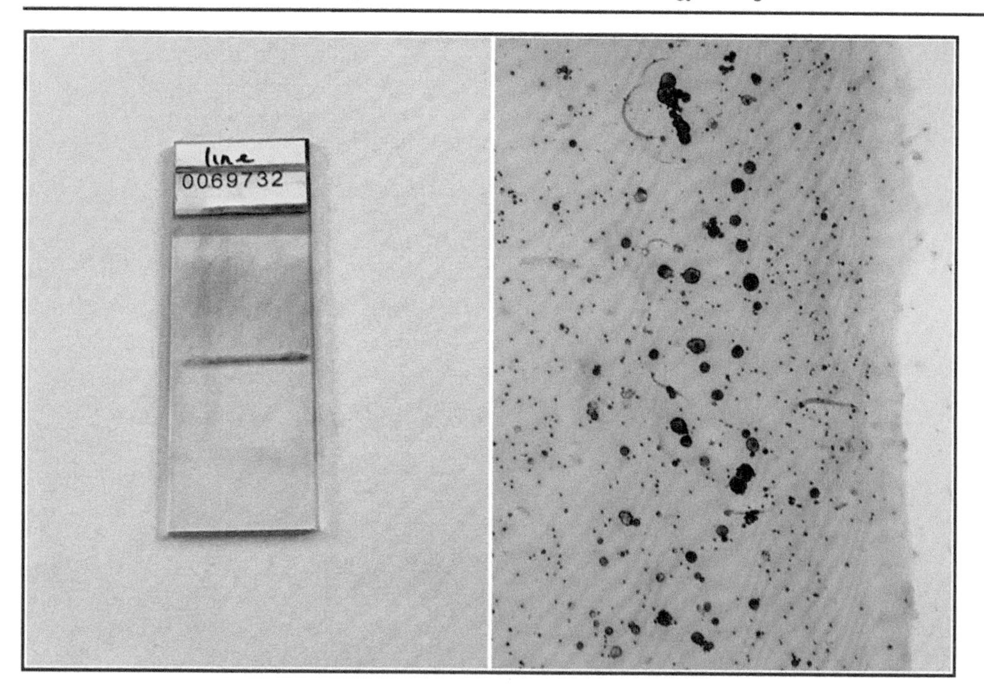

Fig. 1.4. Line smear preparation. (Left) Note the line of concentrated cells in the middle of the smear, instead of a feathered edge. (Right) Microscopic appearance of the concentrated area.

Sediment smear

Use

- Recommended procedure for hypocellular fluids.
- Sediment preparations can also be used to concentrate cells in more cellular fluids when needed.
- Cell estimates are not possible from concentrated smears.

Technique

- Fill a conical-tip centrifuge tube with the fluid. Centrifuge at low speed (~400 g) for 5 min.
- After centrifugation, remove most of the supernatant with a pipette. Resuspend the sediment with the remaining fluid.
- Collect a drop of that fluid with a pipette, and transfer it on to a microscope slide. Use either a line or blood smear technique.
- For hypocellular fluids with a low protein concentration, the use of precoated slides may be considered and would facilitate cell adhesion.

Pearls and Pitfalls

There is often confusion about the relationship between RPM (revolutions per minute) and RCF (relative centrifugal force - also known as G force), and which parameter is most important in centrifugal applications. In a centrifugal process, RCF/G force is what is affecting the sample, so it's important that this is known. To calculate RCF/G force from RPM, the following equation can be used: RCF = 1.1118 x 10^-5 x R x RPM^2. R is radius of the rotor expressed in centimeters. If you would rather not do the calculations yourself, there are online converters available to help.

Buffy coat preparation

Use

- Concentration technique seldomly used in haemorrhagic fluids.

Technique

- Prepare a microhaematocrit tube with the fluid specimen.
- After spinning at high speed with a dedicated centrifuge, break the tube just below the buffy coat area. Expel the buffy coat material on to a slide, and smear it using the blood smear technique.

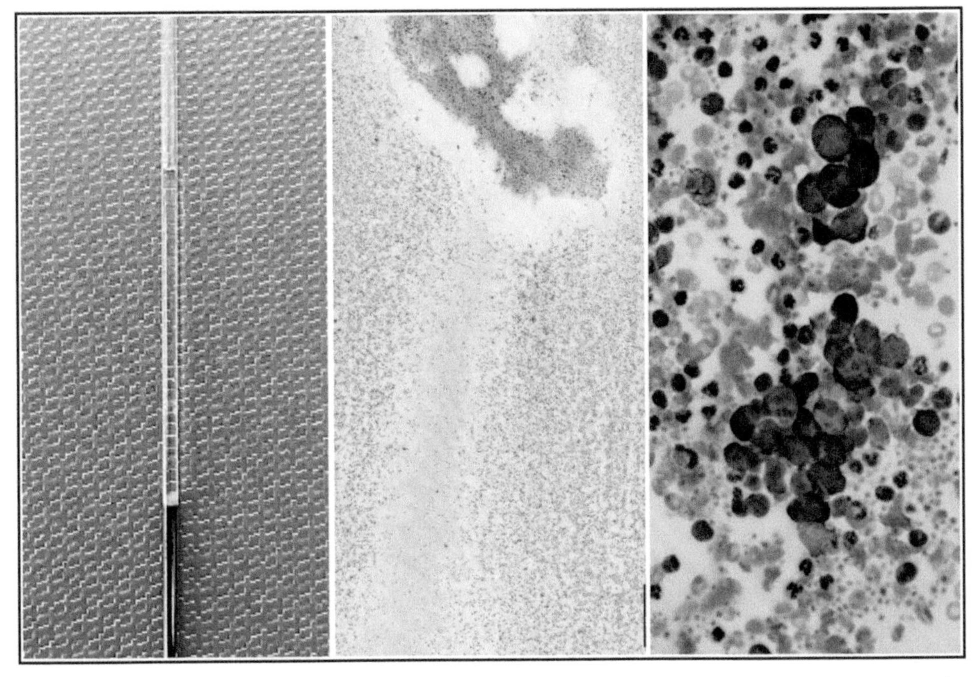

Fig. 1.5. Buffy coat procedure. (Left) Microhaematocrit tube. Note the white area within the tube representing the buffy coat. (Centre, Right) Microscopic appearance of the buffy coat on the smear at low and high magnification.

Cytospin

Use

- Technique often used in referral laboratories to process hypocellular fluids.
- The aim is to concentrate the cellular elements on to a glass slide while maintaining good cellular preservation.

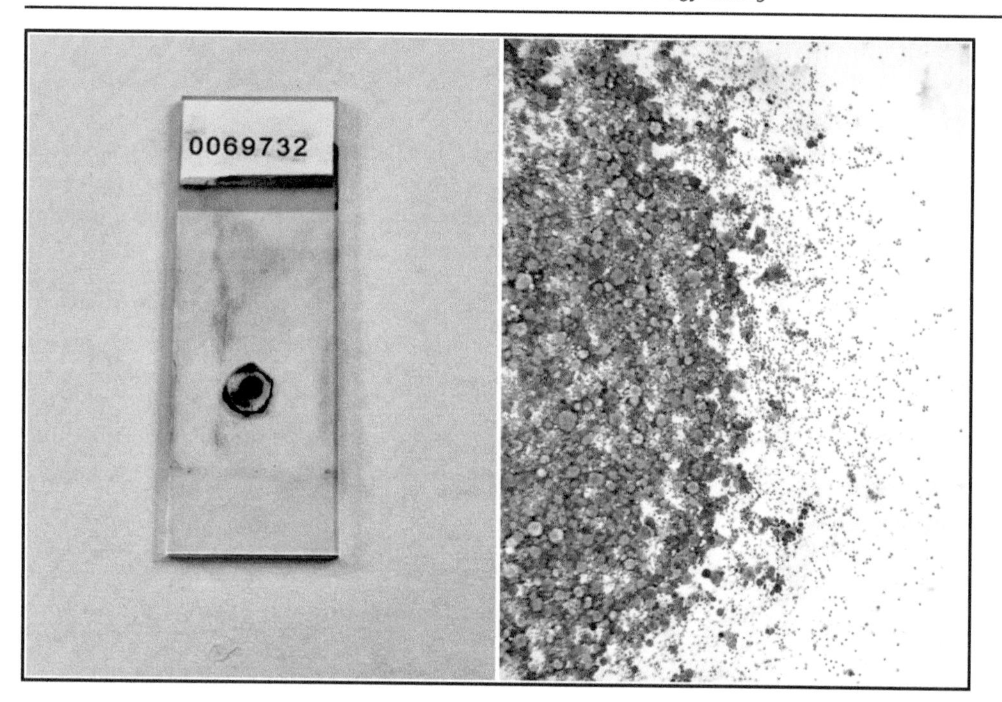

Fig. 1.6. Cytospin technique. (Left) Cytospin preparation. Note the circular area on the slide containing most cells from the fluid sample. (Right) Microscopic appearance of the concentrated area.

1.4 Slide Staining

- Stains most commonly used for cytology fluid specimens are of Romanowsky type and include:
  - Rapid stains: e.g. Diff-Quik.
  - Wright-Giemsa.
  - Modified Wright stains.
- Wright stains provide excellent nuclear detail, including adequate staining of mast cell granules.
- Staining protocols should follow manufacturer recommendations.
- Some stains can be used to highlight the presence of certain organisms (Chapter 9).

Pearls and Pitfalls

Slides must be fully air-dried before any staining procedure is applied. In viscous and thick samples (e.g. synovial fluids), this may take longer. Allow smears to dry by waving them or using a hair dryer or fan in cold settings. No additional fixation is necessary ahead of staining.

1.5 Cell Count

- Nucleated cell count is routinely performed for selected body fluids (e.g. CSF, synovial fluid, body cavity effusions), but not for fluids obtained from the respiratory tract (e.g. nasal flush, tracheal wash, bronchoalveolar lavage), as their cellularity is strongly dependent on the sampling procedure.
- Manual count using a modified Neubauer chamber is the most common method used for CSF and synovial cell count. For most other fluids, nucleated cell count is obtained via an automated haematology analyser.
- Accuracy of automated cell count will vary depending on the analyser and fluid matrix. Fluids with clots or flocculent material will result in inaccurate cell counts (falsely reduced numbers). Cell counts from fluids that are thick and dense may also be inaccurate and can cause blockage of the haematology analyser.
- For some fluids (e.g. synovial fluids), a subjective cell estimate can also be made from the monolayer of a well-spread smear and is discussed in the dedicated chapters.

1.6 Biochemistry Assays

- Biochemistry assays can be performed for most fluids as part of the routine analysis or to answer specific questions.
- The most common biochemistry assay performed on body cavity fluids is total protein.
- Ideally, the fluid sample for biochemistry assays is collected in a plain sterile tube, but most assays can be performed on EDTA samples.
- The biochemistry analysis (dipstick and urine proteine:creatinine ratio) on urine must be performed on plain urine.

1.7 Microbiology Testing in Body Cavity Fluids

Investigations for an underlying infectious disease can be done by different direct and indirect methods.

1.7.1 Direct visualization of bacteria

- Cytological evidence of organisms in fluids has high specificity for the presence of an infection, particularly when associated with inflammation and when intracellular organisms are identified. Unfortunately, this has a relatively low sensitivity as a diagnostic technique, and false-negative results often occur. The presence of commensal flora or environmental contaminants superimposed on sterile inflammation may lead to false positives, which should be carefully interpreted in non-sterile fluids (e.g. free catch urine, nasal flush).

Advantages

- It provides additional context for relevance of the organisms recovered on culture.
- It aids in the differentiation between transient colonization and true infection.
- It aids in identifying the predominant organism in mixed cultures.
- It sometimes allows identification of the pathogens in cases of false-negative cultures that may occur in the following situations:
  - Presence of fastidious or slow-growing organisms.
  - When inhibitors that may preclude bacterial growth have been used prior to sample collection: e.g. antimicrobial therapy.
  - When organisms are present but non-viable.

Limitations

- It does not distinguish between the presence of viable and non-viable organisms.
- In most cases, it does not allow for a definitive and accurate identification of infectious agents involved at a genus/species level.
- It is unable to distinguish between a primary infection caused by obligate pathogens and overgrowth of normal commensal flora or contamination with opportunistic environmental organisms.
- It does not provide information that may guide targeted antimicrobial treatment, and additional tests are required for getting that information.

1.7.2 Special stains

The use of special stains can increase the sensitivity of identification of organisms on cytological specimens. Cytochemical and immunocytochemical stains that can be used to identify different types of organisms are extensively discussed in Chapter 9.

1.7.3 Direct visualization of other infectious organisms

- Fungal organisms can also be found on cytology examination. Presumptive identification on cytology is based on morphology and often aided by the geographical area and anatomical location of the infection.
- Identification of fungal organisms can be challenging using routine stains, and the lack of organisms on cytology does not exclude infection. Special stains, such as periodic acid-Schiff (PAS) and Gomori methenamine silver (GMS), can improve detection of these organisms on cytological examination (Chapter 9).
- Several studies in the human field have revealed overlap in morphology between species of fungal organisms and limitations in cytological identification that may lead to inappropriate antifungal treatment choices. Therefore, confirmatory tests of the presumptive cytological diagnosis are recommended.
- Similarly to bacteria, fungal organisms can represent contaminants from the environment or opportunistic pathogens. Yeasts can be part of the normal commensal flora or may cause infections. Therefore, cytological and clinical information is helpful in interpreting the significance of these organisms when cultured.
- Parasite and protozoal detection on cytology can also be of low sensitivity but is highly specific when present. Identification of these organisms is often sufficient to indicate infection. However, due to the low sensitivity of cytological methods for the detection of these organisms, additional diagnostic tests are recommended when infection is suspected or needs to be excluded.
- Knowledge of the life cycle and physiopathology of the infectious agent is needed to select the best diagnostic modality. As per fungal organisms, cytomorphological overlap between different species can occur; therefore, correlation with clinical findings and risk of exposure may aid in prioritizing differentials.

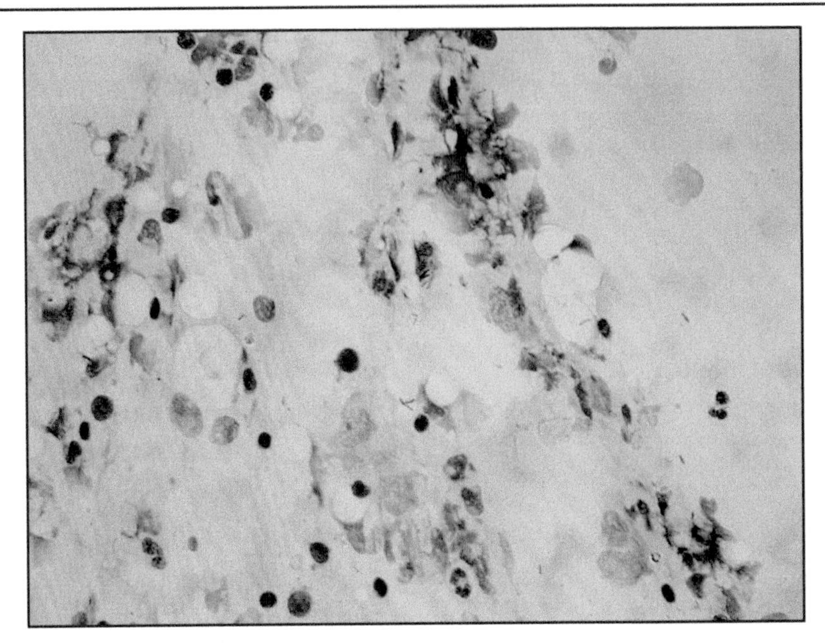

Fig. 1.7. Ziehl-Neelsen stain. Acid-fast bacilli are bright red after staining.

1.7.4 Microbiology culture

As for cytological examination, quality of the sample will influence the diagnostic yield of microbiology assays.

1.7.4.1 General recommendations for collection of samples for culture

- Samples should be collected for culture prior to starting antimicrobial therapy. When this cannot be withheld, a sample should be collected as soon as possible and the initiated therapy mentioned in the submission form.
- Samples should be collected into a sterile leak-proof container (simple plain sterile tubes or tubes with a medium). Where possible, sterile collection is encouraged.
- Ideally, a minimum fluid volume of 1–5 ml should be submitted for culture testing.
- Samples rather than swabs of the fluids are the preferred specimen type to facilitate comprehensive investigation. Use of swabs with transport media can be used when less volume is available or where there is concern for organism viability (e.g. viral culture or anaerobes).
- For selected fastidious organisms (e.g. *Mycoplasma* spp.) or viral culture, special media are recommended. Fastidious organisms are those with complex or specific growth requirements that may not be easily cultured without those specific conditions.
- The use of swabs is not recommended for urine samples, as it does not allow for quantification of organisms. Urine samples have their own set of recommendations that depend on the collection method.
- For selected fluids (e.g. CSF or synovial fluids), the use of blood culture bottles or specific enrichment media can increase the likelihood of identifying a bacterial infection. As for the boric acid, recommended sample volumes should be respected. When lower volumes are used, the sensitivity of the culture is decreased.

- Samples should reach the microbiology laboratory as soon as possible after collection. If not placed in transport medium, samples should be kept moist and refrigerated (except for anaerobes).
- Some organisms have a zoonotic potential (e.g. *Brucella* spp. and *Blastomyces* spp.) and may lead to laboratory-acquired infections. In such cases, immunoassays or molecular testing may be more appropriate than culture. When a zoonosis is suspected clinically, this should always be mentioned in the submission form.

1.7.4.2 Bacterial aerobic culture

- Aerobic cultures should be considered for any sample where a bacterial infection is suspected.
- Selection of culture media and incubation conditions vary depending on the target site and organism(s) of interest.
- For selected organisms such as Mycoplasmas, Actinomyces and Mycobacteria, special media, incubation conditions and culture times differ. Therefore, when the presence of these organisms is suspected (clinically or cytologically), the microbiology laboratory should be informed.

1.7.4.3 Bacterial anaerobic culture

- Anaerobic cultures should be considered for any fluid where anaerobic bacteria may find appropriate conditions for growth (reduced oxygen content). There are several anaerobes that are part of the commensal flora, particularly in the upper and lower gastrointestinal tract.
- In fluid samples, anaerobes are most commonly seen in body cavity fluids or bile.
- Anaerobes can also be of clinical significance in:
  - Any fluid that is associated with penetrating wounds or migrating foreign bodies.
  - In the respiratory tract, if associated with aspiration pneumonia.
- Anaerobic infections are often mixed, either with multiple anaerobes (mixed anaerobes recovered) or with concurrent aerobes and facultative bacteria (e.g. *Pasteurella* spp., *Escherichia coli* or other *Enterobacterales*).
- The volume of specimen influences the stability of the sample. Large volumes of fluid maintain viability of anaerobes for longer. Anaerobes do not survive when exposed to oxygen. Therefore, *in vitro* recovery is increased if contact with air is reduced. This may be achieved by:
  - Collecting a sufficient amount of fluid to fully fill the tube.
  - Using appropriate transport media (recommended).
- Anaerobes are particularly susceptible to delayed analysis, and samples should be processed as soon as possible, ideally within 24 h from collection. Organisms may remain viable in the media up to 48 h. The older the sample, the lower the bacterial recovery.
- Samples for anaerobic culture should ideally not be refrigerated, as oxygen diffuses into cold specimens more rapidly than specimens held at room temperature. However, refrigeration of samples not placed in culture media is preferable for the remaining fluid analysis (including aerobic microbiology).
- Anaerobic culture requires special culture conditions. Anaerobes grow more slowly than aerobes, so results are usually delayed when compared with aerobic culture results.

1.7.4.4 Bacterial identification

Correct bacterial identification to the genus and also to the species level is important to provide a more accurate assessment of the significance of growth. It is also relevant to ensure the correct antimicrobial susceptibility testing is performed and to assess for intrinsic antimicrobial resistance and treatment guidelines.

Bacterial identification can be performed by different methods:

- Presumptive bacterial identification starts with evaluation of growth characteristics of recovered colonies in different media (e.g. haemolysis in blood agar or lactose fermentation).
- Gram staining is used to differentiate between Gram-positive and Gram-negative organisms and between cocci and bacilli (rods).
- Biochemistry reactions (e.g. catalase, coagulase and oxidase) are used for separation into large groups of organisms (e.g. catalase-positive Gram-positive cocci).
- Selective and chromogenic media may be used to presumptively identify specific pathogenic organisms.
- Commercial biochemistry strips or batteries of assays can be used to more fully identify bacteria based on their enzymatic activity or sugar metabolism. Similar automated assays are available and allow for identification of bacteria in 24–48 h. Newer technologies allow for quicker identification of organisms and are becoming more common in veterinary microbiology (e.g. MALDI-TOF-MS).
- MALDI-TOF-MS stands for matrix-assisted laser desorption ionization time-of-flight mass spectrometry. These systems use mass spectrometry to analyse the chemical composition of an organism and allow its accurate and quick identification, providing that there is a reference spectrum for the organism in the database used. Clinical and veterinary databases are constantly being improved, allowing for correct identification of most organisms of interest in routine veterinary microbiology.
- MALDI-TOF methods can be used for anaerobic and anaerobic bacteria and for identification of some yeasts and fungi. The accurate and quick results allow for a shorter turn-around-time and better processing of mixed cultures and samples from non-sterile sites, where commensal or environmental organisms can more easily be differentiated from pathogens. The more accurate identification of the organisms allows the identification of the correct antimicrobial susceptibility breakpoints (e.g. using the correct method of screening for methicillin resistance in different species of staphylococci).
- Identified organisms are then evaluated for significance by taking account of the following:
  - Species of the organism.
  - Species of the patient.
  - Specimen origin.
  - Collection method (sterile *vs* non-sterile).
  - Level of growth (profuse *vs* scant).
  - Growth in mixed *vs* pure culture and predominance of growth in mixed cultures.
  - Additional clinical data, such as clinical history (including prior antimicrobial treatments), cytology results and other diagnostic findings. These are critical points in the evaluation of the results and require experience to provide the best outcome.

1.7.4.5 Antimicrobial susceptibility testing

Glossary and definitions

AMR: Antimicrobial resistance

AST: Antimicrobial susceptibility testing

Clinical breakpoint: Interpretative criteria for the assessment of AST results based on the expected effective concentration of the antimicrobial at the site of infection, following systemic administration at established doses.

CLSI: Clinical and laboratory standards institute

EUCAST: European Committee on AST
MDR: Multidrug-resistant bacteria
MIC: Minimum inhibitory concentration. The lowest concentration of antimicrobial drug that inhibits visible growth of an organism over a defined incubation period, most commonly 18–24 h.
VetCAST: Veterinary committee on antimicrobial susceptibility testing

- AST assesses the *in vitro* likelihood of treatment efficacy of systemic antimicrobial therapy by comparing test results with established guidelines.
- Given the increased recognition of AMR in organisms recovered from veterinary patients and the known impact of AMR in global One Health, AST is essential for best practice in treatment of bacterial infections and appropriate antimicrobial use.
- AST can be performed using dilution or diffusion methods and may provide quantitative (e.g. MIC) or qualitative results (susceptible, intermediate susceptibility and resistant), as established by either CLSI or VetCAST (a subcommittee of the EUCAST).
- The MIC value or area of zone inhibition read by disk diffusion is compared with the clinical breakpoint to determine susceptibility and to classify the organism as susceptible, intermediate or resistant. Different definitions for the qualitative categories are considered, depending on guidelines used. Briefly:
  - Susceptible: an organism that is likely to respond to a standard antimicrobial dose regimen.
  - Intermediate: an organism that may not respond to the standard dose regime, but increased exposure to the antimicrobial (by adjusting the dosing regimen or by increasing the concentration at the site of infection) increases likelihood of therapeutical response.
  - Resistant: an organism is categorized as resistant when there is likely therapeutical failure, even if there is increased exposure.

Exact definitions can be found at https://www.eucast.org and https://www.clsi.org/.

- Clinical breakpoints should be defined for each combination of organism, antimicrobial and species of the patient, and for different target sites, if there are differences in tissue distribution (e.g. concentration of antimicrobial in urine). Unfortunately, this information is not available for many antimicrobials for different species of veterinary interest. In such cases, human or other species' breakpoints might be the only available resource, which may not reflect the efficacy *in vivo* due to interspecies differences in pharmacokinetics and pharmacodynamics. Efforts are under way to expand the number of breakpoints available in veterinary medicine.
- AST results may not be reported for all antimicrobial-organism combinations for several reasons:
  - There are no clinical breakpoints defined for that organism or antimicrobial combination.
  - The organism is intrinsically resistant, and clinical failure is expected even if it appears susceptible *in vitro*. Table 1.1 shows selected intrinsic resistances for organisms commonly reported in veterinary samples.
  - An equivalent antimicrobial is reported and allows for predicted susceptibility (e.g. Enterobacterales susceptible to ampicillin can be considered susceptible to amoxicillin or a single first-generation cephalosporin is tested with results valid for all first-generation cephalosporins). In such cases, the S, I and R categories may be reported without an MIC.
  - For some organisms, growth characteristics preclude routine susceptibility testing in most laboratory settings. In these cases, published reports in medical literature and current consensus recommendations for therapy may be provided.
  - The use of some antibacterial drugs should be restricted to severe MDR infections, and selective reporting can be useful in reducing inappropriate use.

1.7.4.5.1 AST diffusion methods

- Diffusion methods include the following:
  - Disk diffusion methods: these only provide a qualitative result.
  - Gradient diffusion method (also known as Etest): it provides an MIC.
- In disk diffusion techniques, paper disks impregnated with predetermined concentrations of antimicrobial are placed upon an inoculated plate. After incubation, the diameter of the zone of inhibition is read and compared with established breakpoints to classify the isolate as susceptible, intermediate or resistant.
- The Etest involves the use of a plastic strip coated with an antimicrobial gradient on one side and an MIC interpretive scale on the other side. The strip is placed on an inoculated plate, and the antimicrobial drug diffuses into the medium. After incubation, there is an elliptical zone of growth inhibition around the strip. The MIC is read at the point of intersection of the ellipse with the MIC scale on the strip.

1.7.4.5.2 AST dilution methods

- Broth macrodilution, broth microdilution and agar dilution methods can be performed to determine the minimum inhibitory concentration (MIC). Broth microdilution method is the most commonly used system in commercial systems for MIC determination. Bacteria are inoculated on a plate with twofold dilutions of antimicrobials, with concentrations that include clinical breakpoints. The concentration range included varies with the drug and the organism being tested.
- After incubation, the results can be determined visually or by the use of semiautomated or automated instruments.
- Clinical breakpoints are then compared with the obtained MIC to classify the organism into susceptible, intermediate or resistant. The MIC concentration is also reported.

1.7.4.5.3 Interpretation of AST results

- Different combinations of antimicrobials can be reported for different isolates, depending on the organism and site of infection.
- Antimicrobials for which the organism is known to have intrinsic resistance are not usually tested. Table 1.1 shows a basic list of intrinsic resistances that can be noted within common organisms recovered in veterinary microbiology samples. However, this is a general overview, and intrinsic resistances can vary within different species of the same genus. A more comprehensive list is available on EUCAST and CLSI guidelines.

A general guide to interpreting MIC results with examples is provided in Appendix 1.

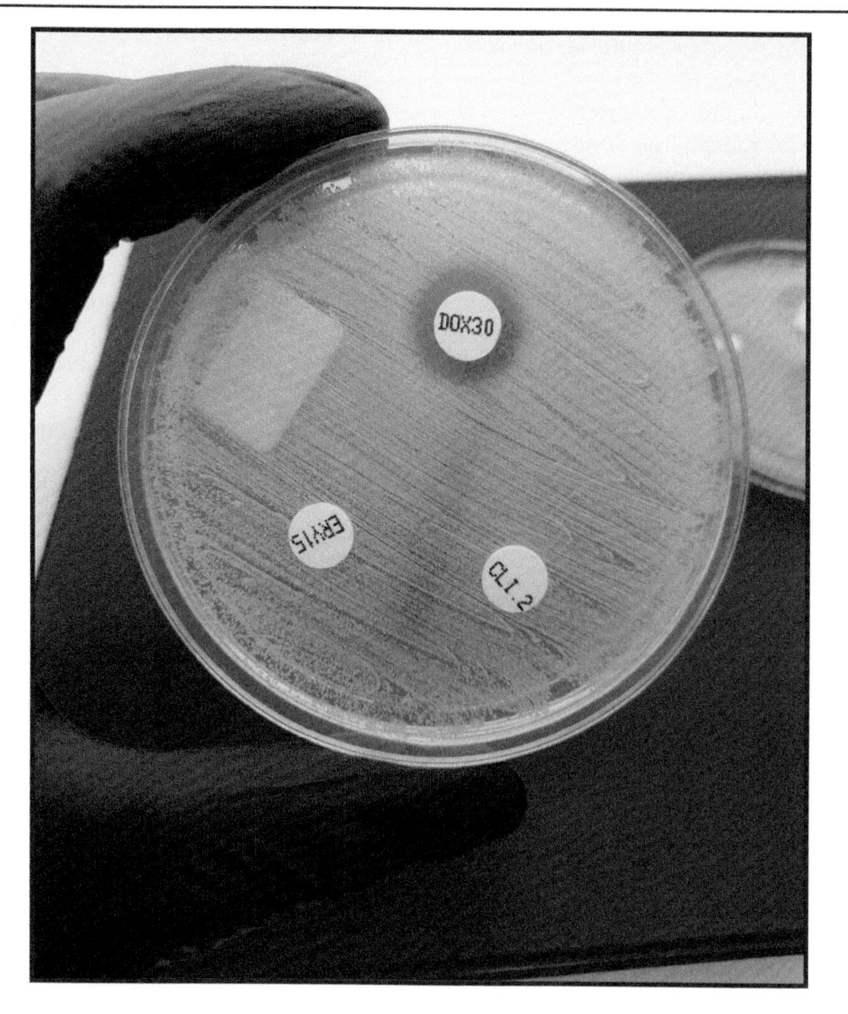

Fig. 1.8. Antimicrobial susceptibility test by disc diffusion showing zone of inhibition.

1.7.4.5.4 Selection of the more appropriate antimicrobial

- Selection of the best antimicrobial is not limited to the AST results, and additional factors must be considered when making this choice:
  - Site of infection.
  - Tissue penetration of the antimicrobial at site of infection:
    - Degree of inflammation and vascular supply may impact tissue penetration.
    - Presence of necrosis and purulent material may limit efficacy of some antimicrobials.
    - The use of topical antimicrobial can achieve much higher concentrations than the ones used to establish the clinical breakpoints; therefore, efficacy of topical treatment is not predicted by AST results.

- Safety and ease of use for the patient:
  - Age.
  - Immunocompetence.
  - Kidney, liver disease or other possible toxic effects.
- Disease severity:
  - Influences choice of topical *vs* oral *vs* parenteral administration.
- Source control:
  - Removal of foreign body, uroliths or implants that can become a nidus for the bacteria to elude both immune system and preclude antimicrobial activity/ penetration.
- Prescribing cascade, local legislation and availability of antimicrobial and cost.

Table 1.1. General overview of intrinsic antimicrobial resistance in common bacterial isolates recovered from clinical samples in dogs and cats.

Organism	Penicillin	Ampicillin, Amoxicillin	Amoxicillin-clavulanic acid	Cephalosporins I: Cefalexin, cephalothin	Cephamycin: Cefoxitin	Cephalosporins II: Cefuroxime	Cephalosporins III: Cefotaxime, Cefovecin, Ceftiofur	Tetracycline:	Doxycycline	Aminoglycosides	Lincosamides	Macrolides	Trimethoprim/trimethop-rim-sulfamethoxazole	Nitrofurantoin (urines only)
Staphylococcus spp.														
Streptococcus spp.										R[1]				
Enterococcus spp.				R[2]	R[2]	R[2]	R[2]			R[2]	R[2]	R[2]	R[2]	
E. coli	R										R	R		
Proteus mirabilis	R							R	R		R	R		R
Klebsiella spp.	R	R									R	R		
P. aeruginosa	R	R	R	R	R	R	R[3]	R	R		R	R		
Acinetobacter spp.	R	R	R	R	R	R	R	R	R		R	R		

Data are based on information from CLSI and EUCAST. This is a summary and information provided by the laboratory should be considered, as individual species within each group may have variations in the intrinsic resistance. These results do not predict susceptibility of individual isolates as acquired resistance may be present. R – resistance. 1 – Low level of resistance. Combinations of aminoglycosides with cell wall inhibitors (penicillin and glycopeptides) are synergistic and bactericidal against isolates that are susceptible to cell wall inhibitors and do not display high-level resistance to aminoglycosides. 2 – For *Enterococcus* spp., cephalosporins, aminoglycosides (except for high-level resistance testing), clindamycin and trimethoprim-sulfamethoxazole may appear active *in vitro* but are not effective clinically and should not be reported as susceptible. 3 – Some third-generation cephalosporins (e.g. Ceftazidime) have anti-*Pseudomonas* activity.

1.7.5 Cytology *versus* culture in the identification of microorganisms in fluid specimens

Discrepancies between cytology and culture results can occur for a variety of reasons.

- Body cavity fluids: a recent retrospective study reported an overall sensitivity and specificity of 63.0% and 89.6%, respectively, of cytology for identification of sepsis. This varied significantly across fluid types, with greater accuracy identified in septic abdominal fluids.
- Bile samples: when the two modalities were compared, bile cytology was found to have similar sensitivity to culture testing.

- Synovial samples: direct culture of joint fluid produces false negative results in approximately 50% of cases that are clinically consistent with septic arthritis. Microorganisms are seen in fewer than 50% of culture positive synovial specimens. Thus, septic arthritis is often a clinical diagnosis based on clinical presentation and the presence of suppurative inflammation.
- BAL samples: comparison of results between cytology and culture in samples from the lower respiratory tract is more challenging, as some of the common organisms recovered from that area are not easily cultured or identified on cytology (e.g. *Mycoplasma* spp.). Moreover, the presence of bacteria does not equate with infection given the frequent oropharyngeal contamination identified in these samples. Furthermore, bacterial infections may be secondary to an underlying pathology (e.g. viral infection, aspiration pneumonia or asthma) and not be responsible for the clinical signs. Integration of full clinical data is often required to interpret culture results.

1.7.5.1 False-negative culture results

Possible causes of false-negative results include:

- Inadequate specimen size.
- Low bacterial load at the site of specimen collection.
- Loss of organism viability. Lack of viability of organisms can occur due to:
  - Prior antimicrobial use.
  - Exposure of the sample to extreme conditions (such as temperature or pH).
  - Absence of media to support growth of more fastidious organisms.
  - Presence of inhibitors within the sample (e.g. excess boric acid).
  - Leucocyte response: this can also lead to false-negative results on culture. In these cases, the presence of high numbers of leucocytes in the sample may phagocytose and destroy the few organisms present during specimen transportation.
- Overgrowth of commensal organisms. In some situations, multiple bacterial species are present within a specimen and one species (e.g. *Proteus* spp.) swarms the plate and obscures the presence of other organisms, or less fastidious organisms overgrow more fastidious or slow-growing organisms.
- The organism is not inoculated on to the correct medium or insufficient time is allowed for growth. Clinicians must consider whether fastidious or slow-growing organisms might be present and inform the laboratory if they are suspected.

1.7.5.2 False-positive culture results

As absence of growth does not indicate absence of infection, growth does not necessarily indicate infection. Not all organisms that are isolated from a clinical case are necessarily the culprits for the clinical signs. This is particularly the case when sampling non-sterile sites or sites where contamination with commensal or environmental flora can occur (e.g. free catch urine samples).

1.8 Molecular Assays

For many organisms, molecular-based methods such as PCR or fluorescent *in situ* hybridization (FISH) are considered an alternative method for detection of infectious organisms. Clinical application of molecular methods of organism identification includes:

- Detection of fastidious organisms of slow growth (e.g. Mycobacteria).
- Detection of organisms for which culture is not possible or easily feasible (e.g. feline haemoplasmas).

- Detection of organisms that are undetectable on microscopic examination of tissues (e.g. viruses).
- Detection of organisms where culture may lead to a significant risk of laboratory-acquired zoonotic infection (e.g. *Brucella* spp., selected fungal organisms).
- Detection of organisms in the presence of inactivating or inhibitory substances (e.g. antimicrobials, EDTA or formalin).
- Identification of an identified organism to species level (e.g. protozoal trophozoites).

1.8.1 PCR

- Samples for PCR include EDTA fluids, plain fluids, fixed samples and, for some assays, even stained smears.
- The presence of heparin or formalin may decrease sensitivity of PCR due to inhibition or degradation of the DNA.
- The swabs used for PCR testing should be dry, not coated with charcoal or any transport medium, as those may interfere with the PCR reaction and could potentially inhibit the amplification of the target genetic material.
- Specific recommendations may vary depending on site and molecular target (e.g. RNA targets degrade more quickly than DNA targets). For most samples that have DNA as a target, refrigeration is recommended for relative short-term storage (up to 72 h), while for longer storage samples should be frozen at −80°C. As RNA is more susceptible to degradation during storage or transport, stabilizing solutions may be provided by the reference laboratory.

Positive PCR results

- A positive PCR result confirms the presence of the organism in question, but does not evaluate its viability.
- Some quantitative RT-PCR assays may provide additional useful information regarding the quantity of genetic material, which can reflect pathogen load.
- Correlation of the positive results with the additional clinical findings is essential for a correct interpretation of the results.

Negative PCR results

- No DNA of the agent in question is present in the speciment at a detectable concentration.
- False negatives can also occur:
  - In the presence of PCR inhibitors (many assays include controls to evaluate for the presence of these substances).
  - When there is a very low load of the pathogen.
  - When mutations to the target sequences have occurred in the pathogen genetic material (e.g. novel viral sequences).

1.8.2 Assays based on nucleic acid probes

- Various nucleic acid probes can be used to detect microorganisms. They react with the target organism DNA present in the sample. The bound probe is then detected via fluorescence, chemiluminescence, radioactivity or colour development.
- For *in situ* hybridization (e.g. FISH), the probe is labelled with a fluorescent or chemical tag, so that the bound probe can be detected. The probe is applied to a tissue specimen on a microscope slide to determine if the organism is present. Location of the organisms within the specimen (e.g. phagocytosed by inflammatory cells, present within clusters) is also facilitated and considered when evaluating results.

1.9 Immunoassays

- Immunoassays rely on the antigen-antibody interactions to identify the presence of organisms or the presence of the host immune response to an infectious organism. Immunoassays are often called serological assays, as many are tested in serum. However, they can be performed on many types of samples, including fluid samples.
- Examples include antigen detection assays (e.g. immunocytochemistry for feline coronavirus [FCoV] in fluid samples from cats with feline infectious peritonitis [FIP]) and measurement of antibody titres, that usually require comparison with serum titres to be of diagnostic use (e.g. distemper antibody titres).
- The preferred sample type for immunoassays is a plain sterile sample, although many can use EDTA samples. The sample can be kept at room temperature, refrigerated or frozen if longer sample storage is required. Sample stability may be different depending if antibodies (generally, if frozen, samples can be stable for long periods of time) or antigens (that may deteriorate more quickly) are tested.

Further reading

Allen, B.A. and Evans, S.J. (2022) Diagnostic accuracy of cytology for the detection of bacterial infection in fluid samples from veterinary patients. *Veterinary Clinical Pathology* 51, 252–257.

Greene, C.E. (2012) *Infectious Diseases of the Dog and Cat.* 4th edn. Elsevier, St. Louis, Missouri.

Marcos, R., Santos, M., Marrinhas, C., Correia-Gomes, C. and Caniatti, M. (2016) Cytocentrifuge preparation in veterinary cytology: a quick, simple, and affordable manual method to concentrate low cellularity fluids. *Veterinary Clinical Pathology* 45(4), 725–731.

Marcos, R., Santos, M., Marrinhas, C. and Caniatti, M. (2017) Cell tube block: a new technique to produce cell blocks from fluid cytology samples. *Veterinary Clinical Pathology* 46(1), 195–201.

Sykes, J.E. (2013) *Canine and Feline Infectious Diseases.* Elsevier, St. Louis, Missouri.

Weese, J.S., Blondeau, J., Boothe, D., Guardabassi, L.G., Gumley, N. *et al.* (2019) International Society for Companion Animal Infectious Diseases (ISCAID) guidelines for the diagnosis and management of bacterial urinary tract infections in dogs and cats. *Veterinary Journal* 247, 8–25.

Web sources

Clinical & Laboratory Standards Institute (CLSI): https://www.clsi.org/

European Committee on Antimicrobial Susceptibility Testing (EUCAST): https://www.eucast.org/

Appendix 1

Minimal inhibitory concentration (MIC) procedure and interpretation of the sensitivity results

Table A.1. MIC procedure and interpretation of the results.

Clinical breakpoints	S	S	S	S	I	R		
Concentration Antimicrobial A (mg/l)	2	4	8	16	32	64	Result	MIC
Organism 1	x						S	4 mg/l
Organism 2							S	< 2 mg/l
Clinical breakpoints	S	S	S	I	I	R	Result	MIC
Concentration Antimicrobial B (mg/l)	0.125	0.25	0.5	1	2	4		
Organism 1	x	x	x	x	x		R	4 mg/l
Organism 2	x	x					S	0.5 mg/l

MIC procedure

- A standard inoculum (number of bacteria) is incubated in serial dilutions of antimicrobials. The dilutions vary depending on the antimicrobials and include the clinical breakpoints. The breakpoints also vary depending on the organism and antimicrobial combinations.
- After incubation, each well is assessed for growth. The MIC is the lowest concentration of antimicrobial drug that inhibits visible growth of an organism.
- The table marks the dilutions where growth is still identified. The lower the MIC, the more susceptible is the isolate to that specific antimicrobial.
- Because different antimicrobials are tested in different concentrations, MIC values of different antimicrobials for the same isolate cannot be compared. Instead, the MIC value (within the range of concentrations tested) should be assessed and compared to the breakpoints for that antimicrobial-organism combination. The further away from the breakpoint, the more susceptible the organism is to that antimicrobial.
- The assessment of the MIC against the clinical breakpoints generates qualitative results.

Assessing results

- The evaluation of an AST panel begins with the assessment of the qualitative results. Antimicrobials (AM) marked as resistant are expected to lead to therapeutical failure.
- Within the susceptible AMs, that which is most appropriate for the site and patient should be used, aiming for a narrow-spectrum and lower tier in the cascade.
- If using drugs where the MIC falls into the intermediate range or close to the clinical breakpoint (one dilution away), adjusting the dose (with concentration-dependent drugs) and/or frequency (with time-dependent drugs) could be considered to increase the tissue concentration and reduce the risk of treatment failure.
- As mentioned above, MIC values between antimicrobials cannot be directly compared. In the example shown in the table above, organism 1 has an MIC of 4 mg/l for both AM A and B, but the interpretation is different:
  - AM A: Sensitive.
  - AM B: Resistant.
- The distance of the MIC to the breakpoint may also be useful. The breakpoint:MIC ratio or index can be taken into consideration in drug selection. With all other factors being equal, antimicrobials with MICs closer to the breakpoint are potentially more vulnerable to treatment failure due to *in vivo* effects (e.g. decrease of the actual tissue concentration in the patient). The further away from the breakpoint, the less likely that is to happen.
- For example, organism 2 is more susceptible to antimicrobial A than organism 1, because it has a lower MIC, but also because the distance between the MIC and the clinical breakpoint is higher for AM A (four dilution steps versus one dilution).

Respiratory Tract Fluids

2.1 Anatomy and Physiology

Anatomically, the respiratory tract is divided into:

- Upper respiratory tract: this includes the organs outside the thorax (nasal cavities, pharynx, larynx and part of the trachea).
- Lower respiratory tract: this includes the structures within the thorax (trachea, bronchi, bronchioles and alveoli).

Functionally, it can be divided into:

- Large conducting system (from the nasal cavities to the bronchi/bronchioles): this serves to warm, filter and conduct the air from the atmosphere to the alveoli.
- Respiratory zone (alveoli): where the gas exchanges take place.

Knowing the microscopic anatomy of these structures is crucial to understand which cell types are expected in the cytology sample obtained from those districts.

- Nasal cavities: extending from the nostril to nasopharynx and separated by the nasal septum. To simplify, the nasal vestibule is lined by keratinized squamous epithelium that transitions to non-keratinized squamous epithelium and ciliated pseudostratified epithelium in the posterior nasal cavity. Interspersed in between the epithelial cells, there are goblet cells (secretory cells), and lymphoid follicles part of the nasal associated lymphoid tissue (NALT). Nasal cavities also contain neuroepithelial, neuroendocrine cells and melanocytes.
- Pharynx: cone-shaped passageway leading from the oral and nasal cavities to the oesophagus and larynx. The digestive surface is lined by non-keratinizing stratified squamous epithelium and the respiratory surface by ciliated columnar respiratory epithelium.
- Larynx: musculocartilagineous portion of the upper respiratory tract that encompasses the vocal folds, arytenoid cartilage and glottis. It is composed of cartilage lined by stratified squamous epithelium with scattered lymphoid follicles.
- Trachea: it extends from the larynx to the carina and is composed of incomplete cartilaginous rings supported by connective tissue and smooth muscle. The epithelium is ciliated and pseudostratified with interspersed goblet cells.
- Bronchi/bronchioles: structures branching from the trachea with complete bronchial cartilaginous rings. They continue into terminal bronchioles, which lack cartilaginous support. Both are surrounded by smooth muscles and lined by ciliated and non-ciliated cuboidal to columnar epithelium. Serous and mucous secreting cells (goblet cells) are also present. Terminal bronchioles branch into respiratory bronchioles, which lack ciliated cells and further divide into alveolar ducts, alveolar sacs and alveoli.

DOI: 10.1079/9781789247787.0002

- Alveoli: terminal portion of the lower respiratory tract. They are responsible for gaseous exchange (CO_2, O_2). They are a complex structure composed of epithelial lining cells (pneumocytes), macrophages and an extracellular matrix surrounded by capillaries.
  - Type 1 pneumocytes: thin and flat squamous epithelial cells connected by occluding junctions. They cover >90% of the alveolar surface and are involved in the process of gaseous exchange between alveoli and capillaries.
  - Type 2 pneumocytes: cuboidal epithelial cells interspersed between the pneumocytes type 1. They cover only a small proportion of the alveolar surface. They have characteristic apical microvilli and secrete pulmonary surfactant. The surfactant serves to reduce the surface tension, preventing the alveoli from collapsing.
  - Macrophages: resident population of macrophages within the alveoli, named alveolar macrophages. These effector cells of the innate immune system phagocytose bacteria and secrete both proinflammatory and antimicrobial mediators.
  - Capillaries and connective tissue: surround and support the alveoli. Network of connective tissue is composed of reticular, collagenous, elastic fibres and fibroblasts.

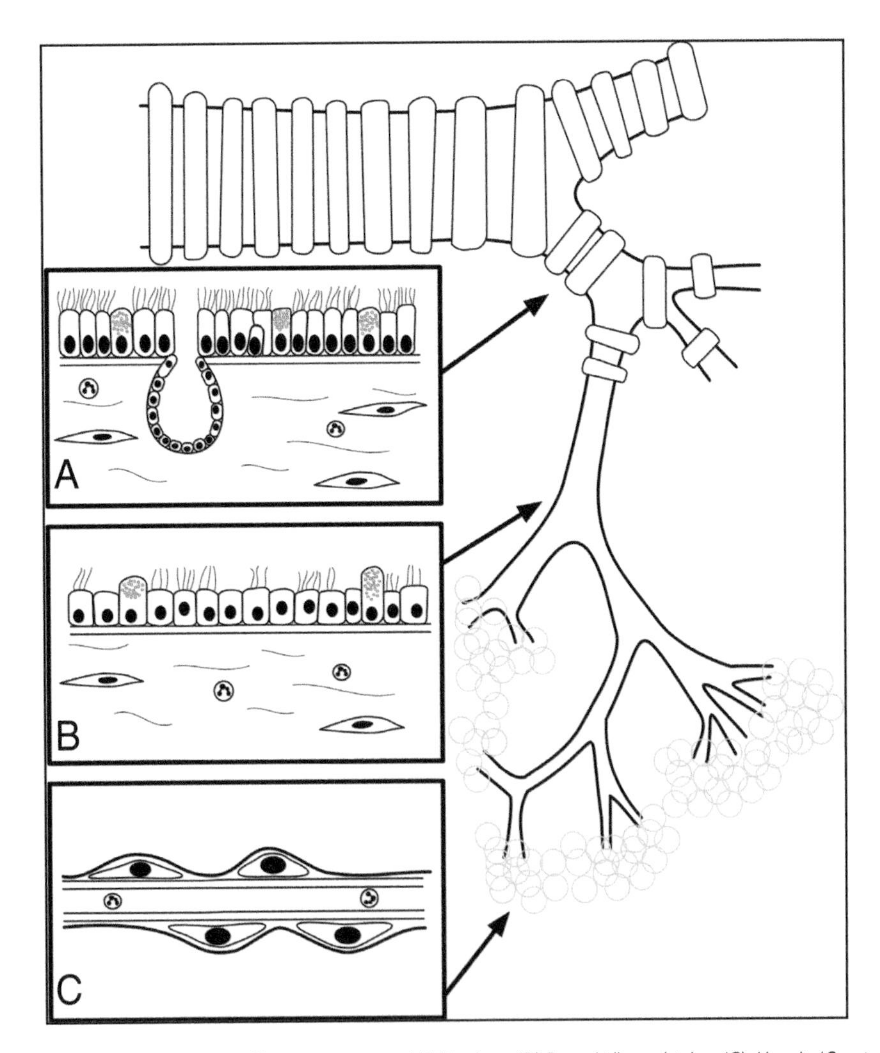

Fig. 2.1. Microscopic anatomy of lower respiratory (A) Trachea. (B) Bronchi/bronchioles. (C) Alveoli. (*Courtesy of Nic Ilchyshyn.*)

2.2 Sampling Techniques

2.2.1 Upper respiratory tract

Indications

Analysis of upper respiratory secretions is recommended when a disease of the nasal cavity is suspected. The first recommended diagnostic steps include thorough inspection of the external and internal upper respiratory tract, starting from the nose and oral cavity. This may be accompanied by imaging studies and sampling techniques aiming to collect samples for cytological and/or histological examination and culture.

Materials

- Disinfectant and sterile gloves.
- Sterile dry swab (for nasal swab procedure).
- Sterile soft catheter with syringe (20–35 ml) and sterile physiologic saline or lactated Ringer's solution (for nasal flush).
- 21–25 G needle and 2–10 ml syringe (for fine-needle aspiration).
- Endoscope and endoscopic brush (for brush cytology).
- Endoscope, alligator biopsy forceps or Tru-Cut disposable biopsy needle (to collect solid biopsy for imprint cytology and/or histopathology).
- Tubes (EDTA and plain) for nasal flush samples.
- Glass smears.

Patient preparation

- Most of these techniques are performed with the animal under general anaesthesia.
- Gauze padding of the oropharynx and tilting the animal head downward help protecting against aspiration during sampling.

Techniques

Nasal swab

- Superficial swab: insert the swab within the nasal cavity to collect any material that may be present in the nasal cavities.
- Deep swap: rub the wall of the nasal cavities with a swab.
- Gently roll the swab across a glass slide.
- This is a non-invasive and non-traumatic procedure but often does not provide sufficient information on the underlying primary process causing the nasal pathology.
- Although often submitted for culture, this type of sample is more likely to reveal overgrowth of normal commensal flora.
- It can also be used for PCR testing for infectious organisms (e.g. respiratory viruses).

Nasal flush

- Insert the catheter into the external nares and flush sterile physiologic saline or lactated Ringer's solution (5–10 ml) with a syringe (20–35 ml) through the nasal cavity.
- A traumatic variant of this technique can be obtained by cutting an angle of the catheter to create a rough surface that helps to dislodge tissue. As the fluid enters the cavity, the catheter can be moved back and forth in attempt to obtain tissue fragments.
- An alternative method involves directing a Foley catheter into the oral cavity and retroflexing around the soft palate into the nasopharynx, inflating the bulb and lavaging with saline so that the fluid passes through the nasal cavity and out of the external nares for collection.

- Nasal flushes can also be used for bacterial and fungal culture and may be useful in the identification of nasal aspergillosis.
- PCR for respiratory pathogens can also be performed with this type of sample.

Fine-needle aspiration

- This is the most rewarding technique in the presence of a solid mass lesion, which can be visible from outside or identified by imaging techniques.
- Insert within the mass a 21–25 G needle and redirect it multiple times in different directions. If the needle is attached to a syringe (2–10 ml), apply gentle suction (aspiration technique).
- Expel the material on to a labelled glass slide and smear to create a monolayer area that could easily be evaluated under the microscope.

Imprint and brush cytology

- Both techniques are usually performed under endoscopic guidance.
- Brush cytology: it requires the use of an endoscopic brush that is rolled on the nasal mucosa and then on a glass slide for cytology.
- Imprint cytology: it can be performed from a tissue biopsy collected for histopathological examination. The biopsy sample can be obtained with alligator biopsy forceps (pinch biopsy sample) or using a Tru-Cut disposable biopsy needle (core biopsy sample). The collected tissue is then rolled on a glass slide or used to make touch imprints, before placing it into formalin. Biopsy remains the gold standard for diagnosing most nasal tumours.

Complications

- Haemorrhage: common sequalae due to damage of the rich venous plexuses underlying the nasal mucosa. This may hinder both imaging and cytological interpretation and should therefore be limited as much as possible.
- Penetration through the cribriform plate into the cranial vault: uncommon complication that can be avoided by measuring the distance from the external nares to the medial canthus of the eye.

2.2.2 Lower respiratory tract

Indications

Analysis of lower respiratory secretions is recommended when a disease involving the respiratory tree is suspected.

The techniques commonly performed to obtain respiratory samples for cytology and/or culture discussed in this chapter include:

- Tracheal wash (TW) obtained as transtracheal wash (TTW) or transoral tracheal wash (TOTW).
- Bronchoalveolar lavage (BAL) with or without bronchial brushing.
- Transthoracic lung aspiration.

Materials

- Disinfectant and sterile gloves.
- Sterile needle (for transtracheal wash).
- Sterile soft catheter with syringe (20–35 ml) and sterile physiologic saline or lactated Ringer's solution.
- Endoscope (for endoscopic-guided BAL sampling).
- Tubes (EDTA and sterile plain tubes).
- Glass smears.

Patient preparation

- All these procedures except for the transtracheal wash are performed with the animal under general anaesthesia.

Techniques

Tracheal wash

This is a procedure used to sample the larger airways (trachea, mainstem bronchi) and can be performed as transtracheal or transoral TW.

- TTW: minimally invasive procedure that can be performed in awake animals under light sedation and with local anaesthesia. It is usually reserved for larger dogs or patients that are at high risk for general anaesthesia. This procedure bypasses the oral cavity, avoiding risks of oropharyngeal contamination and making the sample more suitable for culture testing.
  - Place the patient in sternal recumbency or in sitting position with the neck extended and the nose elevated. The local area should be shaved, aseptically scrubbed and infused subcutaneously with local anaesthetic (2% lidocaine).
  - Palpate the cricothyroid ligament and place the needle of the catheter bevel down through the ligament or between two tracheal rings just distal to the larynx, until the tracheal lumen is reached.
  - Angle the needle down 45° and advance the catheter into the tracheal lumen approximately to the level of the carina (fourth intercostal space). No or minimal resistance should be encountered. Once the catheter is in place, the needle is removed from the trachea.
  - Attach to the catheter a preloaded syringe with warm sterile saline (0.1–0.4 ml/kg body weight) and infuse it into the trachea. The fluid will induce coughing and should then be aspirated back into the syringe. Usually, only 10% or less of the infused volume of saline is recovered. If necessary, the procedure can be repeated.
  - Remove both syringe and catheter in a smooth motion. A soft, padded bandage should be placed over the catheter site for approximately 1 h to minimize formation of subcutaneous emphysema.
- TOTW: procedure particularly recommended in fractious animals and in smaller patients (small dogs and cats), in which the small tracheal lumen diameter precludes placement of a large needle between tracheal rings. This procedure is easy to perform and requires minimal equipment. However, it is more prone to oropharyngeal contamination and can yield less sample volume that TTW, since the cough reflex is suppressed by the anaesthesia.
  - It is performed in lateral recumbency and in general anaesthesia, preventing any cough reflex and resulting in a sample that is more representative of the lower airways.
  - Insert a rubber catheter through the inflated endotracheal tube, up to the carina (this corresponds externally to the level of the fourth intercostal space). Care must be taken not to contaminate the tip of the endotracheal tube in the oropharynx.
  - Infuse saline and re-aspirate, as described earlier and similar to the BAL technique.

Bronchoalveolar lavage

- This procedure requires general anaesthesia and a preliminary clinical risk assessment for lower airway disease.
- Patients should be preoxygenated for at least 5–10 min before the induction of the anaesthesia and should continue for at least 5 min to 20 min after the procedure to reduce the

risks of hypoxia. Preliminary bronchodilator therapy may be considered in feline patients. Topical lidocaine and sterile lubricant can be considered to avoid laryngospasm and arytenoid trauma, and the use of a mouth gag will protect bronchoscope from trauma in case of the patient awakening during the procedure.

- The amount of warm sterile saline to be infused is controversial with different published recommendations. In dogs, aliquots of 15–25 ml per wash or 1–2 ml/kg have been recommended. In cats and owing to their smaller volume, aliquots of 3–10 ml per site or 3–5 ml/kg are often used.
- Bronchoalveolar lavage can be performed with endoscopic-guided or endotracheal/blind technique. Advantages of the endoscopic procedure is the ability to visualize the airways, choose the lobe to be lavaged, biopsy lesions and even remove foreign bodies (therapeutic BAL), when present.
    - Endoscopic-guided technique:
        - Place the anaesthetized and intubated patient in sternal or lateral recumbency. Orientation and access to lung segments varies depending on the species and the recumbency and are beyond the purpose of this chapter.
        - Pass the bronchoscope through an endotracheal tube or directly through the larynx in small patients, to allow visualization of trachea and main bronchi.
        - Pass the bronchoscope into each long lobe to allow visual examination.
        - Instil sterile warm saline with a syringe through the biopsy channel in a single bolus or divided into two or three aliquots. This is followed by immediate suction with the scope in the same wedged position. Aspiration can be manual or mechanical with suction pump. It may be helpful to follow the saline infusion with 3–5 ml of air to make sure all the fluid reaches the lungs. If no saline is retrieved, it may be because of collapsing of the airways and less negative suction should be applied to the syringe. Procedure may be repeated with a second aliquot of saline.
        - Multiple lobes may be lavaged by repeating the same procedure.
        - In dogs, median recoveries of 42–48% of the infused saline have been reported; in cats, retrieval of 59–75% of BAL fluid were recorded in a retrospective study of 68 cats. Fluid retrieval may be increased by tilting the head of the patient downward and rotating the patient with the lavage lung area uppermost to encourage fluid drainage.
    - Endotracheal tube or blind technique:
        - Introduce through an endotracheal tube a flexible catheter, long enough to reach up to the level of the 11th rib.
        - To optimize recovery of fluid from a BAL, the tube should be wedged into the bronchi. To achieve this, advance the tube until it stops; withdraw it a few centimetres, rotate gently and readvance until resistance is felt at a consistent level.
        - Instil warm sterile saline with a syringe and re-aspirate it without visualization of the airway.

Tracheobronchial brushing

- This procedure allows cytological evaluation of visible tracheo bronchial lesions. Specimens are obtained with an endoscopic brush passed through the biopsy channel of the endoscope and moved back and forth along the bronchial wall.
- Alternatively, a sterile culture swab or cytology brush can be introduced directly through the oral cavity into the trachea for sample collection. This procedure should be considered a valid adjunct to BAL cytology and can be useful if the BAL sample is suspected hypocellular. It can also be used when a bronchoscope of appropriate size for the lower airways is unavailable.

Transthoracic lung aspiration

- This technique goes beyond the purpose of this textbook, which is focused on fluid cytology.
- It is an excellent diagnostic method for obtaining material from the lung parenchyma and is particularly useful for those processes that do not communicate with the respiratory tree.

Table 2.1. Advantages and disadvantages of different techniques used to obtain respiratory fluids.

	Advantages	Disadvantages
Transtracheal wash (TTW)	• Readily performed with minimal equipment • No need of general anaesthesia • Sample suitable for culture testing as less risk of oropharyngeal contamination	• Sample representative of trachea and large bronchi only • Lack of standardized cytology criteria for sample evaluation
Transoral tracheal wash (TOTW)	• Readily performed with minimal equipment	• General anaesthesia required • Risk of oropharyngeal contamination • Sample representative of trachea and large bronchi only • Lack of standardized cytology criteria for sample evaluation
Bronchoalveolar lavage (BAL)	• Sample representative of the lower respiratory tract • Sample suitable for culture testing • Extensive literature available and defined cytology criteria for sample evaluation	• General anaesthesia required • Need for special equipment and expertise • Risk of oropharyngeal contamination
Tracheobronchial brush cytology	• Sampling of directly visualized tracheo-bronchial lesions • Allow sampling of selected multiple and selected lung regions	• General anaesthesia required • Need for special equipment and expertise • Lack of standardized cytology criteria for sample evaluation • Risk of oropharyngeal contamination
Transthoracic lung aspiration	• Allow sampling of tracheobronchial lesions, even if not in communication with the respiratory tree (e.g. interstitial inflammatory processes, neoplasms)	• General anaesthesia required • Risk of pneumothorax • Risk of transient needle tract metastasis in case of neoplasia

Complications

- These are rare and include subcutaneous emphysema, pneumomediastinum, haemorrhage, transient hypoxia, needle tract infection, transient haemoptysis and bronchoconstriction.
- Gastric dilation-volvulus in large, deep-chested dogs may also be a concern with rotation of these anaesthetized patients during the procedure.

2.3 Sample Handling, Analysis and Slide Preparation

Samples from upper and lower parts of the respiratory tract are handled similarly.

2.3.1 Sample handling

- 'Standardization' is the keyword for both collection, handling and analysis in particular of TW/BAL fluids and is crucial to obtain results that are accurate and repeatable.
- Fluid sample should be collected and aliquoted in the following tubes:
  - EDTA tube: used for cytology preparations. This anticoagulant avoids clotting formation and preserves cell morphology. However, due to its bacteriostatic activity it should not be used for culture purposes. It can be used for PCR.
  - Plain sterile tube: used for culture/sensitivity testing and PCR.
  - Specific media preparations: used when selected infectious agents are suspected (e.g. Mycoplasma and virus isolation).
- For best results, fresh cytology samples should be prepared at the time of collection, ideally within 1 h, to avoid cell morphology deterioration. If this is not possible, the sample should be refrigerated at 4°C and processed as soon as possible.
- Prolonged storage of BAL specimens (>24 h) has been reported to decrease the percentage of neutrophils and cause variation of eosinophil numbers in both dogs and cats, with a possible impact on the final cytological interpretation.

2.3.2 Sample analysis

- Routine TW/BAL examination includes:
  - Macroscopic evaluation.
  - Cytological evaluation.
  - Other tests.

Macroscopic evaluation

- TW and BAL from healthy animals are clear and transparent fluids.
- White, stable foam is often present on the surface of BAL samples. This reflects sampling from the alveolar district and the presence of surfactant.
- Increased cellularity due to pathological conditions often results in increased turbidity and change in colour of the fluid.
- When blood is present (or products of its degradation), a red to orange-tinged colour is often noted.

Cytological evaluation

- This is considered the most crucial step of TW/BAL analysis and the one able to provide most diagnostic information. Details are described in the following section.
  - Slide preparation:
    - Direct smear: recommended for samples that appear turbid and are likely to have a high cellularity. Preparation of direct smears from clear and transparent samples is usually unrewarding for cytological examination. If small mucoid particles are found suspended in the fluid, a squash preparation is also recommended.
    - Cytocentrifuge preparation: obtained with use of a cytocentrifuge. It yields yields superior cell concentration, more homogenous cell distribution and better preservation than traditional centrifugation. However, cytocentrifugation of canine

BAL samples has been reported to underestimate the number of small lymphocytes and overestimate the neutrophils present; 100 μl or 200 μl is suitable for turbid or clear BAL samples, respectively.

- Smear of the fluid sediment: the fluid should be centrifuged for 10 min at 500–600 *g*, the supernatant discarded and the cell pellet resuspended in the small amount of fluid remaining in the tube (at least 50–100 μl).

Microbiology, antigen and PCR testing

- For the identification of infectious agents that may or not be apparent on cytological samples.

Pearls and Pitfalls

- If a BAL needs to be repeated, this should be done immediately after the first sampling or after 48 h. This is because the sterile saline used for the wash procedure can induce a localized neutrophilic response that peaks 24 h after the procedure.
- Some authors recommend discarding the first aliquot, as this has been reported containing fewer epithelial cells and higher numbers of polymorphonuclear cells. However, this is unlikely to significantly affect clinical interpretation; therefore, different aliquots from the same lobe can be combined.
- Measurement of the total cell count (TNCC) and protein concentration (TP) in TW/BAL fluids is of limited diagnostic value and is discouraged, since the volume of saline infused and retrieved in the respiratory tract is highly variable and the technique used for sample collection may differ between institutions.
- Cell clumping due to the presence of mucus further limits the accuracy of the TNCC. However, it can be used to establish the adequacy of the sample and can be performed on a standard cell counting chamber or by using an automated cell counter.
- Studies assessing BAL cell counts in healthy animals often report values <500 cells/μl.
- Neutrophils and macrophages may phagocytize red blood cells and extracellular bacteria in vitro. This often occurs overtime when analysis is delayed and can result in erroneous diagnosis of septic inflammation or haemorrhage.

Further reading

Dehard, S., Bernaerts, F., Peeters, D., Detilleux, J., McEntee, K. *et al.* (2008) Comparison of bronchoalveolar lavage cytospins and smears in dogs and cats. *Journal of American Animal Hospital Association* 44(6), 285–294.

DeLorenzi, D., Masserdotti, C., Bertoncello, D. and Tranquillo, V. (2009) Differential cell counts in canine cytocentrifuged bronchoalveolar lavage fluid: a study on reliable enumeration of each cell. *Veterinary Clinical Pathology* 38(4), 532–536.

Finke, M. (2013) Transtracheal wash and bronchoalveolar lavage. *Topics in Companion Animal Medicine* 28(3), 97–102.

Nafe, L.A., DeClue, A.E. and Reinero, C.R. (2011) Storage alters feline bronchoalveolar lavage fluid cytological analysis. *Journal of Feline Medicine and Surgery* 13(2), 94–100.

Ybarra, W.L., Johnson, L.R., Drazenovich, T.L., Johnson, E.G. and Vernau, W. (2012) Interpretation of multisegment bronchoalveolar lavage in cats. *Journal of Veterinary Internal Medicine* 26(6), 1281–1287.

Zhu, B.Y., Johnson, L.R. and Vernau, W. (2015) Tracheobronchial brush cytology and bronchoalveolar lavage in dogs and cats with chronic cough: 45 cases (2012–2014). *Journal of Veterinary Internal Medicine* 29(2), 526–532.

2.4 Cell Types

Cytology of the upper and lower airways reflect the microscopic anatomy of these structures. Understanding the 'normal' cytological findings of these samples is crucial to appreciate and recognize any pathological change.

Respiratory epithelial cells

- Ciliated columnar epithelial cells:
  - They cover part of the posterior nasal cavity, nasal pharynx, trachea, bronchi and bronchioles. This cell type prevails in samples from the trachea and main bronchi.
  - They are elongated or cone-shaped. They exfoliate individually or in variably sized clusters. They have small, round hyperchromic nuclei at the basal end of the cell and a moderate amount of lightly basophilic cytoplasm. On the apical part of the cytoplasm (opposite to the nucleus), there are small cilia. Occasionally, the cilia may show a more eosinophilic/pink tint.
- Cuboidal epithelial cells:
  - These cells are more numerous in samples from bronchiolar areas.
  - They are characterized by a squared (cubical) morphology and do not have cilia. The nuclei are small and round and the cytoplasm is scant and pale to moderately basophilic.
- Squamous epithelial cells:
  - They are a normal finding in samples from the nasal cavity, oropharynx and larynx.
  - Large polygonal and angular flat epithelial cells with abundant pale basophilic cytoplasm. Nuclei, when present, are round, often central, small and with granular chromatin.
  - In TW and BAL samples, squamous epithelial cells are usually an indicator of oropharyngeal contamination and are often associated with bacteria (including *Conchiformibius* spp., formerly *Simonsiella* spp.) located in the background or on their surface.

Goblet cells

- They are mucus producing epithelial cells.
- They are columnar, without apical cilia and contain intracytoplasmic mucin granules. The granules have variable tinctorial characteristics. They can be red, purple, blue or clear. They are often variable in size. Free granules, as a result of cell rupture, may be seen in the background.

Alveolar macrophages

- They consist of large mononuclear cells and derive from the respiratory alveoli.
- They prevail in BAL samples (>70%) and are useful indicators that the alveolar space has been adequately washed.
- Morphologically, they are similar to macrophages seen in other tissues. They have a moderate to abundant, pale basophilic cytoplasm. Nuclei are variably located within the cells, and range from round to bean shaped, with granular chromatin and poorly visible nucleoli. When activated, their cytoplasm increases in size and becomes highly vacuolated. They can also contain phagocytized material. Binucleated cells may be observed.

Neutrophils

- Segmented polymorphonuclear cells, similar to those observed in the peripheral blood. They are present in low numbers in nasal, TW and BAL samples from healthy animals and may be increased in the presence of inflammation.

- If the sample is not processed immediately, their nucleus and cytoplasm can swell up due to prolonged suspension in fluid, mimicking degenerative changes. Other signs of delayed processing include pyknosis (the nucleus becomes condensed, round and hyperchromatic) or karyorrhexis (the nucleus is fragmented).

Eosinophils

- Segmented polymorphonuclear cells, similar to those observed in the peripheral blood.
- They are present in very low numbers in TW and BAL samples from healthy animals.
- They have a lobulated nucleus as in neutrophils but are usually slightly larger and less segmented. Their cytoplasm contains distinctive orange or pink intracytoplasmic granules.
- In cats, the granules are slender, rod shaped and pale pink in colour. In dogs, the granules are round.

Lymphocytes

- Small mononuclear cells, similar to those observed in the peripheral blood.
- They are present in variable numbers in the respiratory washes and their presence is generally clinically not significant. They may also be seen in samples from the nasal cavities, as part of the NALT.
- They have a small cytoplasmic rim and a small, round, hyperchromic nucleus. Occasionally, they may appear reactive, with increased amounts of basophilic cytoplasm and slightly larger nuclei.
- Immunophenotypic studies in dogs have shown that lymphocytes from the lower respiratory tract are primarily T-cells with a greater proportion of CD8+ cells than in the peripheral blood.
- A distinct population of lymphocytes that can rarely be found in BAL samples is represented by the globule leucocytes. They are characterized by containing variable numbers of intracytoplasmic eosinophilic granules.

Mast cells

- Mononuclear cells characterized by multiple, fine purple intracytoplasmic granules, often obscuring the nuclei. When cells undergo rupture, free granules may be seen in the background (not to be confused for mucin granules).
- Mast cells may be seen in very low numbers in TW and BAL samples from healthy dogs and cats.

Erythrocytes

- Their presence indicates true or iatrogenic haemorrhage (iatrogenic trauma during the sampling).
- They may be present free in the background or within macrophages, as intact erythrocytes or products of their degradation (e.g. haemosiderin and haematoidin).

Other leucocytes

- Plasma cells are rarely seen in respiratory secretions and washes. They are round to oval cells with deeply basophilic cytoplasm, round eccentric nucleus and often a typical perinuclear pale halo.
- Basophils have a segmented, lobulated nucleus and intracytoplasmic, purple (dog) or lilac (cats) granules.

Neoplastic cells

- These vary in shape, size and morphology depending on their origin.
- Their presence is not very common in lavages from the respiratory tract, unless the neoplasm (primary or metastatic) has involved the respiratory tree. They will be described in the following sections.

Other elements

- Mucus.
  - Variably basophilic amorphous material forming strands and ribbons that are often twisted and whorled.
  - Curschmann's spirals are mucous casts of small bronchioles that appear as spiral aggregates of mucus. They may be seen in disorders that result in chronic, excessive production of mucus and are indicators of bronchiolar obstruction.
- Mucin granules.
  - Small round purple/basophilic structures present in the background as result of goblet cell breaking.
- Exogenous material.
  - This includes vegetable material (e.g. pollen), maize starch (from glove powder), lubricant material, lipid material, barium sulfate, etc.
- Infectious agents.
  - They include bacteria, protozoa, fungi, yeasts and parasites. Bacteria, fungi and yeasts may be either contaminants (oropharyngeal flora) or pathogens.

Pearls and Pitfalls

In cases of delayed sample processing, the cilia can detach from the respiratory epithelial cells and be found free in the background. Care should be taken not to mistaken them for bacteria.

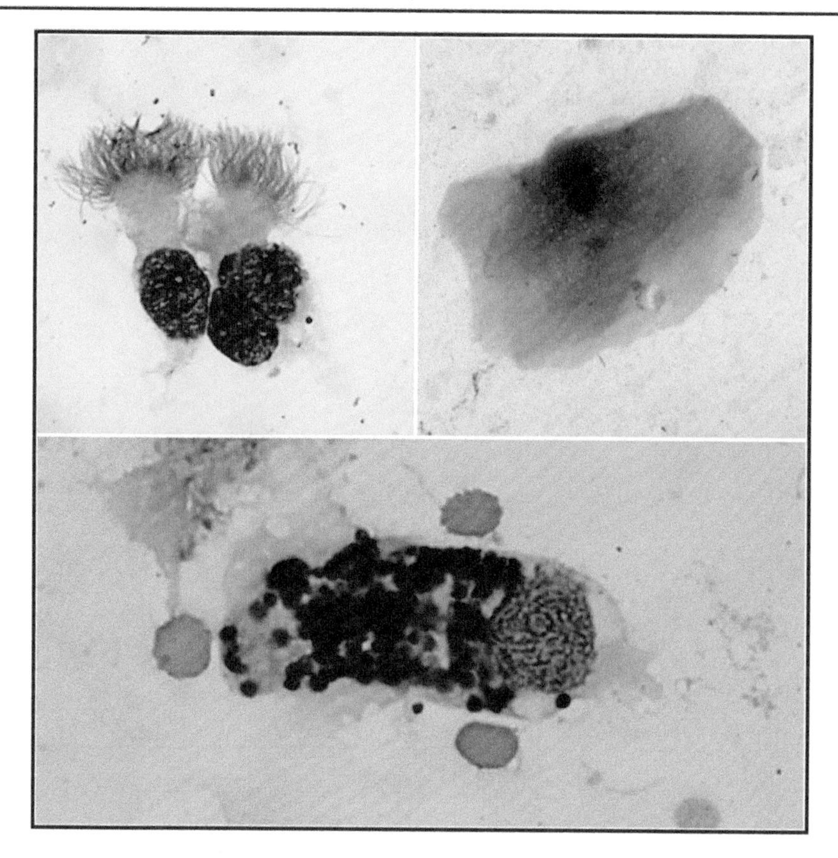

Fig. 2.2. Ciliated columnar epithelial cell (top left). Squamous epithelial cell (top right). Goblet cell (bottom). Wright-Giemsa.

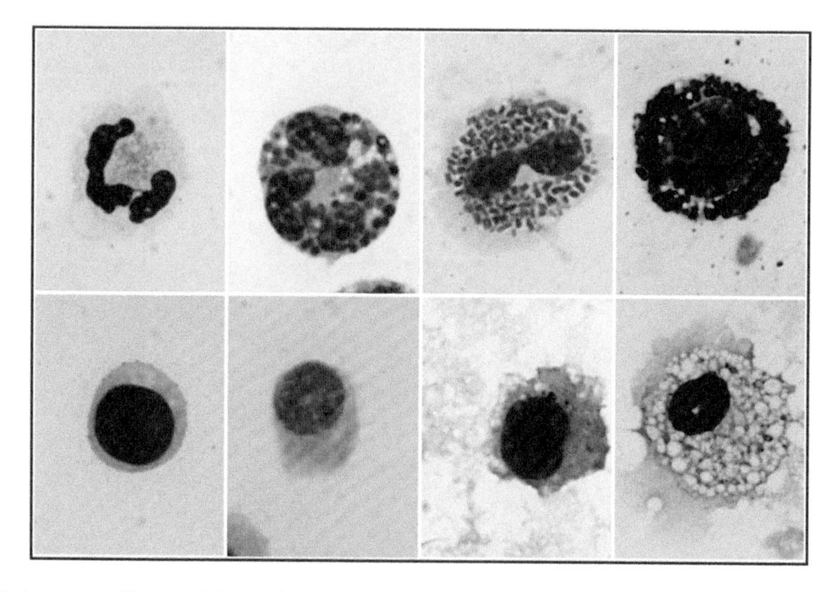

Fig. 2.3. Leucocytes. From top left to right bottom: Neutrophil, canine eosinophil, feline eosinophil, mast cell, small lymphocyte, plasma cell, alveolar macrophage, foamy alveolar macrophage. Wright-Giemsa.

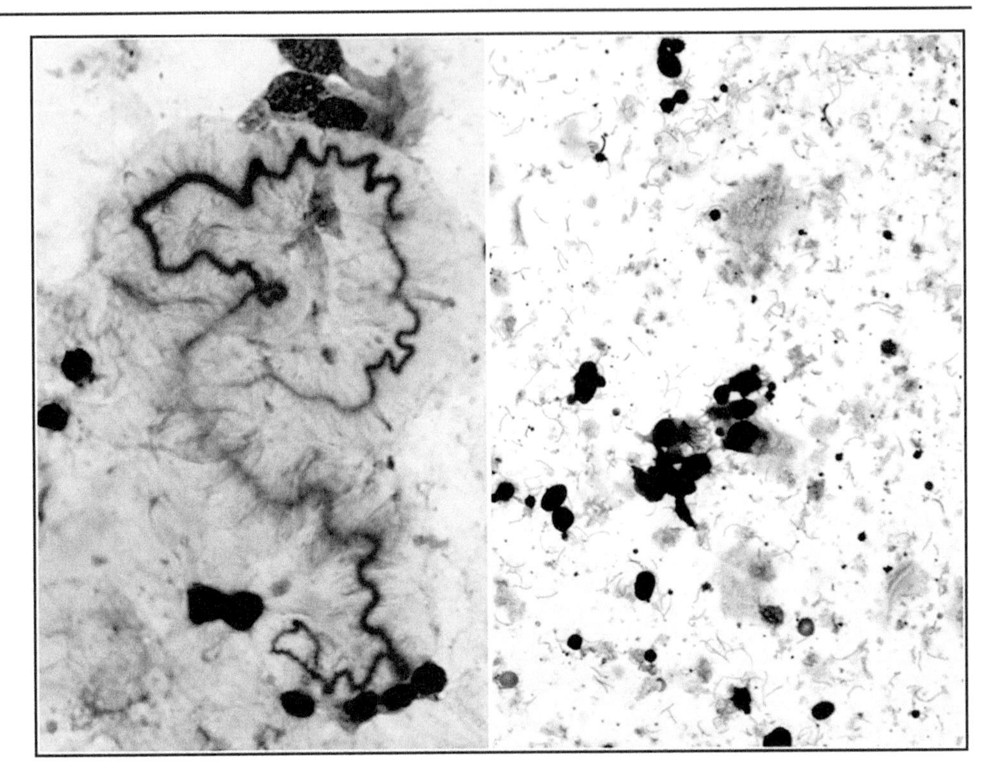

Fig. 2.4. Dog. BAL. Curschmann spiral (left), free cilia (right). Wright-Giemsa.

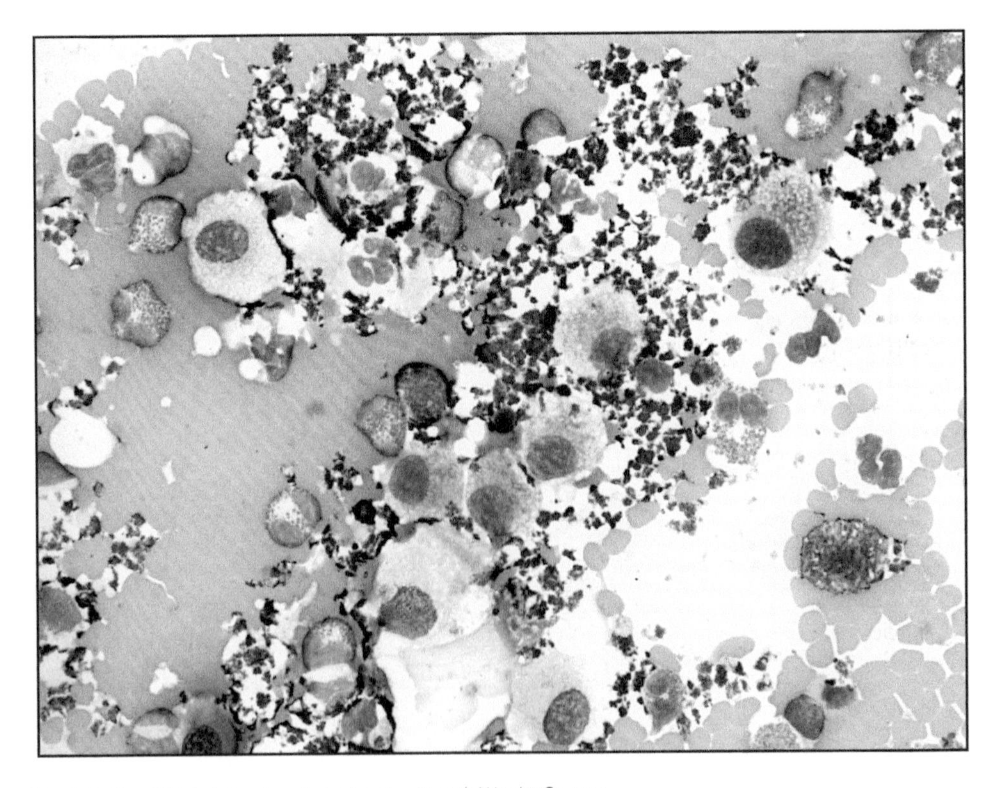

Fig. 2.5. Dog. BAL. Lubricant material (contaminant). Wright-Giemsa.

2.5 Normal Cytology of the Respiratory Tract

Upper respiratory tract

Samples obtained from the upper part of the respiratory tract (nasal swabs and flushes) of healthy dogs and cats may contain the following elements:

- Squamous epithelial cells from the anterior nasal cavity. These are often individual, sometimes arranged in clusters and may be associated with bacteria.
- Ciliated columnar respiratory epithelial cells from the posterior nasal cavity and paranasal sinuses. These are either individual or arranged in clusters, often with palisading arrangement.
- Cuboidal epithelial cells from the caudoventral vestibule, lateral meatus, distal ends of turbinates and nasal septum. They are not seen often and tend to form small cohesive clusters.
- Goblet cells with characteristic intracytoplasmic secretory granules.
- Lymphoid cells, mostly small lymphocytes, from the NALT. Intermediate/large lymphoid cells and plasma cells may also be present especially in reactive processes.
- Red blood cells as result of iatrogenic contamination or true haemorrhage.
- Mucus, present in variable amounts and appearing as amorphous basophilic material.
- Mixed population of extracellular bacteria representing normal flora, often lying on the surface of the squamous epithelial cells.

Lower respiratory tract

Tracheal wash

- In healthy animals, samples obtained by TW harvest low numbers of nucleated cells, almost entirely ciliated and non-ciliated columnar respiratory cells.
- Lower percentages of macrophages, goblet cells and other leucocytes are seen.
- Neutrophils usually account for <5–10% of all leucocytes.
- Small flecks of mucoid material may also be present.
- A recent study showed that cytological findings in TW samples obtained by endotracheal and transtracheal methods were very similar; however, the percentage of hypocellular and non-diagnostic samples was higher for the endotracheal technique.

Tracheobronchial brushing

- Samples from healthy dogs obtained with this technique almost entirely consist of epithelial cells, mainly ciliated and columnar.
- Leucocytes range from 0% to 2% of all nucleated cells and neutrophils are only rarely seen.

Bronchoalveolar lavage

- In healthy animals, alveolar macrophages are the main cell type accounting for >70% of all nucleated cells. Other cell types found in lower numbers include small lymphocytes, neutrophils, eosinophils and mast cells. Epithelial cells and goblet cells are only rarely seen since bronchoalveolar lavage (BAL) should reflect sampling from terminal bronchioli and alveolar space only.
- Nucleated differential count is often performed on 100–200 nucleated cells. However, in a recent study, adequate reproducibility of all cell populations was reached by counting a minimum of 500 cells.

- Differential count can be performed either on all nucleated cells or only on the leucocytes, since the epithelial component should comprise <1% of the entire cell population. However, if the epithelial cells are present in large numbers as individual elements or clusters, they should be described in the cytology report but excluded from the differential count.
- Overall, the data found in the literature regarding the percentages of cells found in BALs of healthy animals vary depending on the source. This may depend on the inclusion criteria used to define 'healthy animals', the process of fluid preparation and microscopic assessment.
- The average of mean percentage cell types from a number of studies of BAL samples from healthy dogs and cats are indicated in the table below (excluding the epithelial cells).
- Percentages of neutrophils as high as 20% have been reported in both healthy dogs and cats. The most significant variability involves eosinophils. In a few studies from North America, they accounted for up to 23% of all nucleated cells in BAL samples from apparently healthy cats and up to 11% in healthy dogs. A possible correlation between percentage of eosinophils and previous parasite exposure, prophylactic anthelmintic treatment and indoor/outdoor state has been suggested.

Table 2.2. Expected percentage range for cell types in BAL samples from clinically healthy dogs and cats.

	Macrophages	Neutrophils	Eosinophils	Lymphocytes	Mast cells
Dog	70-80%	<5%, rarely up to 20%	Typically <5%, but up to 11%	Typically < 11%, but up to 17%	<2%
Cat	70-80%	<7%, rarely up to 20%	Typically < 10%, but up to 23%	<5%	<2%

Pearls and Pitfalls

- Percentages of each cell type in BAL samples and reference values may vary among laboratories and publications. This depends on multiple variables, including biological variation.
- In thick areas where cells are aggregated and often associated with the mucus, it might be difficult to distinguish eosinophils from neutrophils. This is because eosinophil granules may change in colour and become less visible, while neutrophils may stain a diffuse, uneven, light-pink colour.

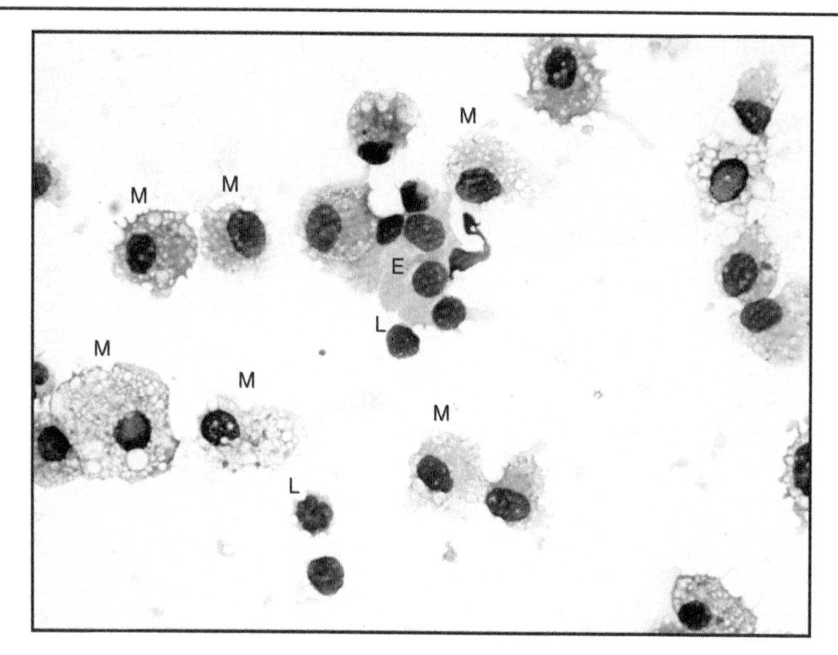

Fig. 2.6. Dog. BAL. Unremarkable findings. Prevalence of alveolar macrophages (M), rare columnar epithelial cells (E) and small lymphocytes (L). Wright-Giemsa.

Further reading

Andreasen, C.B. (2003) Bronchoalveolar lavage. *Veterinary Clinics of North America; Small Animal Practice* 33(1), 69–88.

Baudendistel, L.J., Vogler, G.A., Frank, P.A., Zanaboni, P.B. and Dahms, T.E. (1992) Bronchoalveolar eosinophilia in random-source versus purpose-bred dogs. *Laboratory Animal Science* 42(5), 491–496.

DeLorenzi, D., Masserdotti, C., Bertoncello, D. and Tranquillo, V. (2009) Differential cell counts in canine cyto-centrifuged bronchoalveolar lavage fluid: a study on reliable enumeration of each cell. *Veterinary Clinical Pathology* 38(4), 532–536.

Finke, M. (2013) Transtracheal wash and bronchoalveolar lavage. *Topics in Companion Animal Medicine* 28(3), 97–102.

Graham, A.M., Tefft, K.M., Stowe, D.M., Jacob, M.E., Robertson, J.B. *et al.* (2021) Factors associated with clinical interpretation of tracheal wash fluid from dogs with respiratory disease: 281 cases (2012–2017). *Journal of Veterinary Internal Medicine* 35(2), 1073–1079.

Hawkins, E.C., DeNicola, D.B. and Kuehn, N.F. (1990) Bronchoalveolar lavage in the evaluation of pulmonary disease in the dog and cat. *Journal of Veterinary Internal Medicine* 4(5), 267–274.

Lecuyer, M., Dube, P.G., DiFruscia, R., Desnoyers, M. and Lagace, A. (1995) Bronchoalveolar lavage in normal cats. *Canadian Veterinary Journal* 36(12), 771–773.

2.6 Upper Respiratory Tract

2.6.1 Sterile inflammation

Sterile inflammation may occur in the upper respiratory tract alone or concurrently with involvement of the lower airways. Main leucocyte cell type depend on the cause of the inflammation.

Sterile neutrophilic rhinitis

Clinical features

- Clinical signs include sneezing, nose rubbing and head shaking.
- May be secondary to nasal foreign bodies. These are often inhaled but can also penetrate through the palate. Clinical signs are usually acute and nasal discharge is unilateral.
- Underlying neoplasia may be associated with inflammation, also due to the presence of concurrent necrosis. Clinical signs often begin as a unilateral, but progress to bilateral involvement.
- Secondary bacterial infection may occur.

Causes

- Foreign bodies (e.g. plant awns, foxtails and twigs).
- Underlying neoplasia.
- Inhalation of irritant gases or dust particles.

Cytological features

- Neutrophils are often non-degenerate, unless there is concurrent necrosis, in which case they may appear karyolitic. They may be associated with variable numbers of macrophages (pyogranulomatous inflammation).
- Other elements that may be present include red blood cells (haemorrhage) and foreign material (e.g. plant material or fibres), which can be extracellular and/or intracellular.

Differential diagnoses

- Infectious rhinitis (infectious agents are not always visible on cytology)

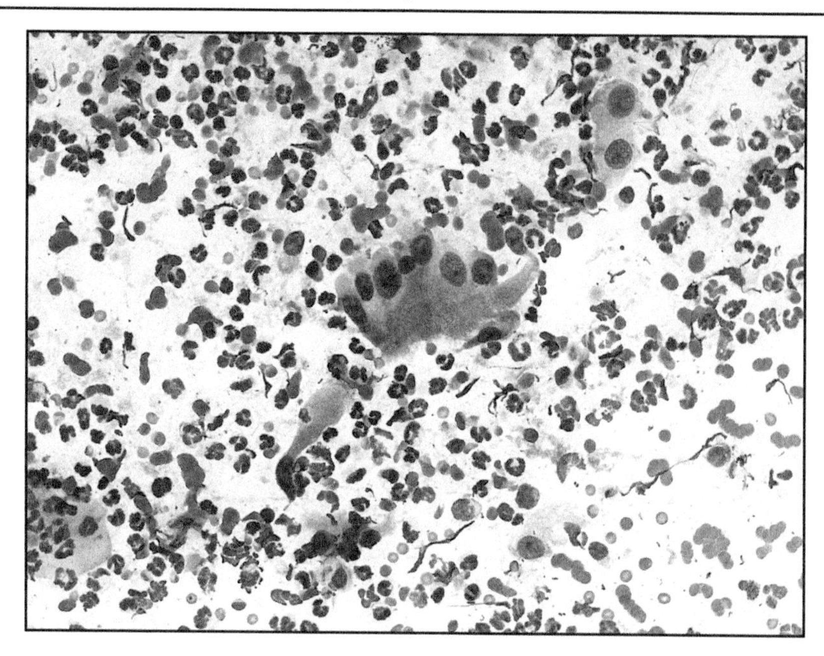

Fig. 2.7. Dog. Nasal flush. Neutrophilic rhinitis, high numbers of neutrophils and a few ciliated columnar respiratory epithelial cells. Wright-Giemsa.

Sterile eosinophilic rhinitis

Clinical features

- Clinical signs may include ocular discharge, sneezing, nose rubbing and head shaking.
- It can be seasonal, depending on the causative allergen.

Causes

- Hypersensitivity type I against variable allergens (allergic rhinitis).
- Paraneoplastic inflammation triggered by underlying neoplasia (e.g. mast cell tumour).

Cytological features

- Eosinophils are often the predominant cell type. They may be accompanied by lower numbers of non-degenerate neutrophils, macrophages and/or granulated mast cells.
- Goblet cells and increased amounts of mucus can be present.

Differential diagnoses

- Infectious rhinitis (fungi, parasites)

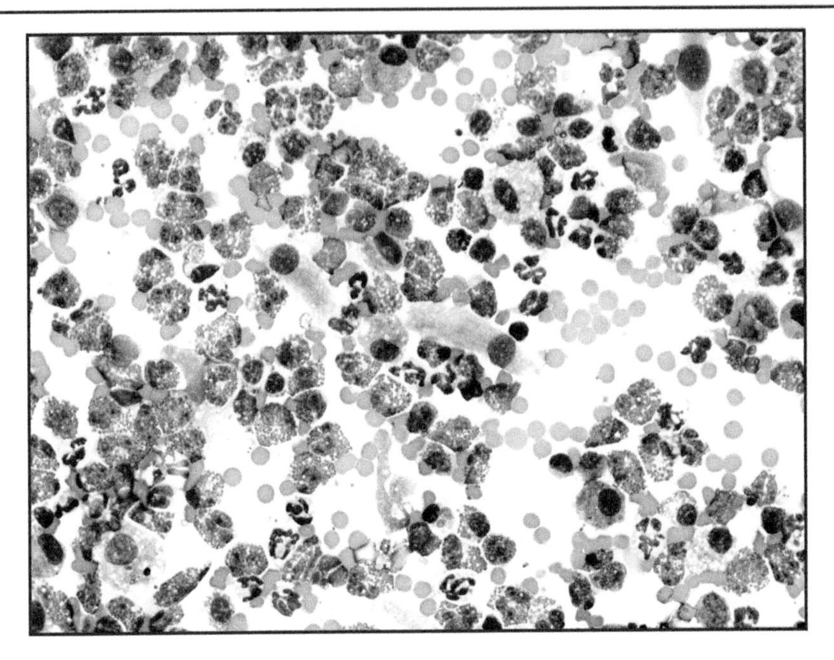

Fig. 2.8. Dog. Nasal flush. Eosinophilic rhinitis, high numbers of eosinophils and scattered columnar respiratory epithelial cells. Wright-Giemsa.

Sterile lymphoplasmacytic rhinitis

Clinical features

- Most common type of rhinitis in dogs rhinitis in dogs.
- Unilateral or bilateral nasal discharge with respiratory signs.
- Increased amount of mucus production and diffuse or polypoid thickening of the mucosa. Turbinate destruction can occur.

Causes

- Idiopathic lymphoplasmacytic rhinitis.
- Chronic inflammation caused by foreign bodies or neoplasia.

Cytological features

- Small lymphocytes are often the predominant cell type. Plasma cells may be present in lower numbers.
- Abundant mucus can be present.
- Rafts of epithelial cells often accompany the inflammation and may also be associated with squamous metaplasia and/or dysplasia.

Differential diagnoses

- Chronic inflammation due to bacteria or fungal infection
- Nasopharyngeal polyps (cats)
- Small cell lymphoma

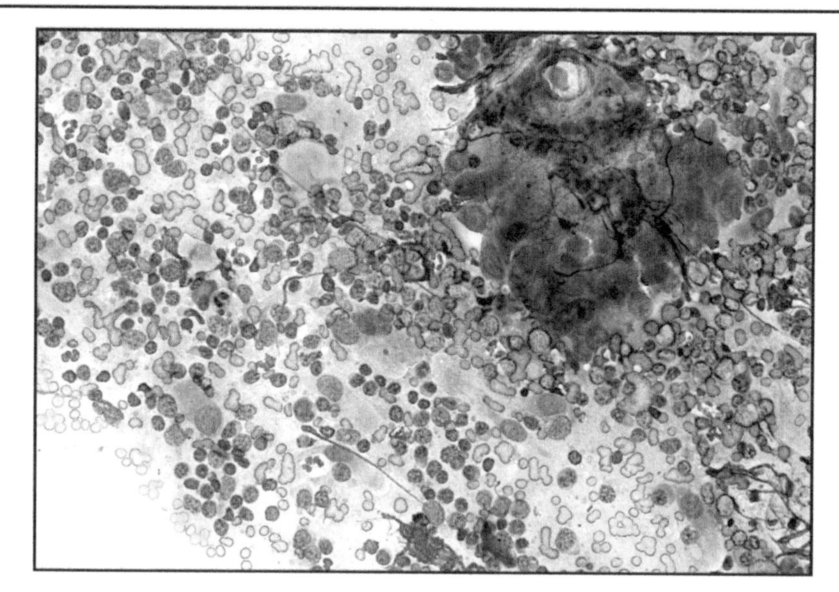

Fig. 2.9. Cat. Nasal flush. Lymphoplasmacytic rhinitis, prevalence of lymphocytes, mostly small, and occasional neutrophils. Respiratory cuboidal epithelial cells are present individually and in small clusters. Wright-Giemsa.

Pearls and Pitfalls

- Idiopathic lymphoplasmacytic rhinitis is a condition most commonly described in dogs (in particular young to middle-aged dolichocephalic large breeds) and less frequent in cats. It can be associated with an increased mucus production, turbinate destruction and diffuse or polypoid thickening of the mucosa. Causes and pathogenesis are unknown.
- Nasal polyps represent a hyperplasia of the mucus membranes or exuberant proliferation of fibrous connective tissue. They appear as pedunculated masses originating from the nasopharyngeal region, Eustachian tube or middle ear. They are particularly common in young cats but have been reported also in dogs. A mixed inflammation is of often present mostly including lymphocytes and plasma cells with lower numbers of macrophages and neutrophils.
- A variant of the feline nasal polyps of the nasal turbinates, called *inflammatory polyp*, has been described. This consists of fibrous tissue covered by columnar epithelial cells. It often contains a prominent inflammatory infiltrate, mainly composed of lymphocytes and plasma cells. However, macrophages and neutrophils are not uncommon.
- Morphological features of atypia observed in association with epithelial metaplasia and dysplasia can mime neoplasia, suggesting exercising caution in the cytological diagnosis of neoplasia, especially if there is inflammation and in absence of a mass.

Further reading

Cohn, L.A. (2020) Canine nasal disease: an update. *North American Small Animal Practice* 50(2), 359–374.

2.6.2 Infectious causes

Septic upper airway inflammation may be caused by various infection agents, such as bacteria, viruses, fungi, yeasts, algae, protozoa and/or parasites. Cytological evidence of these organisms, especially when intracellular and associated with the inflammatory cells, is considered proof of infection. The absence of microorganisms on the smear does not rule out infection. Therefore, additional diagnostic investigations (e.g. culture testing, serology and PCR) may be considered in selected cases.

Bacterial infections

Clinical features

- Primary bacterial rhinitis is very uncommon in both dogs and cats, particularly when unilateral. Therefore, evaluation for possible underlying causes should always be considered and addressed even when bacterial sepsis is identified.
- More often secondary to other infectious agents, foreign bodies, dental disease, oronasal fistulation, underlying neoplasia and/or trauma.

Bacteria that more commonly colonize the upper respiratory tract include:

- Dogs: *Bordetella bronchiseptica*, *Pasteurella multocida*, *Streptococcus canis* and *Streptococcus equi* subspecies *zooepidemicus*, *Pseudomonas aeruginosa*, *Staphylococcus* spp., *Actinomyces* spp. and *Nocardia* spp.
- Cats: *Bordetella bronchiseptica*, *Chlamydophila felis*, *Mycoplasma* spp., *Pasteurella multocida*, *Streptococcus canis* and *Streptococcus equi* subspecies *zooepidemicus*, *Pseudomonas aeruginosa*, *Staphylococcus* spp., *Actinomyces* spp. and *Nocardia* spp.

Cytological features

- Often characterized by the presence of numerous neutrophils, which may show signs of degeneration and may contain intracellular bacteria.
- Other inflammatory cell types may also be present.

Viral infections

Clinical features

- Often manifests as an acute and transient inflammatory process, unless a secondary opportunistic bacterial infection develops.
- May result in turbinate damage and epithelial/glandular hyperplasia.

Upper respiratory tract may be affected by selected viruses. These include:

- Dogs: distemper, adenovirus, herpesvirus, influenza/parainfluenza, coronavirus and reovirus.
- Cats: herpesvirus, calicivirus, coronavirus, influenza, reovirus, feline leukaemia virus (FeLV) and feline immunodeficiency virus (FIV).

Cytological features

- Non-specific, with variable numbers and types of inflammatory cells.
- Viral inclusions within epithelial cells are rarely seen. (e.g. distemper).

Fungal, protozoal and algal infections

Clinical features

- More common in dogs than cats, in particular young to middle-aged adults. They can be primary or secondary/opportunistic diseases.
- Discharge associated with fungal rhinitis often begins as a unilateral, but often progresses to bilateral involvement.
- Conditions that may predispose to fungal nasal infections include foreign body penetration, underlying neoplasia and immunodepression.
- As certain fungi can be present in the environment or could be contaminants or inhabitants of the nasal cavity of healthy patients (e.g. *Aspergillus* spp., *Penicillium* spp. and *Alternaria* spp.), the diagnosis of fungal rhinitis should be supported by appropriate clinical findings and by the presence of an inflammatory response.

Causes and cytological features

- Most common aetiological agents of fungal rhinitis are *Aspergillus* spp., *Penicillium* spp. (dogs) and *Cryptococcus* spp. (cats). Some fungi such as *Blastomyces* spp., *Coccidioides* spp. and *Histoplasma* spp. are endemic only in certain geographical areas and are rare or absent in others, making the likelihood of infection dependent on geographical location and travel history. Phaeohyphomycosis is often associated with the presence of foreign bodies.
- Cytology samples typically show a mixed inflammatory response with neutrophils, sometimes eosinophils and macrophages. Multi-nucleated giant inflammatory cells may also be present.
- Fungal elements can be found extracellularly or phagocytosed by the macrophages.

Aspergillus spp.

- This is the most common cause of fungal rhinitis in dogs, together with *Penicillium* spp., from which it is morphologically indistinguishable.
- Nasal aspergillosis is often characterized by the formation of white plaques visible on rhinoscopy. Sampling from these areas increases the chance to obtain a diagnosis, compared to nasal flushing. Local bone lysis is not uncommon and may affect nasal turbinates and other local bony structures.
- Involvement of the lower respiratory tract has also been reported.
- German Shepherd dogs and dolicocephalic/mesocephalic dogs seem to be predisposed to this infection.
- Cytologically, *Aspergillus* spp. presents as 2–5 μm diameter, parallel-walled, dichotomously branching at 45° angles and septate hyphae with globose terminal ends, often staining intensely basophilic with a thin clear outer cell wall. Organisms may be seen within macrophages and/or extracellular. Round to oval basophilic fungal spores may also be found.
- Inflammation is often present and varies from neutrophilic to macrophagic, sometimes with increased numbers of eosinophils. Concurrent lymphoplasmacytic rhinitis may occur.
- PCR testing or culture may help to further speciate Aspergillus spp. and to differentiate this from Penicillium spp.

Cryptococcus spp.

- Dimorphic fungus, cause of fungal rhinitis in both dogs and cats. It may also result in systemic disease with neurological involvement.
- Most common species are:
  - *Cryptococcus neoformans* reported in both dogs and cats. It is less virulent than other species and may result in colonization of the nasal cavity with no clinical signs, in particular in dogs.

  - *Cryptococcus gattii*, more virulent species. It is particularly common in cats where infection is more often restricted to the upper respiratory tract.
- Organisms of both species are characterized by pink to blue-purple and slightly granular round yeasts with a thick clear capsule. Size is very variable and can reach 40 µm. A characteristic narrow-based budding may be seen. Capsule size may vary in some strains and be absent or less apparent in areas of necrosis. Their morphology should not be assessed in areas of necrosis.
- Inflammation is often present and is mainly neutrophilic and/or macrophagic, with variable numbers of eosinophils.
- Cryptococcus antigen test is a useful method of diagnosis in suspected cases in which the organism is not identified by other means. This test can also be used as a method of monitoring response to treatment.

Rhinosporidium seeberi

- Sporadic cause of rhinitis in dogs and less commonly in cats, often secondary to contact of the nasal mucosa with contaminated standing water. It mainly causes formation of polypoid masses in the nasal cavity.
- Cytologically, samples contain variable numbers of inflammatory cells, associated intracellular and extracellular organisms. These are round, oval and cigar-shaped structures, 3–5 µm wide and 5–9 µm long, and may be surrounded by a clear halo, resembling a capsule.

Other less common fungal diseases described in the upper respiratory tract include *Sporothrix schenckii* and *Alternaria* spp.

Algae (e.g. *Prototheca* spp. and *Entamoeba* spp.) and protozoa (e.g. *Leishmania* spp.) have also been rarely reported.

Parasitic infections

Rare cause of rhinitis.

Parasites that can be identified cytologically in upper respiratory tract include:

- *Pneumonyssoides caninum* (dogs).
- *Eucoleus* spp. (dogs and cats).
- *Linguatula serrata* (dogs).
- *Protists* (e.g. *Entamoeba* sp).

Pneumonyssoides caninum

- Mite causing rhinitis in dogs and most commonly reported affecting dogs in the Scandinavian countries.

Eucoleus spp. (formerly known as *Capillaria* spp.)

- Nematode that may affect the nasal cavity of both dogs and cats. Ova may be seen in nasal secretions and appear as ovoid structures, 50×35 µm, with two asymmetrical terminal plugs.
- The two main species are *E. boehmi* and *E. aerophilus*.

Linguatula serrata

- Wormlike arthropod that can inhabit the nasal cavity and frontal sinuses of dogs. It causes sneezing and nasal discharge.

Protists

- These are a group of organisms characterized by their ability to survive freely in the environment, to move via pseudopods and to phagocytize organic material. The transmission to the host occurs via direct contact or through fomites. These organisms are considered opportunistic; they may be isolated from healthy animals but may also result in clinical manifestation of disease. A recent case of *Entamoeba gingivalis* in the nasal flush of a dog with respiratory signs and dental disease has been reported.

Pearls and Pitfalls

- The presence of nasal signs, in particular when acute or associated with systemic disease or epistaxis, may also be due to a disease of not primary nasal origin.
- Because the nasal passages of healthy dogs are not sterile and because primary bacterial rhinitis is rare, bacterial culture from dogs with nasal disease is of little use.
- Fungal culture may be useful. The sensitivity of culture testing for dogs with sinonasal aspergillosis can be as high as 80% if samples are collected from areas containing rhinoscopically visible plaques but is likely to be lower from samples collected blindly.

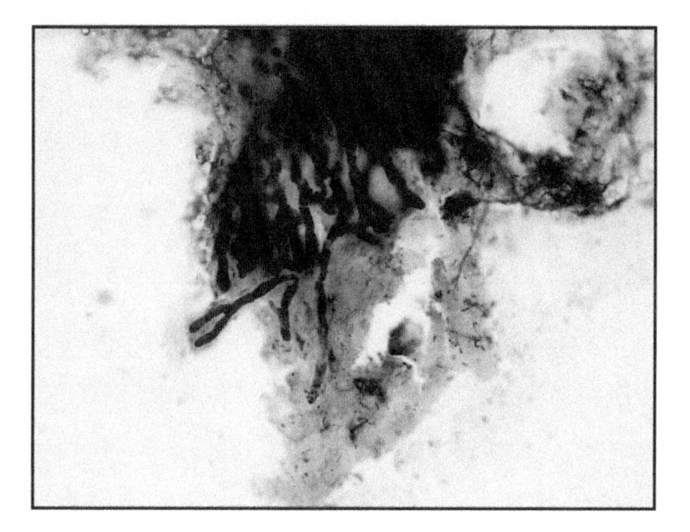

Fig. 2.10. Dog. Nasal flush. *Aspergillus* spp. Intensely basophilic, septate and branching fungal hyphae. Wright-Giemsa.

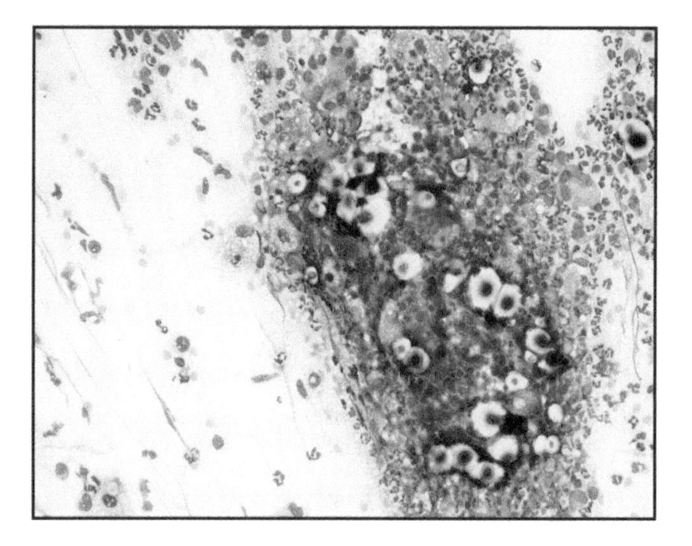

Fig. 2.11. Cat. Nasal flush. *Cryptococcal rhinitis*. Numerous yeast forms with distinctive non-staining, thick, capsule, admixed with leucocytes, mostly neutrophils. Wright-Giemsa.

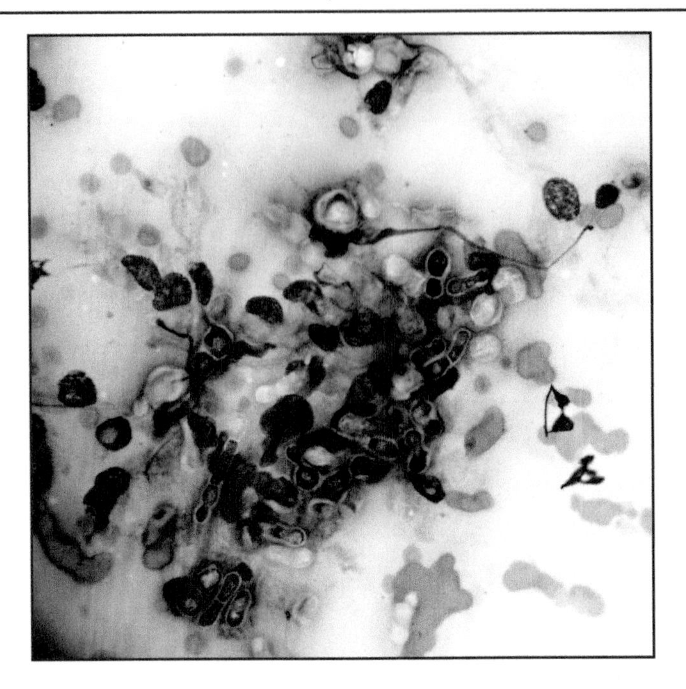

Fig. 2.12. Dog. Nasal flush. *Alternaria* spp. Fungal organisms are pale staining and round with septate hyphae. Wright-Giemsa.

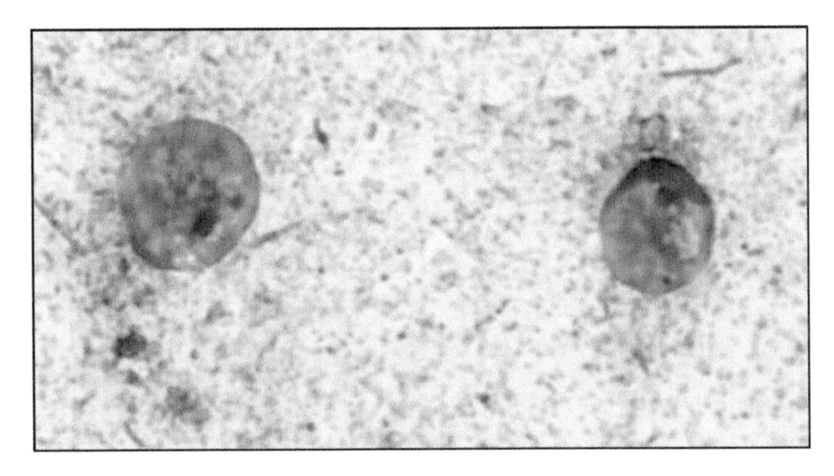

Fig. 2.13. Dog. Nasal flush. Protist colonisation. Two round and individualized organisms (trophozoites) are seen. They have pale basophilic cytoplasm and a small paracentral nucleus. Further speciation was not performed. The background contains numerous extracellular-mixed bacteria. Wright-Giemsa.

Further reading

Cohn, L.A. (2020) Canine nasal disease: an update. *North American Small Animal Practice* 50(2), 359–374.

Lappin, M.R., Blondeau, J., Boothe, D., Breitschwerdt, E.B., Guardabassi, L. *et al.* (2017) Antimicrobial use guidelines for treatment of respiratory tract disease in dogs and cats: antimicrobial guidelines working group of the International Society for Companion Animal Infectious Diseases. *Journal of Veterinary Internal Medicine* 31(2), 279–294.

Randolph, N.K., McAloney, C.A., Ossiboff, R., Hernandez, B., Cook, M. *et al.* (2022) Nasal colonization by *Entamoeba gingivalis* in a 13-year-old Italian Greyhound. *Veterinary Clinical Pathology* 51(2), 269–272.

2.6.3 Neoplasms

Tumours in the upper respiratory tract are most commonly primary. Neoplastic cells do not exfoliate in nasal flush samples and the diagnosis may be more easily achieved by fine-needle aspiration (or solid biopsy) of the mass.

- Upper respiratory neoplasms in dogs and cats are relatively uncommon, representing 2% and 8% of all tumours, respectively.
- They arise from any of the tissue types found in the nasal cavity, rarely from paranasal sinuses, but also pharynx, larynx and nasal planum.
- They are most frequently malignant. Diagnosis can be achieved by cytology, depending on the sample quality and cellularity.
- Confounding factors such as inflammation, hyperplasia of the NALT, necrosis and/or haemorrhage may complicate the diagnostic process.
- Discharge associated with either nasal neoplasia or fungal rhinitis often begins as a unilateral problem but progresses to bilateral involvement.
- In dogs, the most common tumour of the upper respiratory tract is nasal adenocarcinoma; in cats, lymphoma and squamous cell carcinoma (SCC) are the most frequent.
- Over-represented canine breeds: dolichocephalic breeds are 2.5 times more likely to develop nasal neoplasia than mixed-breed dogs. Large dogs are more likely to have nasal neoplasia than small breeds.
- Age: adult and old dogs are more commonly affected.

Epithelial neoplasms

Clinical features

- Both benign and malignant tumours can arise in the upper respiratory tract, but malignant forms are more frequent.
- Most common tumours include papilloma, adenocarcinoma, SCC, transitional cell carcinoma and anaplastic/undifferentiated carcinomas.
- In dogs, nasal adenocarcinoma is the most common type. It mainly arises in the caudal two-thirds of the nasal cavity and may extend to the surrounding tissues/structures. It can metastasize to regional lymph nodes and other organs. This tumour typically has a slow growth rate. At time of diagnosis, metastases are uncommon.
- In cats, SCC is the most common epithelial neoplasm of the upper respiratory tract. It often involves the nasal planum. Ultraviolet radiation is a strong cofactor, and feline papillomavirus may also play a role in it.
- Nasal tumours in both species are more commonly observed in adult/old patients, but they have also been reported in young animals.
- Clinical signs are variable and often related to the slow and insidiously to an often slowly and insidiously expanding space occupying lesion, occasionally causing invasion and destruction of adjacent structures, in particular the bone. They may include cough, sneezing, dyspnoea and ocular discharge. Neurological signs may also occur indicating CNS involvement.
- Over-represented canine breeds: Airedale Terrier, Basset Hound, Old English Sheepdog, Scottish Terrier, Collie, Shetland Sheepdog and German Shorthaired Pointer.

Cytological features

- Cellularity is variable, often high.
- Background: variably haemodiluted. It may contain extracellular bacteria and keratin squames (contaminants).
- Adenocarcinoma: cells are round to columnar and/or cuboidal and arranged in clusters. Acinar-like arrangements may occasionally be observed. Cells may have apical cilia and may also contain clear secretory vacuoles. Occasionally, the vacuoles can be large, displacing the nucleus to the periphery (signet ring cells).
- Squamous cell carcinoma: cells may show a wide range of maturation, in particular polygonal elements with abundant glassy and basophilic cytoplasm, angular borders and centrally placed round nuclei and cuboidal cells with increased nucleus:cytoplasm ratio. Mature cells are often individualized. Less differentiated cells tend to exfoliate in cohesive clusters. Asynchronous nucleus:cytoplasm maturation is not uncommon, and cells may contain perinuclear clear vacuoles.
- Transitional carcinoma: cells are non-keratinized, cuboidal to polygonal and resemble the transitional epithelium of the urinary tract. They often form clusters and may show palisading arrangement. Areas of squamous differentiation may be noted.
- Anaplastic carcinomas: cells are often very pleomorphic, frequently resembling round cells. They can form cohesive but variably disorganized clusters or may exfoliate individually.
- Cytological features of atypia are often prominent and include anisocytosis, anisokaryosis, prominent and multiple nucleoli, mitotic figures.
- In the absence of significant criteria of malignancy, and especially if a concurrent inflammatory process is present, cytological differentiation between well-differentiated carcinoma, benign epithelial neoplasia and epithelial hyperplasia may not be possible.
- Concurrent inflammation is common and is usually neutrophilic. Necrosis can be present.

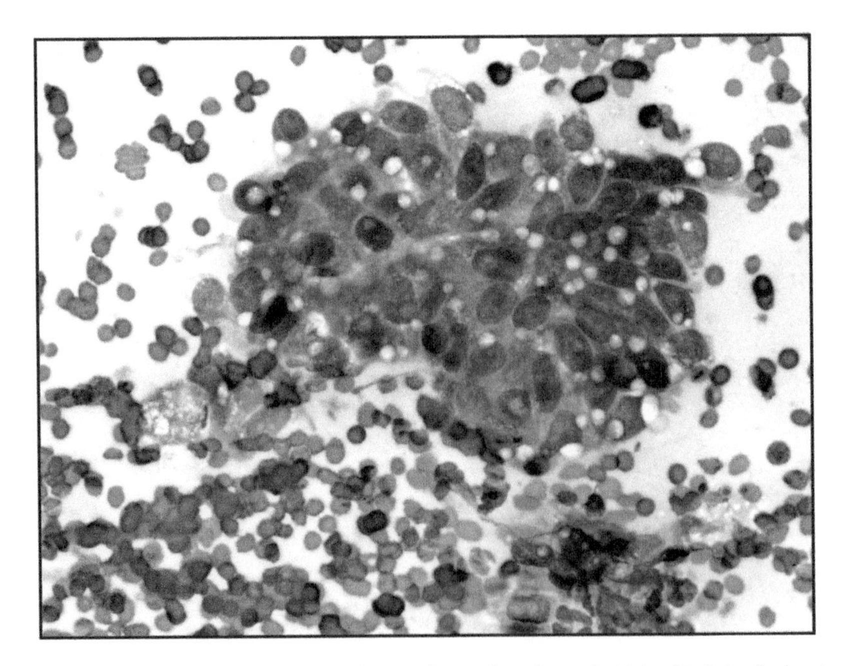

Fig. 2.14. Dog. Nasal flush. Nasal carcinoma, clusters of irregular, often cuboidal epithelial cells showing some degree of micro/macro vacuolations and some signs of atypia. Wright-Giemsa.

Mesenchymal neoplasms

Clinical features

- They include fibroma/fibrosarcoma, chondroma/chondrosarcoma, osteosarcoma, leiomyoma/sarcoma and rarely other sarcomas, including undifferentiated forms.
- They are significantly less common than epithelial and round-cell tumours in both species. In the dog, mesenchymal neoplasms account for approximately 18% of all nasal tumours, with chondrosarcoma being the most common form, in particular in young and medium-to-large canine breeds.
- Sarcomas arising from these districts have a low tendency to cause distant metastases.

Cytological features

- Cellularity is often low Cells usually do not exfoliate in nasal flushes and require fine needle aspiration of the mass or a biopsy for the diagnosis.
- Background: variably haemodiluted. It may contain extracellular bacteria and keratin squames (contaminants).
- Aspirates are composed of variably shaped mesenchymal cells, which exfoliate individually or in aggregates, sometimes associated with pink amorphous material (matrix). Morphological features are similar to those observed in sarcomas arising in other anatomical locations. Cytological features of atypia vary from mild to prominent.
- Chondrosarcomas: there is often abundant amorphous, homogeneous, eosinophilic to magenta amorphous material (cartilage) admixed with variable numbers of mononuclear cells (chondrocytes). The presence of a large amount of matrix often causes the understaining of the neoplastic cells, causing loss of details. Binucleation is possible.
- Osteosarcomas: the neoplastic cells (osteoblasts) are often individualized, round to oval. Occasionally, they may be found in small non-cohesive groups. They have round to oval, eccentric nuclei, finely stippled chromatin, prominent single or multiple nucleoli, and a moderate amount of basophilic cytoplasm. This may contain irregularly shaped pink granules. Multi-nucleated cells (osteoclasts) and amorphous eosinophilic to magenta amorphous material (osteoid) can also be present.

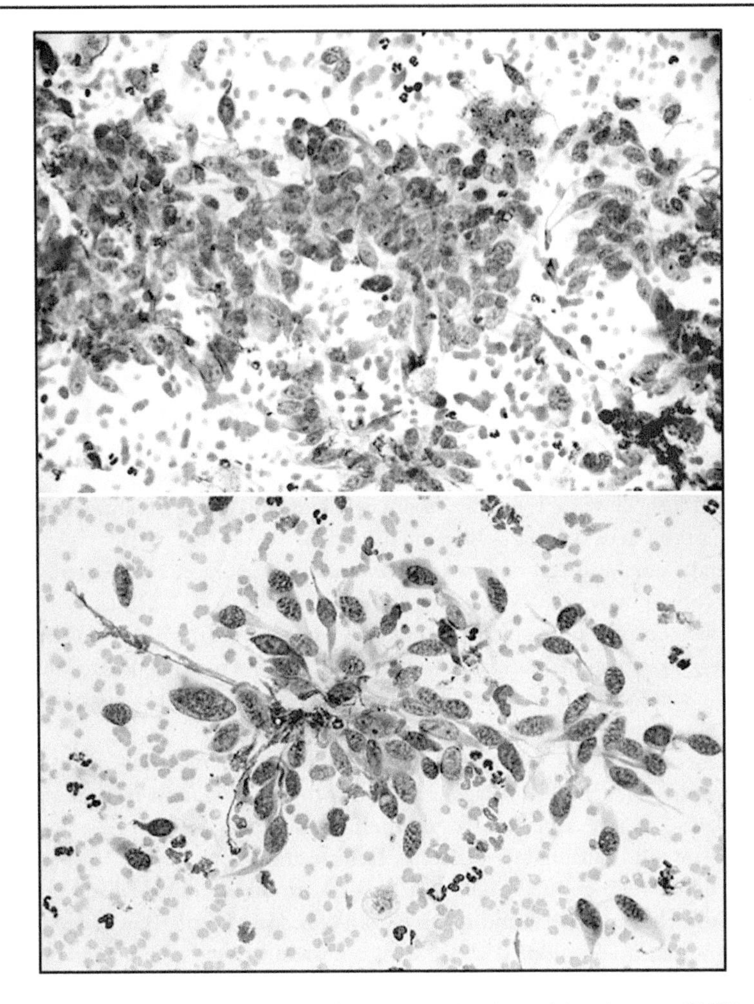

Fig. 2.15. Cat. Nasal mass. Soft tissue sarcoma confirmed as peripheral neural sheath tumors (PNST) on histopathology and immunohistochemistry. Mesenchymal spindle cells either individualized or forming poorly cohesive groups with storiform arrangement, admixed with neutrophils. Wright-Giemsa.

Neuroendocrine/neuroepithelial neoplasms

Clinical features

- These tumours include:
  - Neuroendocrine carcinoma (NEC): rarely described in the nasal cavity of dogs and arising from the neuroendocrine cells present in this location, which originate from the endododerm.
  - Olfactory neuroblastoma (ON): rarely described in both dogs and cats and originating from the neuroendocrine cells of neuroectodermal origin. It is also known as esthensioneuroblastoma.
- Due to the paucity of reported cases in the literature, the clinical behaviour of these neoplasms is not well defined but, in the long term, the prognosis is believed to be poor.
- Both types of tumours are locally infiltrative, sometimes with invasion of the brain. They both have the potential for widespread metastases, though it has been rarely reported in ON with a few more individual cases reported for NEC.

Cytological features

- Cellularity is variable; cells are often disrupted (bare/free nuclei). Since neoplastic cells usually do not exfoliate in nasal flushes, fine needle aspiration or solid biopsy of the mass is often needed.
- NEC and ON share similar cytological features. Morphological differentiation between these two tumours often requires histopathology and immunohistochemistry.
- Cells range from round to polygonal and may exfoliate either individually or in variably cohesive clusters. Occasional rosette-like structures may be found.
- Nuclei are round, variably sized and eccentric, with granular chromatin and poorly visible nucleoli. The cytoplasm is often scant and basophilic.
- Cytological features of atypia from mild to marked and include anisocytosis, anisokaryosis, mitotic figures and cell cannibalism.

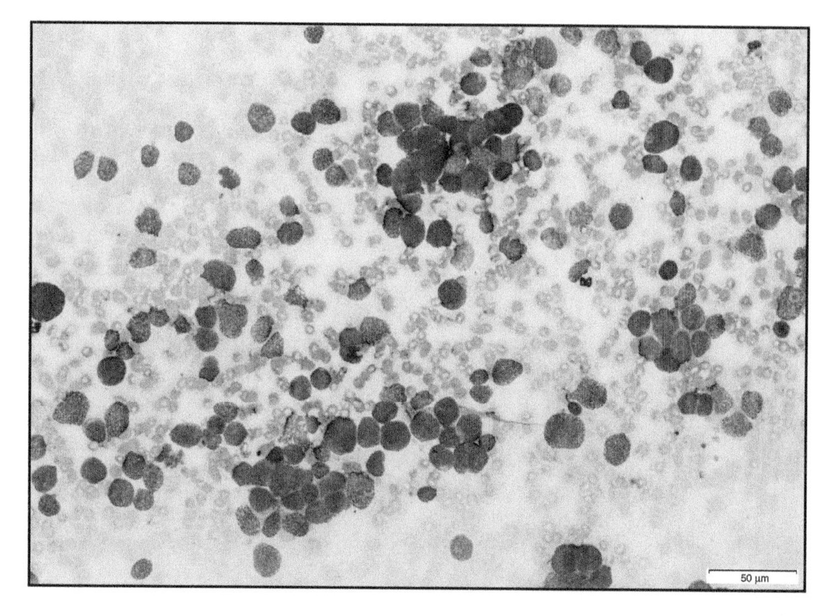

Fig. 2.16. Dog. Olfactory neuroblastoma. Large cells, often disrupted, with tendency to form small variably cohesive clusters. Wright-Giemsa. (*Courtesy of Paola Cazzini.*)

Differential diagnoses

- Carcinoma (e.g. adenocarcinoma, poorly differentiated carcinoma)
- Other poorly differentiated neoplasms

Lymphoma

Clinical features

- Lymphoma represents the most common upper respiratory neoplasm in cats. Nasal lymphoma is rare in dogs.
- Male cats and domestic shorthaired (DSH) subjects seem predisposed. Association with FeLV is controversial.
- In cats, most upper respiratory tract lymphomas are large B-cell lymphomas.
- It is usually localized in the nasal cavity, but a small proportion of cases arise in the nasopharynx or in both anatomical compartments.
- It is an aggressive neoplasia with shorter survival times, if not treated. Involvement of regional lymph nodes, other organs and bone marrow/peripheral blood may occur, especially in advanced stages.

Cytological features

- Cellularity is variable, often high.
- Background: variably haemodiluted. It often contains variable numbers of lymphoglandular bodies (cytoplasmic fragments of lymphoid cells).
- Neoplastic lymphoid cells are most often medium-large in size with high mitotic activity. Forms composed of a prevalence of small- to medium-sized lymphocytes may also occur.

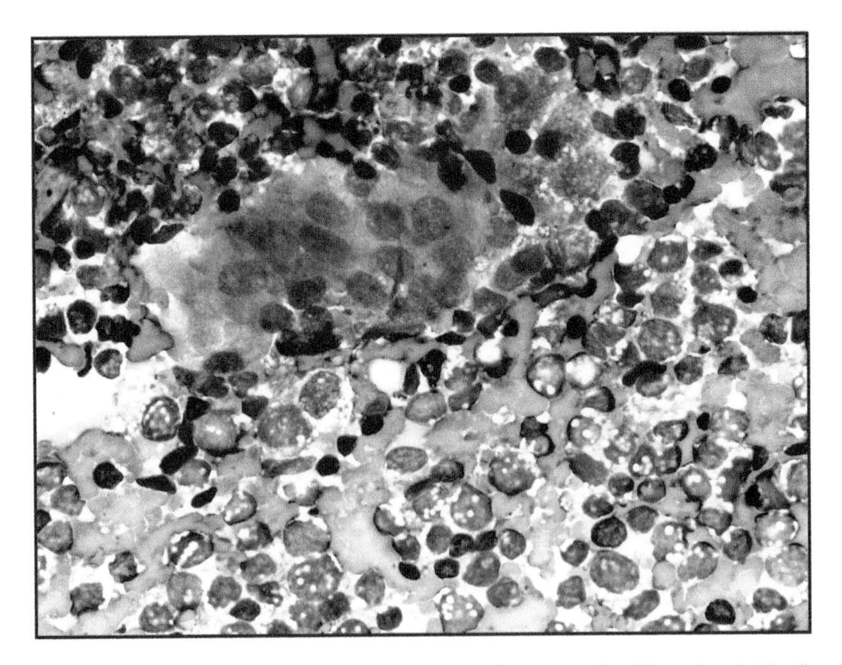

Fig. 2.17. Cat. Nasal flush. Nasal lymphoma. Main population of vacuolated and large lymphoid cells admixed with a few clusters of epithelial respiratory cells. Wright-Giemsa.

Transmissible venereal tumour

Clinical features

- This tumour has a histiocytic origin.
- It most frequently occurs in intact stray and wild young dogs (2-5 years of age) that exhibit unrestrained sexual activity. It is transmitted through direct skin-to-skin contact. Male dogs may be predisposed to develop the nasal form.
- Macroscopically, the mass can be variably sized, often cauliflower-like, pedunculated, nodular, papillary, or multi-lobulated. It is often firm but friable It is most commonly found in the external genitalia, but it may also occur in the nasal, oral and conjunctival mucosae.
- Clinical signs include sneezing, nasal bleeding, and unilateral/bilateral nasal purulent haemorrhagic discharge. Skull infiltration, formation oronasal fistulas within the hard palate and facial asymmetry may occur.
- Diagnosis is usually achieved by impression smears and/or fine needle aspiration of the nasal masses.
- It is most commonly found in the external genitalia, but it may also occur in the nasal, oral and conjunctival mucosae.
- Nasal TVT often has good response to chemotherapy or radiotherapy. Spontaneous regression may also occur. Metastatic spread has also been reported.

Cytological features

- Cellularity is variable, often high.
- Background: often basophilic and variably haemodiluted.
- Neoplastic cells are round and discrete with distinct cytoplasmic borders.
- Nuclei are almost perfectly round, paracentral to eccentric, with coarse chromatin. Single or multiple, round nucleoli may be seen.
- The cytoplasm is moderate to abundant and lightly basophilic. It often contains punctate clear, intracytoplasmic vacuoles. These are often located along the cells borders.
- Cytological features of atypia are variable, up to moderate. They include anisocytosis and anisokaryosis. Mitoses can be frequent.
- Small lymphocytes are often observed in the regressing phase. Reactive fibroblasts associated with collagen bundles may also be observed.
- Neutrophils may be present in ulcerated lesions.

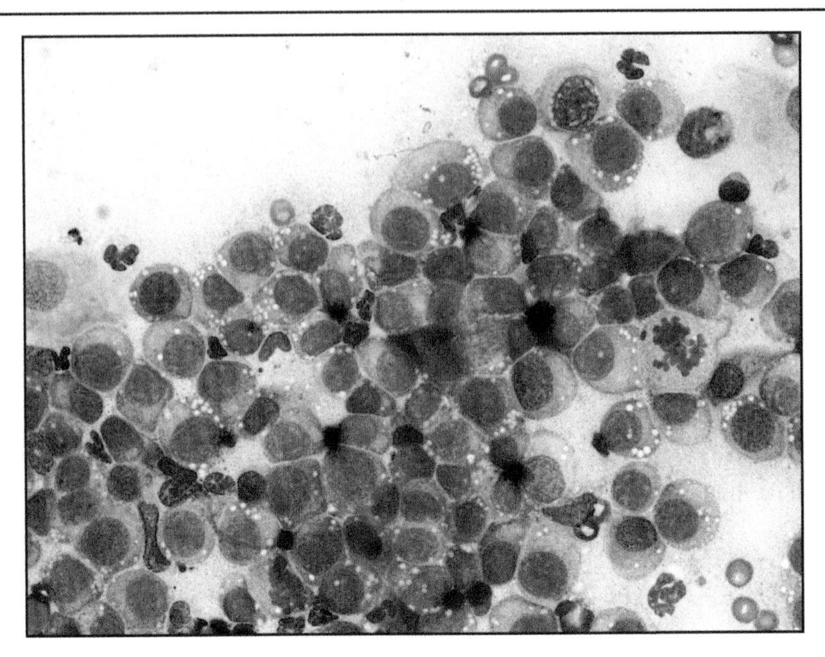

Fig. 2.18. Dog. Nasal imprint. Transmissible venereal tumour (TVT), population of histiocytic like discrete cells with distinct clear vacuoles, sometimes arranged along the cell borders. Wright-Giemsa.

Pearls and Pitfalls

- Anaplastic epithelial cells may appear round and individualized, resembling lymphoid cells or other cell types (e.g. neuroblastomas, neuroendocrine tumours, undifferentiated sarcomas and amelanotic melanomas). However, small areas in which the cell cohesion is preserved can be found. Nevertheless, further investigations (e.g. immunocytochemistry, immunohistochemistry) may be needed for a definitive diagnosis.
- To avoid non-cellular cytological smears, aggressive sampling that yields multiple tissue cores is suggested. From these, impression smears may be made.
- Diagnosis of lymphoma is often based on the presence of a monomorphic population of lymphoid cells, either small or large in size. Cytological diagnosis can be complicated by the concurrent presence of lymphoid hyperplasia of the NALT, which could make the overall lymphoid population appear mixed.
- TVT has mainly been reported in countries with a high population of stray animals. However, due to the increased migration processes, sporadic cases can also occur in countries that do not have stray dogs.

Further reading

Cazzini, P., Bęczkowski, P., Millins, C., Sharman, M., Hammond, G. *et al.* (2019) What is your diagnosis? Fine-needle aspirate from a nasal mass in a dog. *Veterinary Clinical Pathology* 48(2), 367–369.

Cohn, L.A. (2020) Canine nasal disease: an update. *North American Small Animal Practice* 50(2), 359–374.

Ganguly, B., Das, U. and Das, A.K. (2013) Canine transmissible venereal tumour: a review. *Veterinary Comparative Oncology* 14(1), 1–12.

Ignatenko, N., Abramenko, I., Soto, S. *et al.* (2020) Nasal transmissible venereal tumours in 12 dogs – a retrospective study. *Tierarztl Prax Ausg K Kleintiere Heimtiere* 48(3), 164–170.

Santagostino, S.F., Mortellaro, C.M., Boracchi, P., Avallone, G., Caniatti, M. *et al.* (2015) Feline upper respiratory tract lymphoma: site, cyto-histology, phenotype, FeLV expression, and prognosis. *Veterinary Pathology* 52(2), 250–259.

2.7 Lower Respiratory Tract

2.7.1 Not representative sample

This may occur when:

- TW or BAL do not harvest any intact nucleated cells.
- BAL sample contains a prevalence of columnar epithelial cells and no alveolar macrophages. This indicates that only the upper airways and not the alveolar space have been sampled.

2.7.2 Oropharyngeal contamination

Oropharyngeal contamination usually occurs during the passage of the catheter/endoscope through the oropharynx.

General information

- The presence of oropharyngeal contamination may alter the cytological evaluation and culture results. Depending on the degree of contamination, in the presence of neutrophils and/or bacteria, it could be difficult to establish if the bacteria are all contaminants of if there is a true infection, unless the bacteria are found phagocytosed by the neutrophils.
- In cases of recurrent aspiration of pharyngeal material or in bronchoesophageal fistula, the cytological findings may mimic iatrogenic oropharyngeal contamination.

Cytological features

- Squamous epithelial cells from the oral cavity and/or upper respiratory tract. They are large and polygonal cells (as described above) and do not show cytological features of atypia. They are often associated with bacteria.
- Neutrophils: often observed in samples from the oral cavity in particular when in the presence of inflammatory processes (e.g. dental disease).
- Bacteria: mixed population of cocci and/or rods. They are extracellular, free in the background or lying on the surface of the squamous epithelial cells.
- *Conchiformibius* spp. (formerly *Simonsiella* spp.): these are non-pathogenic bacteria that divide lengthwise, lining up in parallel rows. This gives the impression of a single large bacterium barcode shaped. They may adhere on the surface of squamous epithelial cells or be present in the background.

Pearls and Pitfalls

Contaminant bacteria are often found in association with the squamous epithelial cells and tend to be more mixed. In case of true infection, bacteria are distributed more evenly in the sample, they can be found phagocytes by the neutrophils, and tend to be less mixed in morphology.

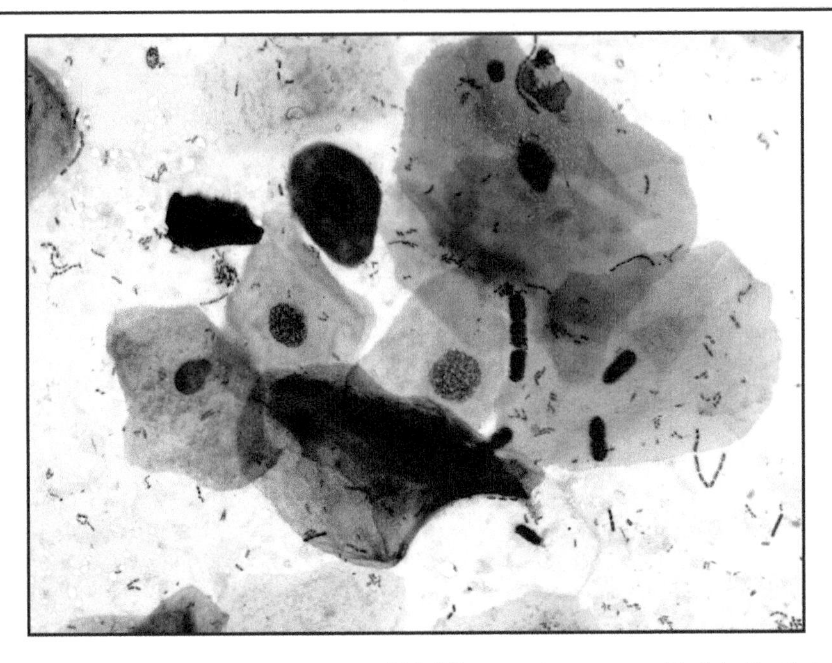

Fig. 2.19. Dog. BAL, oropharyngeal contamination. Well-differentiated squamous epithelial cells admixed with numerous bacteria and ***Conchiformibius*** spp. Wright-Giemsa.

2.7.3 Non infectious causes

2.7.3.1 Neutrophilic inflammation

Neutrophils are involved in innate cell-mediated immunity.

Causes

- Allergic airway inflammation (admixed with eosinophils).
- Aspiration pneumonia (e.g. inhaled barium or sucralfate).
- Underlying neoplasia.
- Idiopathic pulmonary fibrosis.
- Bromide-associated broncho-interstitial lipid pneumonia.
- Bronchiectasis.
- Bronchomalacia.
- Tracheal collapse.
- Microlithiasis (calcifications).

Cytological features

- Neutrophilic inflammation is diagnosed when neutrophils are typically >5% and >7% in dogs and cats, respectively.
- Samples are characterized by the presence of variable numbers of neutrophils which are usually non degenerate.
- Depending on the cause, exogenous material may be seen in the background or within the inflammatory cells.
- Neutrophilic inflammation may be associated with other leucocyte types, in particular macrophages. An increased amount of mucus and sometimes hyperplasia of the goblet cells may also be present.

Differential diagnoses

- Bacterial infections
  - Aspiration pneumonia of ingesta
  - Foreign body
- Fungal infections
- Viral infections
- Protozoal infections

Pearls and Pitfalls

- In BALs and TWs, careful examination is required to distinguish eosinophils from neutrophils, especially in areas where cells are in thick aggregates and/or associated with mucus. Sometimes, the cytoplasm of neutrophils may diffusely or unevenly stain faintly pink.
- The presence of degenerate neutrophils in BAL samples should prompt bacterial and fungal culture, even if organisms are not noticed on microscopy.

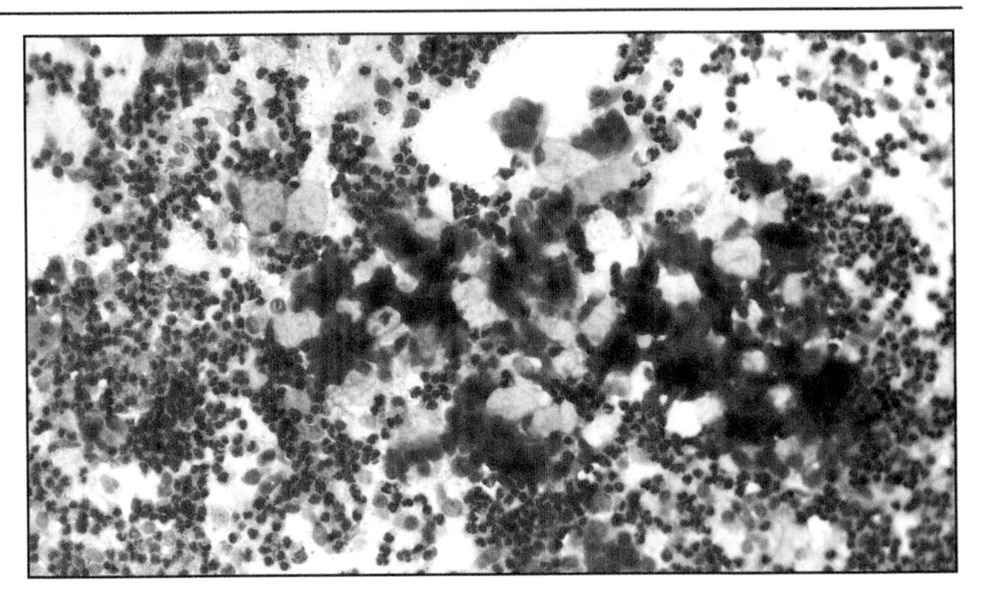

Fig. 2.20. Dog. BAL. Neutrophilic inflammation. Large numbers of segmented neutrophils admixed with ciliated columnar respiratory cells and Goblet cells. Wright-Giemsa.

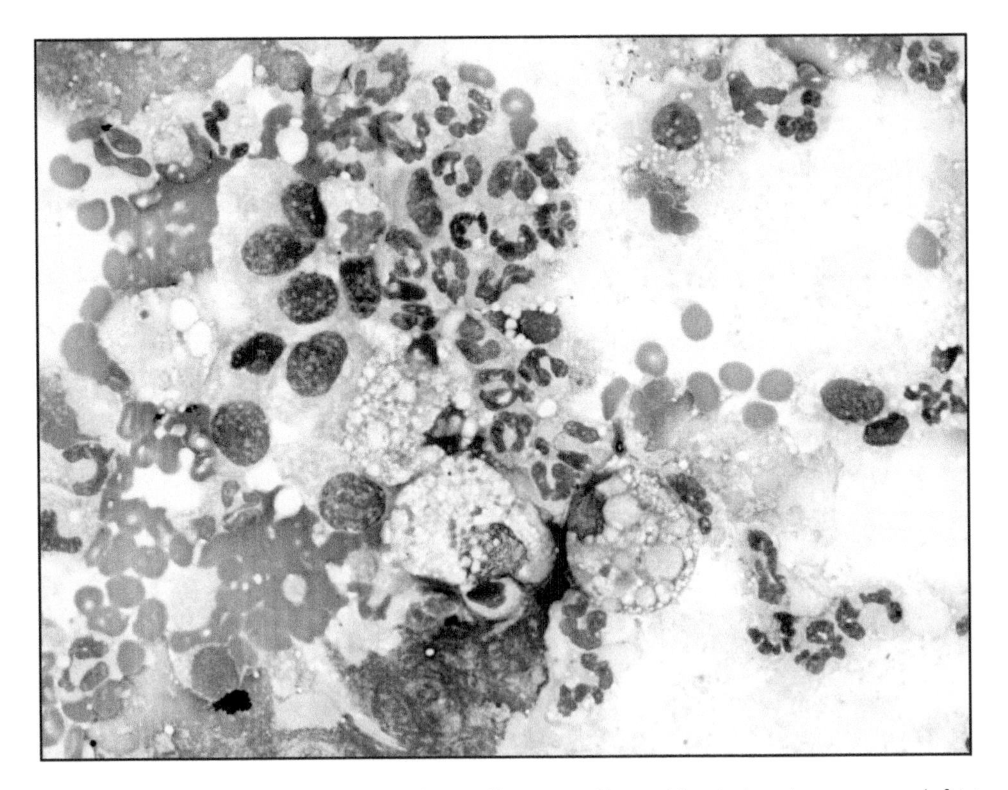

Fig. 2.21. Dog. BAL. Neutrophilic and macrophagic inflammation. Neutrophils cytoplasm have an unevenly faint pink appearance. Wright-Giemsa.

2.7.3.2 *Macrophagic inflammation*

Macrophages are involved in innate cell-mediated immunity. They are commonly seen in established or chronic inflammatory processes.

Causes

- Necrosis.
- Atelectasis.
- Lung lobe torsion.
- Haemorrhage.
- Neoplasia.
- Inhalation pneumonia.
- Lipoid pneumonia.
- Aspiration pneumonia.

Cytological features

- Macrophagic inflammation is diagnosed when there are variable percentages of macrophages, which appear reactive. Reactive changes include the presence of:
  - Bi- and multinucleated cells: usually with abundant and vacuolated cytoplasm. This may contain amorphous phagosomes or could display leucophagia.
  - Epithelioid macrophages: characterized by variably basophilic and poorly/no vacuolated cytoplasm and tendency to form clusters.
- Macrophages may contain red blood cells or products of their degradation (e.g. haemosiderin and haematoidin crystals) in haemorrhagic events.
- In lipoid pneumonia, macrophages contain small clear, punctate vacuoles of lipid origin.
- Macrophagic inflammation is often accompanied by increased numbers of other leucocyte types, in particular neutrophils. In those cases, it may be referred as pyogranulomatous.
- Hyperplastic epithelium, together with increased numbers of goblet cells and mucus, is often seen with chronic events.

Lipoid pneumonia

Clinical features

- Also known as lipid pneumonia, paraffinoma, cholesterol pneumonia and lipid granulomatosis.
- Uncommon condition characterized by intra-alveolar lipid and lipid-laden macrophages in the alveoli, which can have exogeneous or endogenous origin.
- Exogenous lipoid pneumonia is caused by a chronic foreign body reaction to fatty substances in the alveoli, typically after inhalation or aspiration of laxative mineral oils.
- Endogenous lipoid pneumonia (EnLP) has unclear causes and pathogenesis. It may be caused by pneumocyte injury, leading to the alveolar lipid deposition. It has been reported more often in cats in association with obstructive pulmonary diseases. In both dogs and cats, it may also be associated with lung neoplasm.
- Clinical signs are variable and non-specific and vary widely from cough to respiratory distress, lethargy, anorexia and weight loss. Imaging features may also vary.

Cytological features

- Characterized by the presence of lipid droplets in the background and numerous clear lipid vacuoles, within macrophages.
- Lipid material is positive to Oil-Red-O stain. Importantly, air-dried cytology specimens are required rather than methanol-fixed slides because alcoholic fixatives remove the lipid from the sample.

Pearls and Pitfalls

- In low-cellular fluids, especially when only macrophages are seen, a macrophagic inflammation may be difficult to diagnose, as alveolar macrophages are normally present in representative BAL samples, even from healthy animals. The presence of reactive changes helps in the diagnosis when present.
- Samples from healthy or diseased animals living in cities or polluted areas may contain dark or black intracytoplasmic granules consistent with anthracotic pigment.

Differential Diagnosis

- Selected bacterial infections (e.g. *Mycobacterium* sp.)
- Fungal infections (e.g. *Aspergillus* sp, *Blastomyces* sp, *Histoplasma* sp., *Coccidioides* sp.)

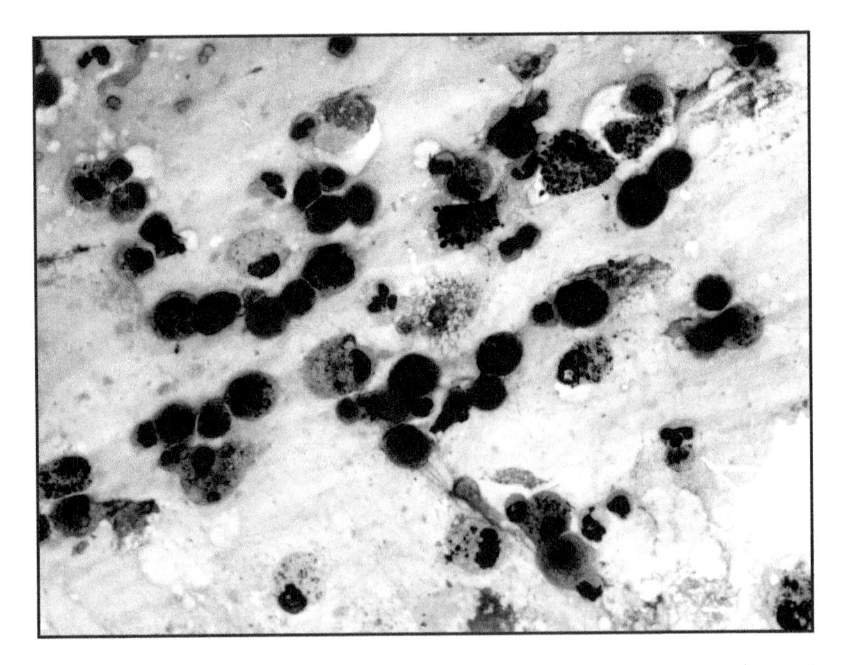

Fig. 2.22. Dog. BAL. Anthracosis. Macrophages cointain dark or black intracytoplasmic granules consistent with anthracotic pigment. Wright Giemsa.

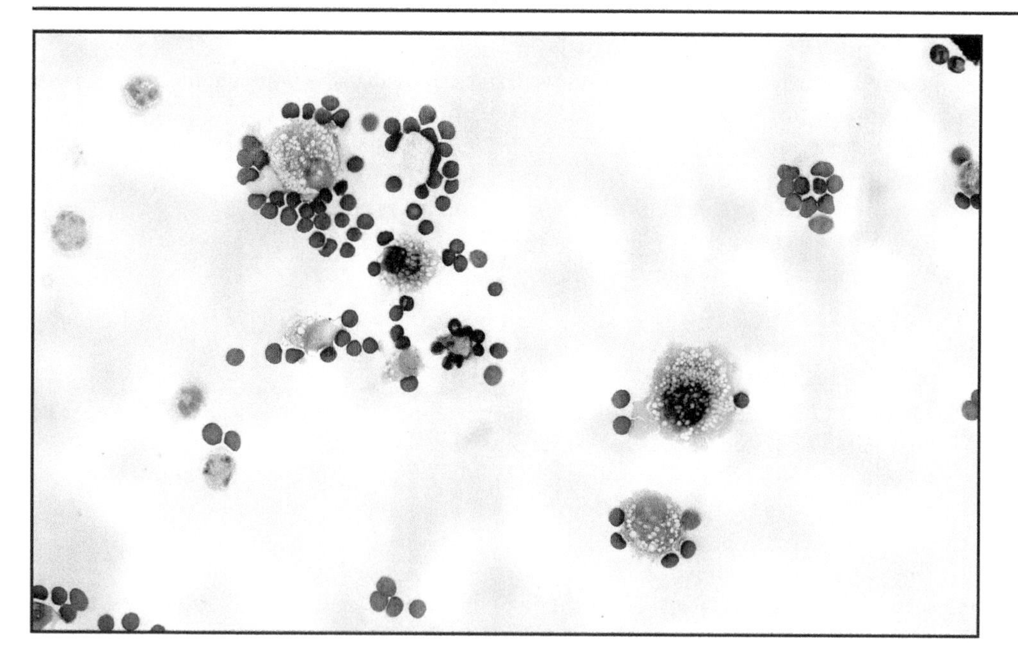

Fig. 2.23. Dog. BAL. Lipoid pneumonia. Macrophages contain small and discrete lipid vacuoles. Wright Giemsa.

Further reading

Perez-Accino, J., Liuti, T., Pecceu, E. and Cazzini, P. (2021) Endogenous lipoid pneumonia associated with pulmonary neoplasia in three dogs. *Journal of Small Animal Practice* 62(3), 223–228.

2.7.3.3 Lymphocytic inflammation

Lymphocytes participate in both the humoral and cell-mediated adaptive immune response. They are also involved in type IV (delayed) hypersensitivity reactions.

Causes

- Immune stimulation due to infectious or non-infectious causes.
- Airway hyperreactivity.
- Airway collapse.
- Viral infections.

Cytological features

- Lymphocytic inflammation is diagnosed when lymphocytes are typically >11% and >5% in dogs and cats, respectively. Higher percentages of lymphocytes have been described in dogs, and can be up to 17% of all nucleated cells in BAL samples from apparently healthy animals.
- Small lymphocytes are present in low numbers in respiratory washes, and their presence is generally clinically not significant.
- Occasionally, low numbers of intermediate and large forms can also be observed. Some of them may have a plasmocytoid appearance with small eccentric round nuclei, moderately basophilic cytoplasm and a paler perinuclear halo.
- Other leucocytes may be seen, including neutrophils and eosinophils.

Pearls and Pitfalls

- Causes of increased percentage of small lymphocytes in BAL samples of dogs and cats are unclear as information on scientific literature is very limited.
- Dogs with selected increase of lymphocytes in BAL fluid were noticed to be more commonly affected by airway collapse than dogs with other types of inflammation. It is possible that cartilage degeneration associated with airway collapse results in release of antigenic material, triggering lymphocytic inflammation.

Differential Diagnosis

- Lymphoma (small cell)

Further reading

Johnson, L.R. and Vernau, W. (2019) Bronchoalveolar lavage fluid lymphocytosis in 104 dogs. *Journal of Veterinary Internal Medicine* 33(3), 1315–1321.

2.7.3.4 *Eosinophilic inflammation*

Eosinophils regulate acute hypersensitivity reactions (type I hypersensitivity) and are typically present in allergen and parasite-mediated inflammatory reactions.

Causes

- Hypersensitive disease/allergy.
- Idiopathic.
- Underlying neoplasia.

Cytological features

- Eosinophilic inflammation is diagnosed when eosinophils are typically >5% and >10% in dogs and cats, respectively. Some studies have reported a higher percentage (up to 23%) of eosinophils in BALs from apparently healthy cats. However, a subclinical hypersensitivity process could not be ruled out in these patients.
- In fluids, careful examination is required to distinguish eosinophils from neutrophils, especially in thick areas and if embedded in mucus. This is because eosinophil granules may change in colour (dark red to brown) and sometimes also be less visible, while neutrophils may stain a diffuse, uneven, light-pink colour.
- Eosinophilic inflammation may be accompanied by other leucocyte types, in particular neutrophils, mast cells and basophils, but also plasma cells and small lymphocytes.

Feline asthma

- Lower airway inflammatory disease affecting 1–5% of the feline population.
- It most likely represents an allergic response to exposure of inhaled aeroallergens.
- Clinically, in the acute forms, this condition presents as asthmatic crisis; in the chronic forms, the most common signs are cough and increased breathing effort.
- Adult cats are more commonly affected, and Siamese cats show a breed predisposition.

Eosinophilic bronchopneumopathy

- Pathologic condition of dogs characterized by eosinophilic infiltrates in the bronchial mucosa and interstitium as result of a hypersensitivity process.
- A breed predisposition in Siberian Huskies has been reported; however, the disease has been diagnosed in various breeds.
- At the time of diagnosis, dogs are generally young and clinical signs include coughing, gagging, retching, exercise intolerance, dyspnoea and nasal discharge.
- It may share similarities with eosinophilic bronchitis and eosinophilic granuloma. Differentiation is based on imaging, clinical, bronchoscopic and BAL fluid cytology findings. Based on a recent study, dogs with eosinophilic granuloma (EG) and eosinophilic bronchopneumopathy (EBP) had higher total nucleated cell count in BAL, higher percentages of BAL fluid eosinophils, and exhibit more frequently peripheral eosinophilia.
- It is also unclear if these various conditions represent distinct processes or share the same aetiopathogenesis. Determining the specific type of eosinophilic lung disease may provide improved treatment modalities and more predictable responses. For example, eosinophilic granuloma often has been given a guarded prognosis, although disease remission has been reported.

Pearls and Pitfalls

- Eosinophils may be trapped in strands of mucus and may only be found in focal areas of the slides, underlying the importance of examining the entire slide.
- Free eosinophil granules may be observed secondary to cell rupture and should not be confused with bacteria, which are darker and basophilic in colour. These granules may also coalesce into a large crystal known as Charcot-Leyden crystal.

Differential Diagnosis

- Parasitic infections
- Fungal infections
- Bacteria infections

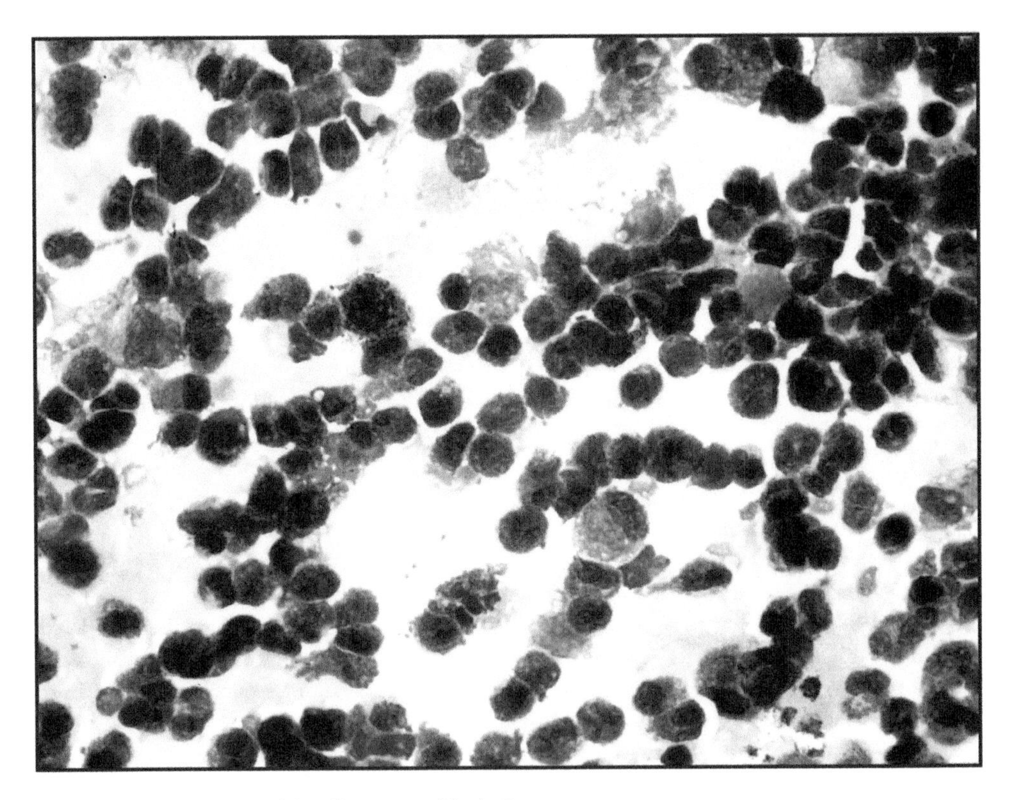

Fig. 2.24. Dog. BAL. Eosinophilic inflammation. Wright-Giemsa.

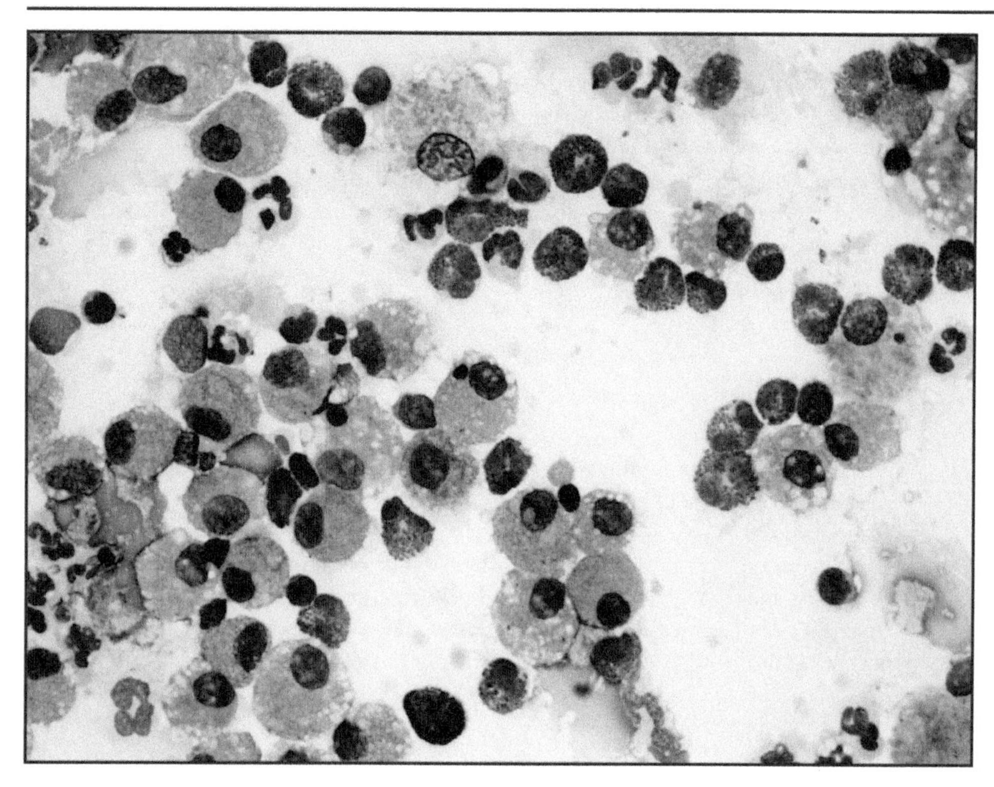

Fig. 2.25. Cat. BAL. Eosinophilic inflammation. Wright-Giemsa.

Further reading

Abbott, D.E. and Allen, A.L. (2020) Canine eosinophilic pulmonary granulomatosis: case report and literature review. *Journal of Veterinary Diagnostic Investigations* 32(2), 329–335.
Johnson, L.R., Johnson, E.G., Hulsebosch, S.E., Dear, J.D. and Vernau, W. (2019) Eosinophilic bronchitis, eosinophilic granuloma, and eosinophilic bronchopneumopathy in 75 dogs. *Journal of Veterinary Internal Medicine* 33(5), 2217–2226.
Trzil, J.E. (2020) Feline asthma: diagnostic and treatment update. *Veterinary Clinics of North America: Small Animal Practice* 50(2), 375–391.

2.7.4 Infectious causes

Lower airway inflammation may be caused by various infection agents, such as bacteria, fungi, yeasts, algae, protozoa and/or parasites. Cytological evidence of these organisms, especially when intracellular and/or associated with inflammatory cells, is considered proof of infection.

The absence of microorganisms in the cytologiacl preparations does not rule out infection. Therefore, additional diagnostic investigations (e.g. culture testing, serology and PCR) may be considered in selected cases.

2.7.4.1 Bacterial infections

Clinical features

- Bacterial bronchitis/pneumonia could be a primary disease of the lung caused by inhalation of food or liquid, or it could be secondary to viral infections, mucosal damage and extension of infection from intrathoracic structures or pleura, or haematogenous spread.
- Clinical conditions that predispose to bacterial infection of the lower airways include pre-existing infection (viral, fungal or protozoal); regurgitation, dysphagia or vomiting; reduced levels of consciousness (general anaesthesia with aspiration, coma, stupor); thoracic trauma or surgery; immunosuppression; functional or anatomical pathology (e.g. laryngeal paralysis, tracheal hypoplasia and primary dyskinesia).

Cytological features

- Cellularity: variable, often high.
- Background: usually pale basophilic and finely granular; may contain mucus, mucin granules or cilia.
- Neutrophils usually predominate. They show signs of degeneration and may contain intracytoplasmic bacteria. Other leucocyte types (e.g. macrophages and eosinophils) may also be increased in numbers.
- In case of aspiration pneumonia, the following can be found in the sample:
  - Squamous epithelial cells from the oropharynx and/or upper gastrointestinal tract.
  - Food material particles.
  - Bacteria: generally mixed. Note that when exclusively extracellular bacteria are present, they may either be true pathogens or reflect sample contamination (e.g. oropharyngeal).

Common bacterial infections of the lower respiratory tract in dogs and cats include:

- Resident microflora of the upper respiratory tract (including *Pasteurella* spp., *Bordetella* spp., *Streptococcus* spp. and *Enterobacterales*, including *E. coli*, etc.).
- *Mycoplasma* spp.: small coccoid-bacillar bacteria, extremely difficult to visualize on cytology because they are at or near the level of light microscopy. Identification is usually based on culture and/or PCR. *Mycoplasma* spp. has been associated with respiratory tract diseases in both dogs (in particular *Mycoplasma cynos*) and cats (*Mycoplasma felis*), but is rarely a primary pathogen.
- *Bordetella bronchiseptica*: rods or coccobacillary structures often associated with the cilia of the columnar respiratory epithelial cells and rarely phagocyted by the neutrophils. This is a common aetiological agent part of kennel cough syndrome in dogs and may also be cause of respiratory disease in cats. Samples obtained by bronchial brushing are more likely to harvest epithelial cells than BAL samples and to contain *Bordetella* spp.

- *Mycobacterium* spp.: negatively stained bacillus, generally located within macrophages, but occasionally present within neutrophils. When present in low numbers, the use of the Ziehl-Neelsen stain may help in their identification. One report of *Mycobacterium bovis* infection in a dog describes the presence of calcospherite-like bodies and caseous necrotic debris in tracheal mucus. Mycobacterial culture or PCR may also be considered for diagnostic purposes, considering its zoonotic potential and related risks in sample handling.
- *Nocardia* spp. and *Actinomyces* spp.: Gram-positive bacilli often related to penetrated wounds. They appear as filamentous, branching structures. *Nocardia* spp. is variably acid-fast, *Actinomyces* spp. is acid-fast negative. Since these species require special culture techniques, laboratory should be alerted if such organisms are suspected.
- *Streptococcus* spp.: Gram-positive cocci. Some species are part of normal upper respiratory flora. They are frequently associated with pneumonia in dogs than in cats. *S. canis* and *S. equi* subsp. *zooepidemicus* are the most pathogenic species with the latter been reported to be associated with outbreaks of haemorrhagic pneumonia in densely housed dogs.

Pearls and Pitfalls

- Culture of BAL fluids increases the chances to identify the presence of a bacterial component. The sensitivity of cytology in identifying bacterial infection is significantly lower than culture testing and ranges between 70% and 90%. Culture testing also allows accurate bacteria identification and antimicrobial susceptibility testing.
- A number of studies have reported Gram-negative bacteria (e.g. *Pasteurella* spp., *Bordetella* spp. and Enterobacteriaceae) as the most common types of bacterial infectious agents in dogs, and in those cases, one single agent was most commonly isolated.

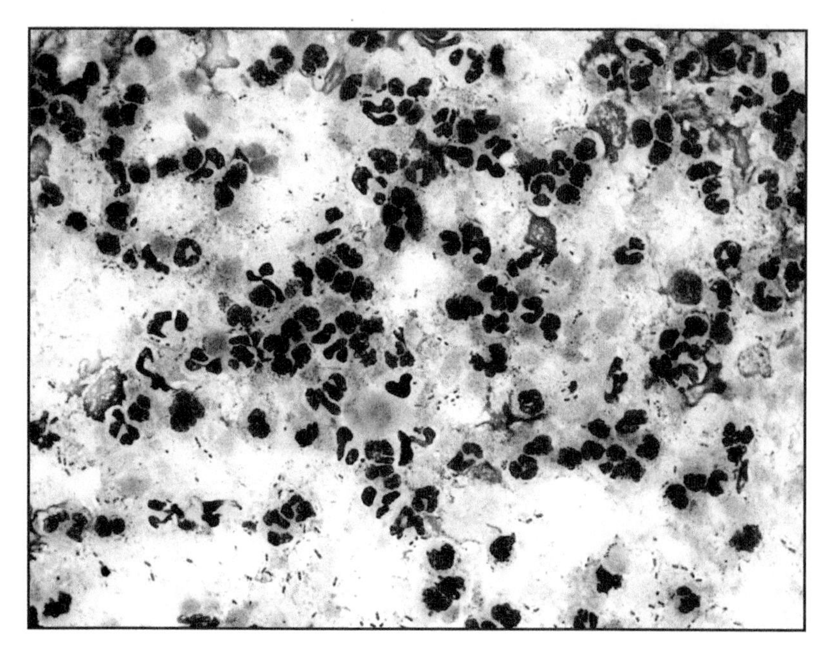

Fig. 2.26. Dog. BAL. Septic neutrophilic inflammation. Numerous segmented neutrophils with intracellular and extracellular bacteria (rods). Wright-Giemsa.

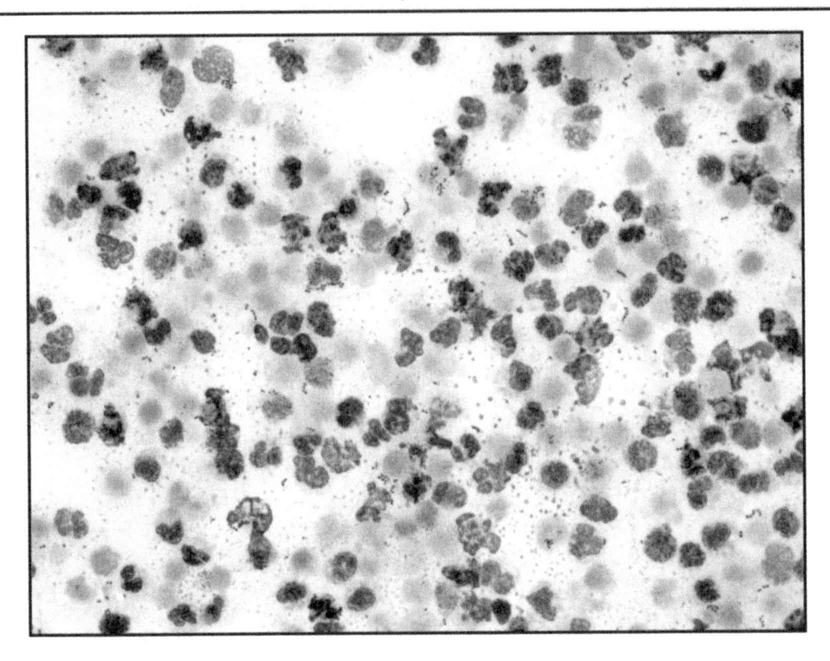

Fig. 2.27. Dog. BAL. Septic neutrophilic inflammation. Numerous highly degenerate neutrophils with intracellular and extracellular bacteria (cocci). Wright-Giemsa.

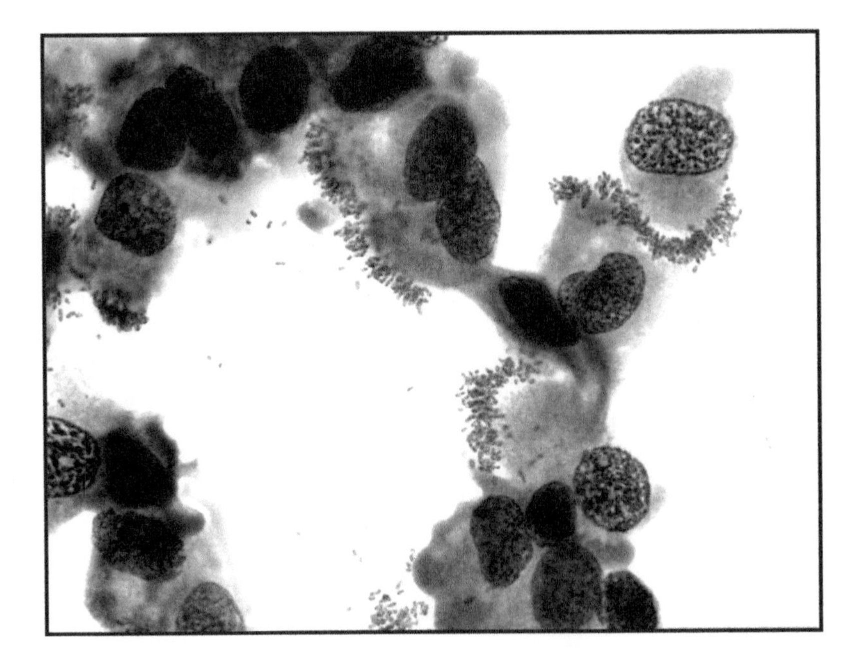

Fig. 2.28. Dog. BAL. *Bordetella* spp. Rods or coccobacillary structures often associated with the cilia of the columnar respiratory epithelial cells. Wright-Giemsa.

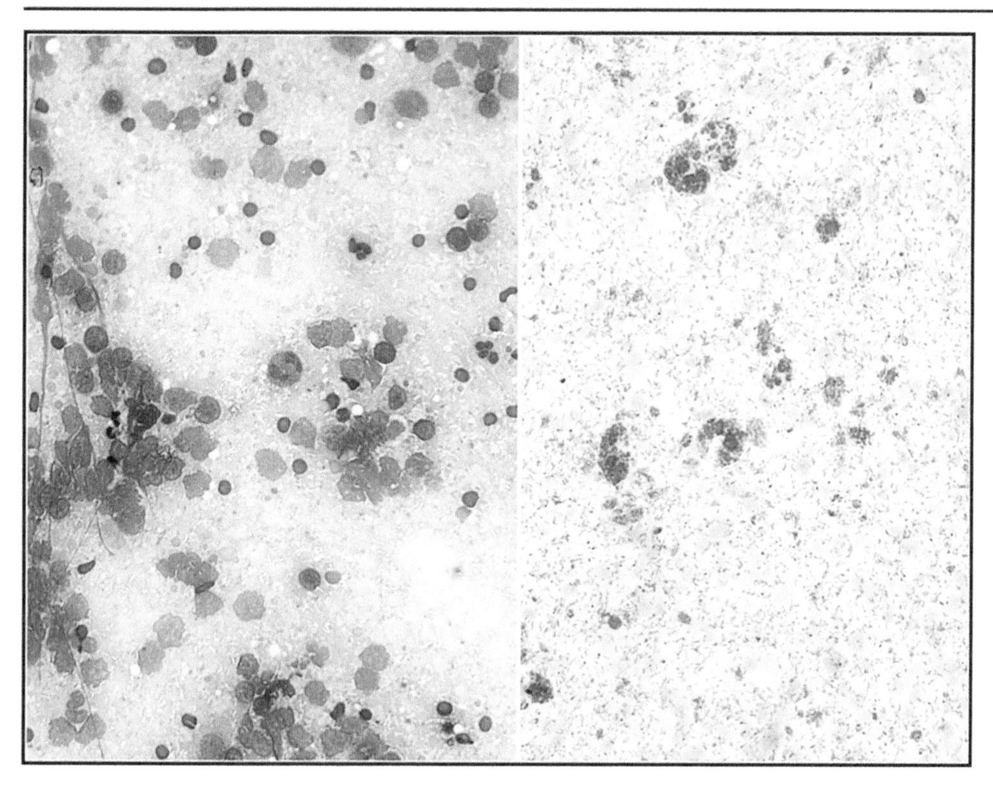

Fig. 2.29. Cat. BAL. (Left) *Mycobacterium* spp. Negatively stained rod-like bacteria within macrophages and free on the background. Wright-Giemsa. (Right) Bacteria appear as red rod-like structures. Ziehl-Neelsen stain. (*Courtesy of Ugo Bonfanti.*)

2.7.4.2 Viral infections

The lower respiratory tract may be affected by selected viruses. These include:

- Dogs: distemper, adenovirus, herpesvirus, influenza/parainfluenza, coronavirus, poxvirus.
- Cats: coronavirus, herpesvirus, cowpox virus, influenza and FIV.

Cytological features

- Viruses are not usually identified on cytological preparations, even if rare reports of viral inclusions have been described in the literature. Diagnosis is largely made by PCR or culture for some viruses.
- Distemper inclusions may occasionally be seen and are variably sized, eosinophilic with methanolic Romanowsky stains, intranuclear or intracytoplasmic. They may be seen either within leucocytes, red blood cells and/or epithelial cells.
- Large amphophilic/basophilic intranuclear inclusions may be seen within bronchiolar epithelial cells in infection with canine adenovirus type 2.
- Acidophilic intranuclear inclusions may be seen in lung tissue of dogs infected with herpesvirus.
- Many of these viruses cause lung damage and may result in secondary bacterial infections, commonly characterized by increased numbers of neutrophils (with variable degree of degeneration) and often bacteria, intracellular and/or extracellular. Anecdotally, lymphocytes may be increased, but this is considered a non-specific finding.

2.7.4.3 Fungal, yeasts, or algae infections

Lavage cytology may provide diagnosis for fungal, yeast and algal infection, some of which may be the cause of systemic infections. Some of the fungal agents are endemic in certain areas of America and are rare/absent in Europe (e.g. *Blastomyces* spp. and *Coccidioides* spp.).

Cytological features

- Cytology samples typically contain increased numbers of leucocytes, mainly neutrophils, sometimes eosinophils, and may contain infectious agents.
- The inflammatory cells are usually localized in the pulmonary interstitium; therefore, direct aspiration of lung parenchyma or nodular lesions may be more rewarding.

Blastomyces spp.

- Fungus found in the environment (in particular in North America/Canada) and cause of infection in dogs (mostly young large-breed) and cats through inhalation. Lung is one of the more common sites for this infection. Disease in dogs can vary with infection site; lethargy, fever, cough and trouble breathing are most common. Skin lesions and other systemic signs (e.g. fever, anorexia, lethargy) are not uncommonly observed.
- Young, large-breed dogs are more commonly affected. Lung is one of the more common sites for this infection.
- The fungal elements are blue, round, medium-sized (5–20 μm) thick double-walled structures (no clear capsule). Broad-based budding may be seen. Hyphae forms may also be rarely encountered. They are most likely found within the dense aggregates of inflammatory cells.
- Urine antigen testing (a quantitative, non-invasive and sensitive method, but with cross-reactivity with *Histoplasma* spp.) and PCR testing (sensitive method if the sample contains organisms) can be used for diagnosis. Serology for diagnosing blastomycosis has low sensitivity. Culture is not recommended since the cultured form is zoonotic.

Coccidioides spp. (Valley Fever)

- Fungus found in the environment (in particular in Southwestern United States, Central and South America) and cause of infection in dogs and cats through inhalation with localisation to the lungs. Often not cause of clinical signs. A variable percentage of subject may develop systemic/respiratory signs. The disease is also known as Valley Fever.
- Sporangia are thick-walled, blue-staining spherical structures of 10–100 μm of diameter and contain the endospores. They are small, round and granular structures of 1–5 μm of diameter and may be free in the background after rupture of sporangia. Since sporangia are very large structures and often not present in high numbers, preliminary slide examination at low power field is recommended.
- Serological testing and PCR are available for diagnosis. Culture is not recommended.

Cryptococcus spp.

- Upper respiratory infection is more common than pulmonary involvement, and cats are more often affected than dogs. It is extensively described in the first section of this chapter (upper respiratory tract).
- Organisms are characterized by pink to blue purple and slightly granular yeasts with thick clear capsule. Size is very variable and can reach 40 μm. Narrow-based budding may be seen.
- PCR and antigen test are available for diagnosis.

Histoplasma spp.

- Dimorphic fungus found in the environment (in particular in North and Central America) and cause of infection in dogs and cats through inhalation. Lung and gastrointestinal tract are the more common sites for this infection and clinical signs depends on the organs involved and can also be non spçcific.
- Dimorphic fungus that infects both dogs and cats.
- Organisms are small (2–4 µm) with a thin, clear halo surrounding a darker staining, round-to-oval, yeast-like organism. These are more commonly noted intracellularly, within macrophages and neutrophils. However, extracellular forms may be seen as result of cell rupture.

Pneumocystis spp.

- Opportunistic fungal pulmonary pathogen, mainly observed in young, small-breed dogs, often affected by immune defects. Clinical disease has also been described in cats.
- Depending on the severity of infection, Pneumocystosis has variable nonspecific respiratory signs ranging from cough to tachypnoea and dyspnoea.
- It often presents as cysts, which are 5–10 µm poorly stained structures with four to eight 1–2 µm intracystic bodies. Trophozoites appear as one or two poorly stained elongated structures, which should not be confused for platelets. This organism cannot be cultured.

Sporothrix spp.

- Fungus found in the environment that affects the skin (by traumatic inoculation), respiratory system (by inhalation) and occasionally other organs. Clinical signs vary accordingly to the organs involved and may include respiratory signs. More frequently observed in cats than dogs.
- The organisms can be intracellular and/or extracellular. They are cigar shaped, 2–7 µm diameter structures with a thin, clear halo slightly eccentric purple nucleus and lightly basophilic cytoplasm.

Aspergillus spp.

- Opportunistic fungus that can occasionally colonise the lung and also become disseminated. Clinical signs of broncopulmonary forms are nonspecific, including depression, fever, and cough.
- When found in BALs, it often represents an environmental contaminant.
- It usually presents in the form of septate and acute angle branching (45° angles) hyphae, with variable uptake of staining.

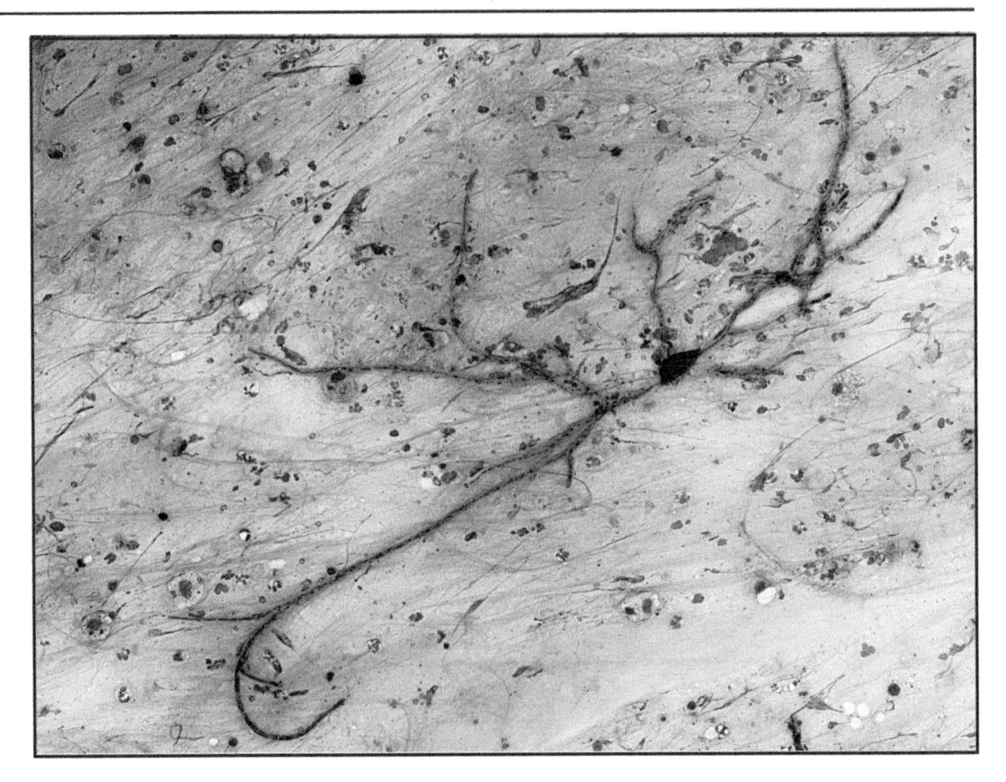

Fig 2.30. Dog. Bronchoalveolar lavage. Fungal hyphae admixed with neutrophils and foamy macrophages. Wright Giemsa.

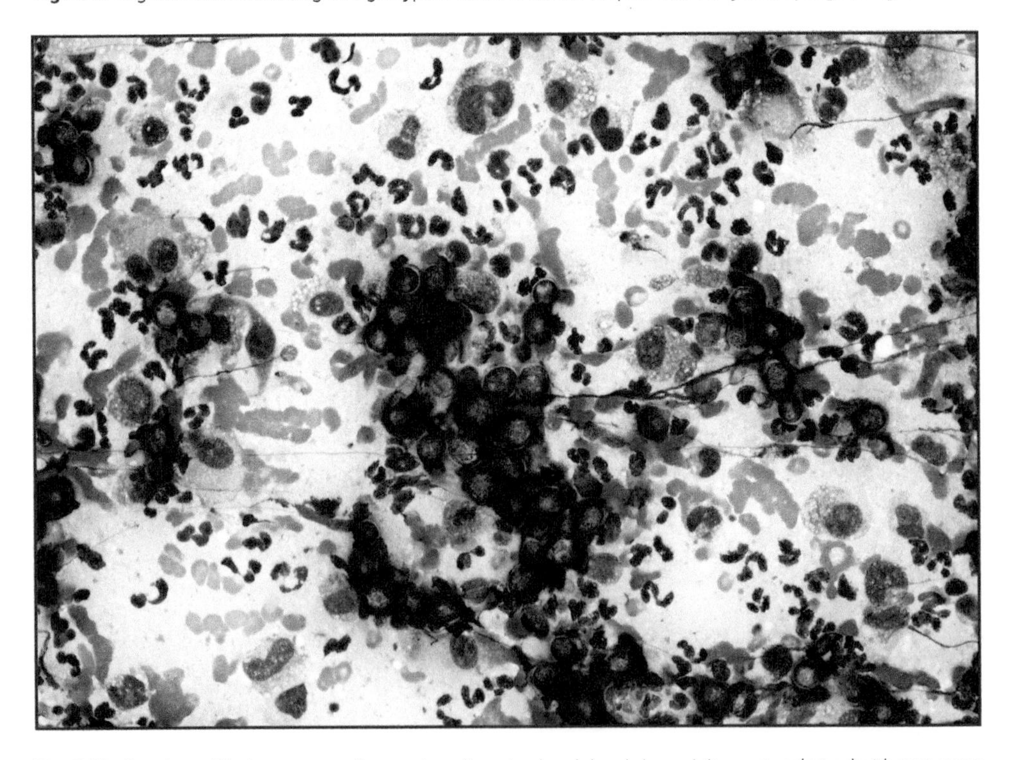

Fig. 2.31. Dog. Lung. *Blastomyces* spp. Frequent medium sized and deeply basophilic yeasts admixed with numerous neutrophils and a few foamy macrophages. Wright-Giemsa. (*Courtesy of Lisa Viesselmann.*)

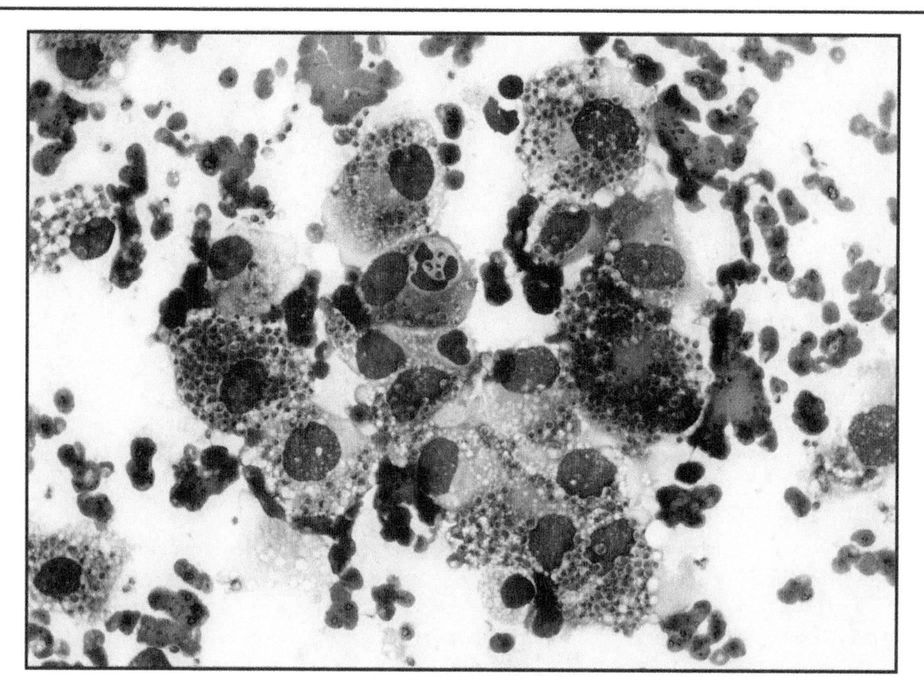

Fig. 2.32. Dog. Lung, *Histoplasma* spp. Macrophages containing high numbers of small, round-to-oval yeasts. These are also noted free within the background. Wright-Giemsa. (*Courtesy of Lisa Viesselmann.*)

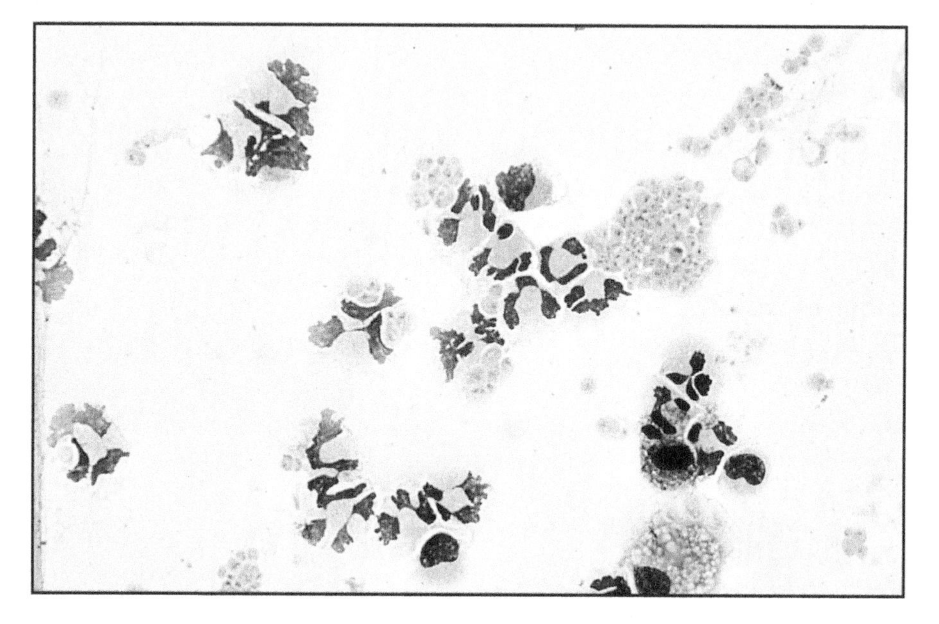

Fig. 2.33. Dog. BAL. *Pneumocystis* spp. trophozoites admixed with neutrophils. Wright-Giemsa.

2.7.4.4 *Protozoal infections*

Cytological features

- BALs are often characterized by increased numbers of neutrophils. Protozoa may be seen in the background or intracellularly, in particular within macrophages.
- Since identification of protozoa on cytology does not allow for differentiation between organisms, full diagnosis requires correlation with serological tests and PCR for definitive organism identification.

Toxoplasma gondii

- This protozoon can cause necrotizing interstitial pneumonia in cats, in particular in immunocompromised subjects. It is rare in dogs.
- In BALs, *Toxoplasma tachyzoites* may be seen intra- or extracellularly. They consist of small (1–4 µm) crescent-shaped bodies with light-blue cytoplasm and dark-staining pericentral nucleus.

Neospora caninum

- It may cause systemic disease, including pneumonia and neurological signs, mainly in young dogs.
- Cytologically, this protozoon morphologically indistinguishable from *Toxoplasma* spp.

Sarcocystis neurona

- It can cause pyogranulomatous pneumonia in dogs.
- Morphologically, it cannot be distinguished from *Toxoplasma* spp. and *Neospora* spp. However, a rosette pattern of radial arrangement of the merozoites may be observed, and this has been noted only in *Sarcocystic* spp. infection.
- Molecular sequencing is required for final diagnosis.

2.7.4.5 *Parasitic infections*

- Airway lavage can be helpful to identify parasite larvae. Accurate identification of the parasite may benefit from examination by a parasitologist with detailed morphology and size evaluation of the parasite. Molecular tests may also be required for speciation.
- Lack of direct parasite detection by microscopy does not rule out infection and may be due to several causes, including intermittent release into the airways. When suspected clinically, appropriate faecal examination, serology or molecular testing should be suggested.

Cytological features

- Overall, parasitic infections affecting the lower airways are accompanied by an inflammatory response, either neutrophilic or eosinophilic.

Parasites that can be identified cytologically in tracheal/lung samples from dogs include:

- *Angiostrongylus vasorum*.
- *Crenosoma vulpis*.
- *Eucoleus aerophilus* (formerly *Capillaria* spp.).
- *Filaroides hirthi* and *milksi*.
- *Oslerus (Filaroides) osleri*.
- *Paragonimus kellicoti*.
- *Toxocara canis*.

Parasites that can be identified cytologically in lung samples from cats include:

- *Aelurostrongylus abstrusus.*
- *Eucoleus aerophilus* (formerly *Capillaria* spp.).
- *Oslerus rostratus.*
- *Paragonimus kellicoti.*
- *Toxocara catis.*
- *Troglostronglylus brevior.*

Angiostrongylus vasorum

- Metastrongyloid nematode found in Europe, the UK and parts of North America, South America and Africa. It is also known as French heartworm or fox lungworm.
- Infection commonly causes respiratory signs (and sometimes bleeding) due to the migration of first-stage larvae into the bronchioles, bronchi and trachea.
- Diagnosis can be achieved by identification of first-stage larvae in respiratory fluid lavages. Larvae are 310–400 μm length and long tail with dorsal notch.
- Diagnosis may also be achieved via identification of larvae and eggs by Baermann faecal flotation test. Other diagnostic tests include PCR on lavages and swabs and antigen detection.

Aelurostrongylus abstrusus

- Metastrongyloid nematode affecting the feline species. Pathogenesis is similar to *A. vasorum.*
- It is generally considered asymptomatic, but it can induce coughing.
- Larvae have 360–400 μm length and a short, kinked tail.

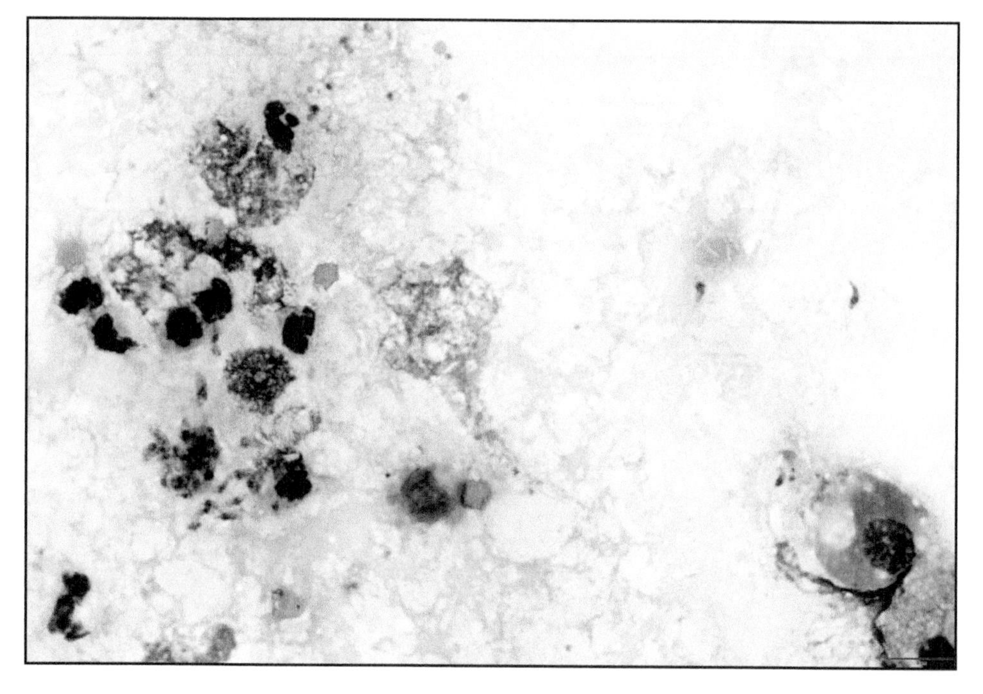

Fig. 2.34. Cat. BAL. *Toxoplasma* spp. tachyzoites characterized by typical crescent-shaped bodies with light blue cytoplasm and dark staining pericentral nucleus, admixed with neutrophils. Wright Giemsa. (*Courtesy of Martina Piviani.*)

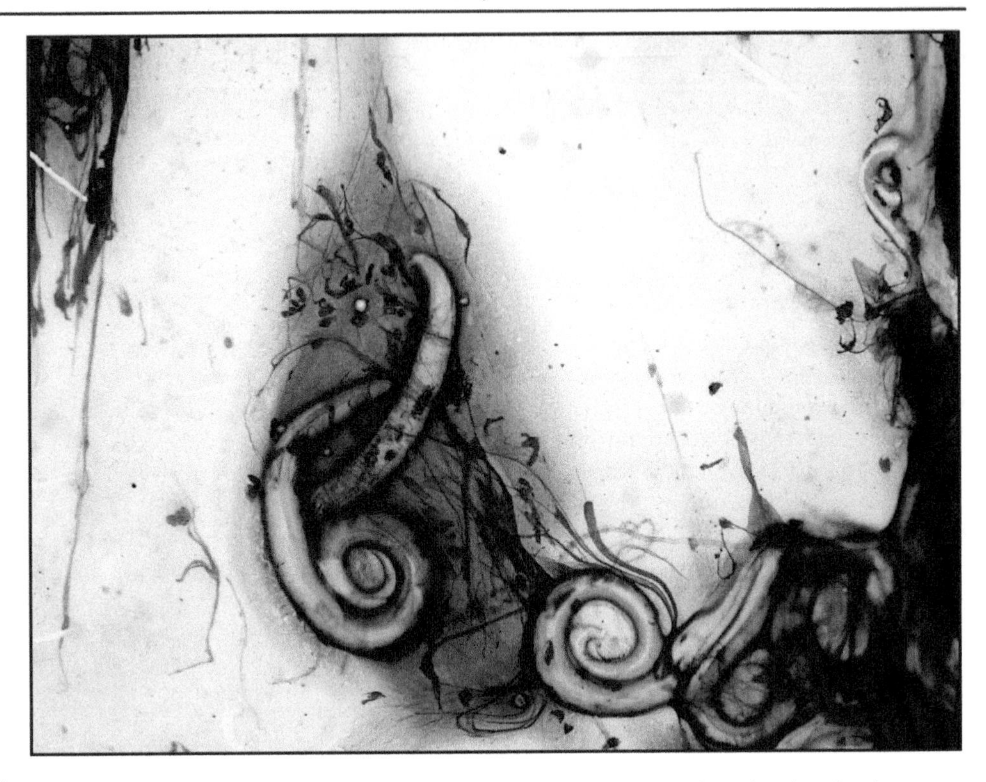

Fig. 2.35. Cat. BAL. *Aelurostrongylus abstrusus* infection. Numerous larvae admixed with a few leucocytes.. Wright-Giemsa. (*Courtesy of Robert Lukacs.*)

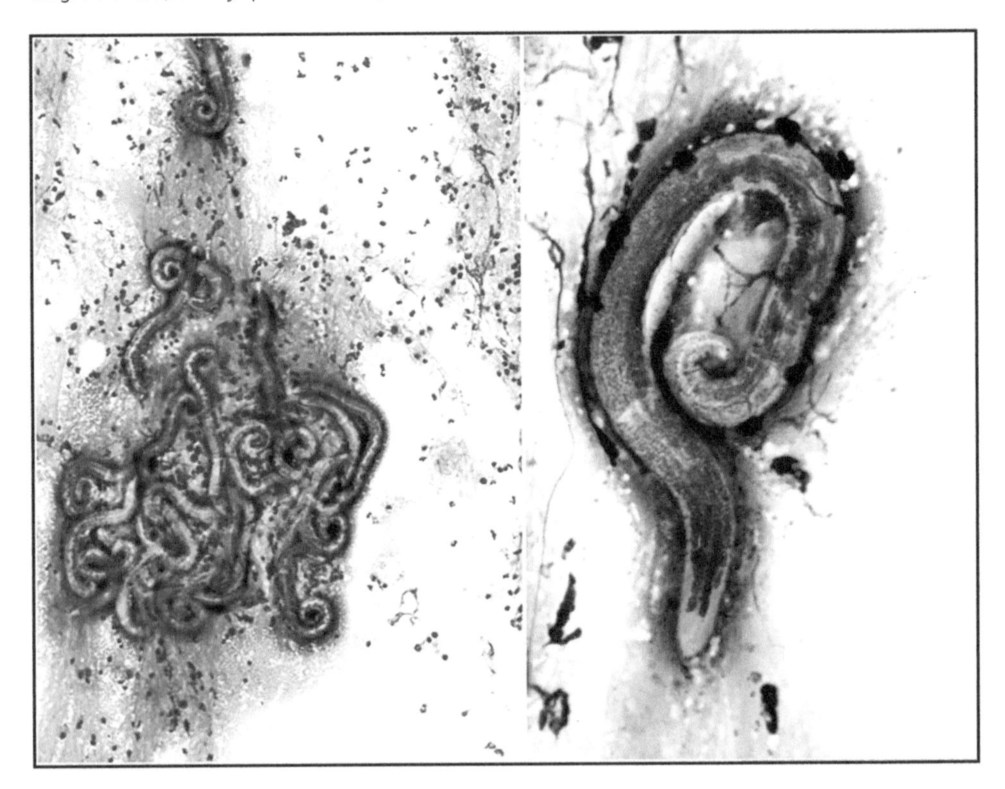

Fig. 2.36. Dog. BAL. ***Angiostrongylus vasorum*** infection. Numerous larvae admixed with leucocytes. Wright-Giemsa.

Further reading

Canonne, A.M., Billen, F., Tual, C., Ramery, E., Roesl, E. *et al.* (2016) Quantitative PCR and cytology of bronchoalveolar lavage fluid in dogs with Bordetella bronchiseptica infection. *Journal of Veterinary Internal Medicine* 30(4), 1204–1209.
Dear, J.D. (2014) Bacterial pneumonia in dogs and cats. *Veterinary Clinical Small Animal* 44, 143–155.
Egberink, H., Addie, D., Belak, S., Boucraut-Baralon, C., Frymus, T. *et al.* (2009) Bordetella bronchiseptica infection in cats. ABCD guidelines on prevention and management. *Journal of Feline Medicine and Surgery* 11(7), 610–614.
Jambhekar, A., Robin, E. and Le Boedec, K. (2019) A systematic review and meta-analyses of the association between 4 Mycoplasma species and lower respiratory tract disease in dogs. *Journal of Veterinary Internal Medicine* 33(5), 1880–1891.
Johnson, L.R., Queen, E.V., Vernau, W., Sykes, J.E. and Byrne, B.A. (2013) Microbiologic and cytologic assessment of bronchoalveolar lavage fluid from dogs with lower respiratory tract infection: 105 cases. *Journal of Veterinary Internal Medicine* 27(2), 259–267.
Lappin, M.R., Blondeau, J., Boothe, D., Breitschwerdt, E.B., Guardabassi, L. *et al.* (2017) Antimicrobial use guidelines for treatment of respiratory tract disease in dogs and cats: antimicrobial guidelines working group of the International Society for Companion Animal Infectious Diseases. *Journal of Veterinary Internal Medicine* 31(2), 279–294.
Lee-Fowler, T. (2014) Feline respiratory disease: what is the role of Mycoplasma species? *Journal of Feline Medicine and Surgery* 16(7), 563–571.
Peeters, D.E., McKiernan, B.C., Weisiger, R.M., Schaeffer, D.J. and Clerck, C. (2000) Quantitative bacterial cultures and cytological examination of bronchoalveolar lavage specimens in dogs. *Journal of Veterinary Internal Medicine* 14(5), 534–5541.

2.7.5 Haemorrhage

Haemorrhage is an escape of blood from a ruptured blood vessel.

Causes

- Iatrogenic: haemorrhage caused during sampling procedure. Extremely common sequela to FNA of the lung parenchyma but also seen in BALs and TWs.
- Intrapulmonary haemorrhage:
  - Pneumonia.
  - Inhaled irritants.
  - Bleeding diathesis.
  - Congestive heart failure.
  - Trauma.
  - Spontaneous pneumothorax.
  - Collapsed trachea.
  - Neurological disease.
  - Pulmonary embolism.
  - Lung lobe torsion.
  - Neoplasm.

Cytological features

- Cytological findings depend of the time on onset of the haemorrhage at the time of sampling:
  - Per-acute haemorrhage (few hours from extravasation):
    - Background: numerous intact red blood cells with/without platelets.
  - Acute haemorrhage (>12–24 h from extravasation):
    - Background: numerous intact red blood cells. Platelets will have dissolved by this time.
    - Macrophages displaying erythrophagocytosis: intact red blood cells are seen within the cytoplasm of macrophages.
  - Chronic haemorrhage (>24–36 h from extravasation):
    - Background: numerous red blood cells, intact or lysed. Cholesterol crystals may form secondary to the erythrocyte membrane dissolution.
    - Macrophages containing the degradation products of the red blood cell breakdown (haemosiderin and/or haematoidin crystals). Haemosiderin appears as dark basophilic-black granules of variable sizes, always within the cytoplasm of the macrophages. Haematoidin crystals are typically rhomboid and yellow/orange. They may be found in the macrophages or occasionally scattered in the background.

Pearls and Pitfalls

- Prussian blue is a special cyto/histochemical stain that can be used to identify haemosiderophages.
- Pulmonary haemosiderosis is more commonly seen in BALs from cats than dogs. The reason may be an increased susceptibility to alveolar haemorrhage or a reduced rate of haemosiderin degradation by the alveolar macrophages.

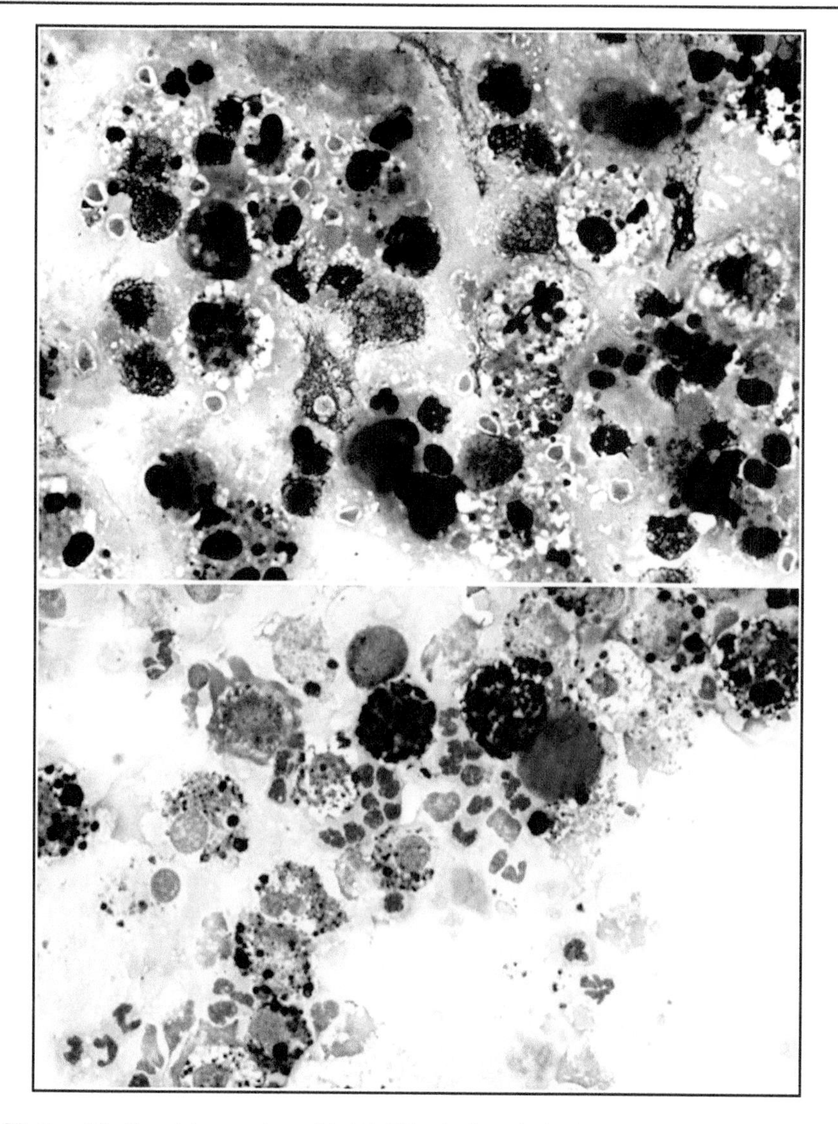

Fig. 2.37. Dog. BAL. Chronic haemorrhage. (Top) Red blood cells in the background and numerous macrophages containing intracytoplasmic dark-pigment compatible with haemosiderin. Wright-Giemsa. (Bottom) Numerous macrophages containing dark-blue pigment indicative of haemosiderin. Prussian blue.

Further reading

Hooi, K.S., Defarges, A.M., Jelovcic, S.V. and Bienzle, D. (2019) Bronchoalveolar lavage hemosiderosis in dogs and cats with respiratory disease. *Veterinary Clinical Pathology* 48(1), 42–49.

2.7.6 Neoplasms

- Primary, neoplastic or systemic neoplasia of the lower respiratory tract may present as solitary or multiple nodules or diffise infiltration. Estimated incidence of tumours of the respiratory system in the canine and feline population is <1%.
- If the tumours involve the bronchial tree, bronchial tree, there are higher chances that the neoplastic cells will be collected by routine washing. Alternatively, diagnosis may be achieved by direct fine-needle aspiration of affected lung areas.

Primary epithelial lung tumours

Clinical features

- Bronchioloalveolar tumours and adenocarcinomas are the most common neoplasms in dogs and cats, respectively.
- Cough is a common clinical sign, but asymptomatic cases can also occur.
- Concurrent pleural effusion is not uncommon.
- In cats, cases of primary pulmonary neoplasia may be discovered by recognition of metastatic disease involving the digits (lung digit syndrome).
- Paraneoplastic syndromes are not very common and are seen mainly in dogs; they include hypertrophic osteopathy and hypercalcaemia.

Cytological features

- Main population of epithelial cells, ranging from cuboidal to columnar or polygonal, depending on the cell type involved, and often forming aggregates/clusters. In the presence of acinar formation or secretory products, glandular origin (adenocarcinoma) is likely. Further differentiation of primary lung tumours or metastatic carcinomas is not possible based on cytology alone.
- Only squamous cell carcinoma has a typical morphology, with cells with abundant keratinized cytoplasm with angular borders and small dense and round nuclei, centrally located. Asynchrony of cytoplasmic and nuclear maturation is common. Basaloid and cuboidal cells arranged in clusters may also be seen.
- Cytological features of atypia are usually marked and include anisocytosis, anisokaryosis, perinuclear vacuolations, nuclear moulding, signet ring formation, bi/multinucleation cell gigantism and cell cannibalism. However, well-differentiated carcinomas where cells do not display significant signs of malignancy may occur.
- Concurrent inflammation is is common, and an increase in neutrophils may be observed. Eosinophilic infiltrate may also accompany bronchoalveolar carcinoma in dogs. Lipid filled macrophages and haemosiderophages have been reported both in dogs and cats.

Differential diagnosis

- Metastatic carcinomas of other origin

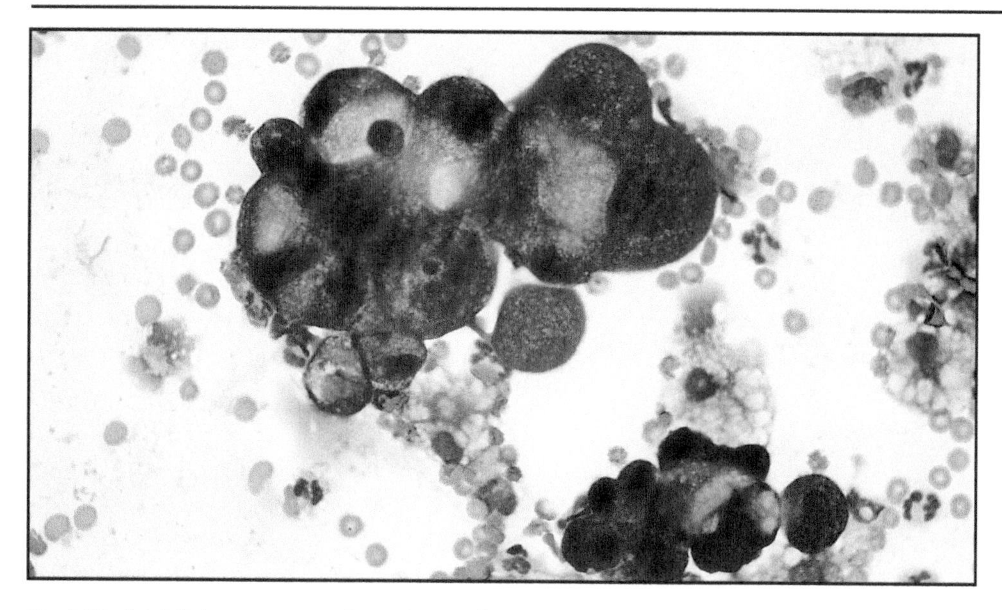

Fig. 2.38. Cat. BAL. Lung carcinoma. Large clusters of epithelial cells with marked signs of atypia and signet ring formation. Wright-Giemsa.

Lymphoma

Clinical features

- It presents as diffuse infiltrative disease or as discrete nodules.
- In a study of 47 dogs with multicentric lymphoma, 66% had pulmonary involvement confirmed on cytology of the BAL collected by bronchoscopy. TW fluid examination was much less sensitive.
- Rare cases of angiocentric inflamed large B-cell lymphoma (formerly lymphomatoid granulomatosis) with primary lung involvement have also been reported in young dogs and very rarely in cats.

Cytological features

- Monomorphic population of intermediate to large lymphoid cells.
- Nuclei are often intermediate to large mainly eccentric, with stippled chromatin, and nucleoli often visible.
- Cytoplasm is usually increased in amount, variably basophilic, with distinct borders, and may contain clear intracytoplasmic vacuoles.
- Mitotic figures are often seen and may be numerous. Atypical forms are not uncommon.
- In angiocentric inflamed large B-cell lymphoma, atypical large B lymphoid cells are admixed with other leucocytes (small lymphocytes, eosinophils, neutrophils, plasma cells). Therefore, definitive diagnosis may not be achieved by cytology and often requires histopathology and/or PARR testing.

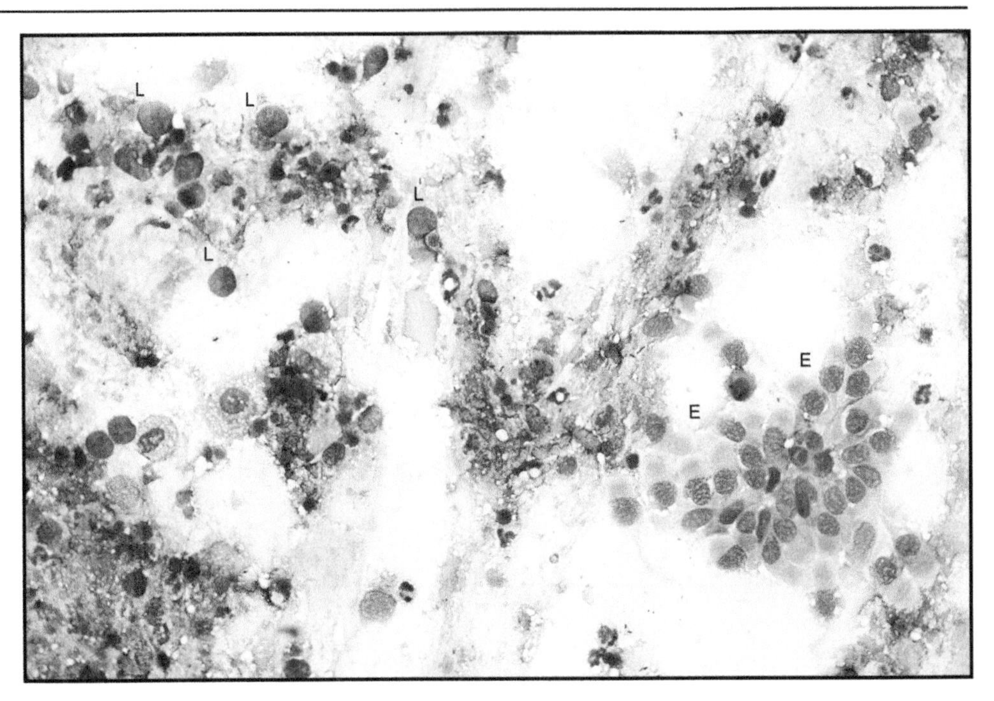

Fig. 2.39. Dog. BAL. Lymphoma. Large lymphoid cells (L) admixed with respiratory columnar epithelial cells (E) and occasional leucocytes. Wright-Giemsa.

Histiocytic tumours

Clinical features

- In dogs, they are represented by histiocytic sarcoma (HS), which can primarily involve the lungs, or it may be part of a disseminated form.
- Over-represented canine breeds: Bernese Mountain Dogs, Rottweilers, Golden Retrievers and Flat-Coated Retrievers. However, the disease can be seen in almost any canine breed.
- In cats, histiocytic disorders may also appear in the form of pulmonary Langerhans cell histiocytosis, an uncommon and fatal disorder that leads to progressive respiratory failure and may involve other organs.

Cytological features

- Pleomorphic population of individualized, round-to-oval and/or slightly elongated cells, which may contain intracytoplasmic vacuoles and show signs of phagocytosis.
- Cells often show marked cytological features of atypia, including bi- and multinucleation and atypical mitoses.

Carcinoid

Clinical features

- Extremely rare tumour in both dogs and cats arising from neuroendocrine cells in the airway epithelium.
- Cases are too rare to define an established typical clinical presentation and biological behaviour. However, indolent forms in dogs have been reported.

Cytological features

- Main population of naked nuclei embedded in a background of pale basophilic/blue cytoplasmic material.
- Few intact cells may be observed and appear round to polygonal with a moderate amount of lightly basophilic cytoplasm. Intracytoplasmic dark granules may be seen.
- Nuclei are round with fine chromatin and occasionally visible nucleoli.

Sarcoma

Clinical features

- Primary sarcomas of the lung are rare but may occur in both dogs and cats. They include osteosarcoma, chondrosarcoma, fibrosarcoma or undifferentiated sarcomas.

Cytological features

- Main population of variably spindle cells, either individualized or forming poorly cohesive groups, sometimes associated with amorphous pinkish material (matrix).
- Features of atypia/malignancy vary but may be marked.

Metastatic tumours

Clinical features

- They include carcinomas of various types (e.g. mammary carcinoma, urotehlial and prostatic carcinoma, etc.), sarcomas, melanomas and rarely TVT.
- They often appear as multiple nodules (in particular at the periphery of lung lobes) or diffuse infiltration. Localization of neoplastic cells is often interstitial; therefore, neoplastic cells often do not exfoliated in TW/BALs, unless the tumour has invaded the bronchial tree. Diagnosis is more often achieved by direct fine-needle aspiration of affected lung areas.

Cytological features

- Neoplastic cell population appearance varies and resembles those seen in primary sites.
- Criteria of atypia/malignancy are often prominent.
- Dogs with mammary gland tumours and radiographic evidence of pulmonary metastasis had significantly higher relative neutrophil counts in bronchoalveolar lavage fluid than dogs with tumours without evidence of metastasis. Bronchoalveolar lavage does not appear to be sensitive for identifying malignant cells.

Pearls and Pitfalls

- In the presence of inflammation, attention must be paid before diagnosing epithelial neoplasia on cytology, since dysplastic or metaplastic changes to epithelial cells may occur and may mimic neoplasia.
- Further differentiation of primary or metastatic carcinomas and sarcomas is generally not possible based on cytology alone and requires histopathology.

Further reading

Choi, U.S., Alleman, A.R., Choi, J.H., Wook Kim, H., Youn, H.J. *et al.* (2008) Cytologic and immunohistochemical characterization of a lung carcinoid in a dog. *Veterinary Clinical Pathology* 37(2), 249–252.

Hawkins, E.C., Morrison, W.B., DeNicola, D.B. and Blevins, W.E. (1993) Cytologic analysis of bronchoalveolar lavage fluid from 47 dogs with multicentric malignant lymphoma. *Journal of American Veterinary Medical Association* 203(10), 1418–1425.

Moore, P.F. (2014) A review of histiocytic diseases of dogs and cats. *Veterinary Pathology* 51(1), 167–184.

Pavelski, M., Correa Leite, N., Pedri, E., Guerios, S.D., De Sousa, R.S. *et al.* (2017) Single-aliquot, non-bronchoscopic bronchoalveolar lavage in the diagnosis of metastatic mammary tumours in dogs. *Journal of Small Animal Practice* 58(3), 168–173.

Body Cavity Effusions

The serosal cavities include the pleural, pericardial and peritoneal spaces. They are lined by a single layer of mesothelial cells and contain a small amount of fluid that functions as lubricant to allow a frictionless movement of the body cavity walls and organs.

An increased amount of fluid within these cavities is always regarded as pathologic and can be associated with a wide range of underlying diseases. The causes that lead to cavity effusions could be either benign or malignant.

3.1 Anatomy and Physiology

3.1.1 Pleural cavity

The thoracic cavity is lined by the pleura, which is a serosal membrane composed of two portions:

- Parietal pleura: outer part of the pleura. It forms the internal lining of the thoracic cavity on each side of the mediastinum.
- Visceral pleura: inner part of the pleura. It surrounds and lines the lungs and dips into the areas separating the different lung lobes.

Between the visceral and parietal pleura, there is a virtual space, which contains a small amount of serous fluid produced by the mesothelial cells. This fluid has two functions:

- Lubricate the surface of the pleurae, allowing them to slide over each other.
- Create a surface tension that keeps the two pleurae together. This means that during respiration, when the thorax expands, the lungs follow by expanding and filling with air.

Both pleurae are composed of a single layer of flat or cuboidal mesothelial cells with small apical microvilli. They are both supported by connective tissue, which is rich in elastic fibres and contains a wide capillary network. The capillary network of the visceral pleura derives from the pulmonary circulation, while that of the parietal pleura arises from the systemic circulation. The parietal pleura also contains numerous lymphatics.

The serous fluid enters the pleural space through the parietal pleura arteriolar capillaries following a net filtration rate. It is removed by:

- Absorptive pressure gradient at the level of the visceral pleural venous capillaries.
- Lymphatic drainage in the parietal pleura.
- Cellular mechanism.

In healthy conditions, the amount of fluid is small, with an average volume of 0.1 ml/kg in dogs and 0.3 ml/kg in cats. This volume results from a balance of liquid *in* and liquid *out* and is governed by Starling forces, the degree of endothelial and mesothelial permeability and the integrity of the lymphatic drainage.

DOI: 10.1079/9781789247787.0003

3.1.2 Peritoneal cavity

The peritoneal cavity is the virtual space between the visceral and parietal peritoneum. It is lined by the peritoneum and, in health, contains a very small amount of fluid (<1 mg/kg bodyweight).

The peritoneum is a semipermeable membrane lined by mesothelial cells and is supported by a thin layer of fibrous tissue. It functions to support the organs contained in the abdominal cavity and contains nerves, blood vessels and lymphatics.

It is composed of two layers:

- Parietal layer: outer leaflet. This attaches to the abdominal and pelvic walls and lines the cavities. It receives blood from the abdominal wall vessels. The venous drainage goes into the caudal vena cava.
- Visceral layer: inner leaflet. It wraps around the abdominal organs. It receives blood from the cranial and caudal mesenteric arteries and drains into the portal vein.

The peritoneum allows a free exchange of water and solutes between the peritoneal fluid and plasma. The production and absorption of the peritoneal fluid is constant, and it follows the same principles described in Section 3.2.1. The rate of this fluid formation follows the Starling laws and depends on the balance between plasma and tissue oncotic and hydrodynamic pressure. The forces promoting fluid filtration out of the capillary on the arteriolar side are slightly higher than the forces regulating fluid absorption from the tissue back into the capillary on the venule side. This leads to a net accumulation of a small amount of fluid in the interstitium, which then diffuses between the mesothelial cells and enters the body cavity. The lymphatic system contributes to the drainage of the excess of fluid.

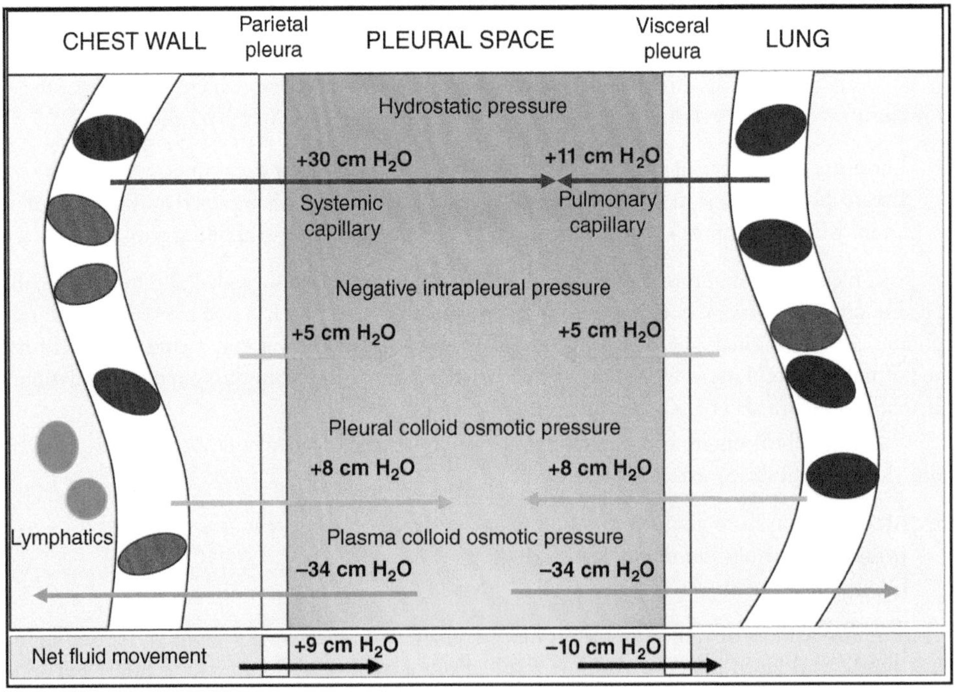

Fig. 3.1. Starling forces.

3.1.3 Pericardial cavity

The pericardial space is the potential space between the two leaflets that compose the pericardium. These consist of:

- Fibrous pericardium: outer layer. It is made of strong connective tissue.
- Serous pericardium: inner layer. It is a serous membrane that wraps the fibrous pericardium, the heart and the root of the major vessels, forming the pericardial space. It is composed of two parts:
  - Parietal serous pericardium: this is fused with the fibrous pericardium.
  - Visceral serous pericardium (epicardium): it lines the myocardium. It is mostly made of a single layer of mesothelial cells.

Between these two leaflets, there is a small amount of fluid that forms following the same principles described later in Sections 3.2.1 and 3.2.2. It is mainly drained by the lymphatic capillary bed.

3.2 Sampling Techniques

3.2.1 Thoracocentesis

Materials

- Clippers and disinfectant.
- Needles: depending on the size of the patient and personal preference, one of these needles can be used:
  - 19G or 22G butterfly catheter.
  - 18G to 22G over-the-needle intravenous catheter.
  - 18G to 22G, 1-in to 1.5-in needle.
- IV extension set connected to a three-way stopcock valve.
- Syringe.
- Kidney dish.
- Tubes:
  - EDTA tube for cytology and total cell count.
  - Plain tube for total protein measurement and microbiology.
- Glass slides.

Patient preparation

- Sedation and local anaesthesia are generally not required and might be contraindicated in severely dyspnoeic patients.
- A standing position or a sternal recumbency is usually adopted.
- Clip the area of insertion of the needle and aseptically clean it.

Technique

- If only a small amount of fluid is to be drained, then attach the syringe directly to the catheter.
- If a larger volume of fluid needs to be removed, then attach the IV extension tube to a three-way stopcock valve. Make sure that the valve is closed.
- Insert the needle with a 45° angle approximately two-thirds down the thoracic cavity, just above the costochondral junction at the seventh or eighth intercostal spaces. To avoid the costal vessels and nerves, the needle should be inserted next to the cranial aspect of the rib.

- Place a small amount of negative pressure on the syringe. If collecting only a small amount of fluid, when this is aspirated, the needle/butterfly and catheter can be withdrawn with the syringe attached.
- Otherwise, drain as much as possible using the three-way stopcock valve, syringe and kidney dish.

Complications

Complications during thoracocentesis are rare and include:

- Pneumothorax by laceration of the pulmonary parenchyma (rare).
- Haemothorax by laceration of the coronary artery (extremely rare).

Pearls and Pitfalls

Patients with chronic effusions may have compartmentalization of fluid, which might be difficult to aspirate. Ultrasound-guided thoracocentesis might help in these cases.

3.2.2 Abdominocentesis

Materials

- Clippers and disinfectant.
- Needles: 20G or 22G, 1-in to 1.5-in needle.
- IV extension set.
- Syringe: 5–10 ml depending on the size of the patient.
- Tubes:
    - EDTA tube for cytology and total cell count.
    - Plain tube for total protein measurement and microbiology.
- Glass slides.
- Kidney dish.

Patient preparation

- Sedation and local anaesthesia are generally not required, although the latter may be used if desired.
- A standing position or a sternal recumbency is usually favoured, although lateral or dorsal recumbency might be adopted.
- Clip the area of insertion of the needle and aseptically clean it.

Technique

- For simple blind abdominocentesis, the needle is inserted caudal to the umbilicus, a few centimeters to the right of the midline, to avoid inadvertent aspiration of the spleen. Ultrasound-guided technique may also be used to insert the needle directly into the a fluid pocket.
- Insert the needle through the skin and apply a light negative pressure in the syringe, prior to advancing the needle into the abdominal cavity. Drain as much as required.

Pearls and Pitfalls

Usually only a very light aspiration of the syringe is required to harvest the abdominal effusion. This prevents the clogging of the needle with the omentum.

Complications

Complications during abdominocentesis are rare and most typically include inadvertent penetration of the spleen. This usually does not cause serious complications, unless the patient is coagulopathic.

3.2.3 Pericardiocentesis

Materials

- Clippers and disinfectant.
- Ultrasound machine.
- Large intravenous catheter: 10–14G. The length of the needle depends on the size of the patient.
- Extension set connected to a three-way stopcock valve.
- Lidocaine 2%.
- Collection container.
- Syringe.
- Tubes:
  - EDTA tube for cytology and total cell count.
  - Plain tube for total protein measurement and microbiology.
- Glass slides.
- Kidney dish.

Patient preparation

- Pericardiocentesis is a sterile procedure. The area of insertion of the catheter must be clipped and aseptically cleaned.
- Lateral or sternal recumbency or standing position.
- It is commonly performed on the right side to avoid injury to the carotid arteries and lungs.
- Sedation might be required, and the patient should be monitored with an ECG.

Technique

- Pericardiocentesis can be performed blind or under ultrasound guidance.
- Prepare the area between the second and eighth intercostal spaces and between the sternum and mid-chest. When the procedure is performed blind, the insertion of the catheter is usually between the third and fifth right intercostal spaces.
- Perform a local block with lidocaine 2% including the skin, intercostal muscle and pleura.
- Depending on the size of the catheter used, a small incision of the skin may help in the procedure.
- The catheter is inserted in the middle of the intercostal space and is advanced slowly and perpendicular to the skin, until the pericardial sac. The pericardial sac is reached when a loss of resistance is felt, and the fluid starts entering the catheter hub.
- Advance the catheter slightly more over the stylet, remove the stylet and connect the catheter to the collecting system.
- Remove all the fluid and then retrieve the catheter.

Complications

- Uncommon complications include:
  - Premature beats.
  - Ventricular tachycardia from myocardial injury by the catheter.
  - Laceration of coronary artery.
  - Ventricular puncture.
  - Pneumothorax.
  - Haemorrhage.

3.3 Sample Handling, Analysis and Slide Preparation

3.3.1 Sample handling

- Fluid samples should be collected and aliquoted into the following tubes:
  - EDTA tube: used for cytology preparations and total nucleated cell count (TNCC). EDTA avoids clotting formation and preserves cell morphology. It can also be used for flow cytometry and PCRs when required.
  - Plain sterile tube: used for measurement of proteins and other biochemistry parameters, such as albumin, bilirubin, creatinine, potassium, triglycerides, cholesterol, lipase and glucose. It is also used for microbiology.
- Fluid should be analysed as soon as possible. Until then, refrigeration at 4°C is recommended.
- When submission to an external laboratory is required, it is better to guarantee the delivery within 24 h from collection. Fluids are naturally rich in nutrients; therefore, there is no need to add solutions such as normal saline or preservative such as formalin. It is also recommended to make a couple of fresh smears to avoid cell deterioration and guarantee the preservation of the cell morphology. If the fluid is poorly cellular, a smear of the fluid sediment should be made to be submitted to the laboratory.

Pearls and Pitfalls

- EDTA has a bacteriostatic activity; therefore, it should not be used for culture, as it may lead to false-negative results.
- A study on the preservation of body cavitary effusion revealed that the cellular composition can change over time with a decrease of TNCC after 24 h and 48 h when stored at room temperature.

3.3.2 Fluid analysis

Routine analysis of body cavity effusions include:

- Macroscopic evaluation.
- Quantitative measurements:
  - Total cell count.
  - Protein measurement.
  - Other biochemistry parameters, such as albumin, bilirubin, creatinine, potassium, triglycerides, cholesterol, lipase and glucose, are measured on selected cases.
- Cytological examination of direct and/or concentrated stained slides.

Macroscopic evaluation

The fluid is evaluated grossly for colour, clarity and other features, such as viscosity.

- Colour: the evaluation of the supernatant provides an indication of the pigmented solutes present in the fluid, e.g.:
  - Yellow to orange, occasionally green: bilirubin.
  - Pink-red, brown: haemoglobin.
- Turbidity: can be associated with a high cellularity, bacteria, lipids, etc.

Quantitative measurements

Protein concentration

- Usually measured on the fluid supernatant.
- Methods:
  - Clinical refractometer: it measures the refractive index of a fluid, which is then displayed on a total protein (TP) or total solids (TS: electrolytes, glucose, urea, etc.) and SG scales. Falsely raised results might be caused by lipaemia of the sample or presence of some solutes in high concentration, such as urea.
  - The refractometer is fairly accurate when the fluid protein concentration is > 25 g/l. It is less accurate for lower concentrations, although the degree of inaccuracy is usually not clinically significant.
  - Chemical analysis: performed on the same instruments used for blood chemistry analysis. These analysers are also used for the measurement of other solutes, such as bilirubin, creatinine, lipase, electrolytes and glucose. The method used to measure TP is colorimetric.

Total nucleated cell count

- Performed on EDTA sample after gently mixing the fluid.
- Methods:
  - Haemocytometer (manual method): not commonly used.
  - Automated count: fluid cell count is most commonly obtained by using a haematology analyser.
- Inaccurate results might be caused by cell clumping, fragmentation and presence of non-cellular particulates in the effusion.

Haematocrit (HCT)/Packed cell volume (PCV)

- Performed on EDTA sample after gently mixing the fluid.
- Methods:
  - PCV: obtained by centrifugation using a microhaematocrit centrifuge.
  - HCT: calculated parameter provided by haematology analysers.

Slide preparation and staining

Slides are prepared from the EDTA sample:

- Slides can be made in different ways depending on the expected cellularity:
  - Direct smear: for highly cellular fluids. It can also be used for a subjective estimation of the cellularity of the fluid (low or high), if the TNCC is not readily available.
  - Fluid sediment and cytospin preparations: recommended for low-cellular fluids.
  - If particulates are present in the fluid, they can be used to make a squash preparation.
- Slides are air-dried and stained with Romanowsky stains.
- More information on the different techniques to prepare smears from a fluid can be found in Chapter 1.

Further reading

Maher, I., Tennant, K.V. and Papasouliotis, K. (2010) Effect of storage time on automated cell count and cytological interpretation of body cavity effusions. *Veterinary Records* 167(14), 519–522.

3.4 Classification of Cavitary Effusions

Effusion can be classified based on:

- Characteristic of the fluid (total protein and nucleated cell count).
- Underlying cause (pathophysiology).

The most common criteria used in veterinary medicine to classify effusions are based on:

- Total cell count and protein concentration:
    - Traditional classification scheme:
        - Transudates.
        - Modified transudates.
        - Exudates.
    - Most recent classification scheme:
        - Transudates:
            - Protein-poor.
            - Protein-rich.
        - Exudates.
- Pathophysiology: based on the underlying aetiology causing the effusion:
    - Transudates.
    - Exudates.
        - Septic.
        - Non-septic.
    - Effusion from cell exfoliation.
        - Neoplasia.
        - Reactive mesothelium.
    - Effusion from ruptured or leaky vessels or viscera.
        - Haemorrhagic effusion.
        - Bilothorax and bile peritonitis.
        - Urothorax and uroabdomen.
        - Chyle.
        - Gastrointestinal perforation.
        - Others.
- A recent study investigated the lipid pattern of pleural and abdominal effusions in dogs and cats with known underlying pathologies. This study identified two different patterns, based on the amounts of very-low-density (VLDL), intermediate-density (IDL) and high-density (HDL) lipoproteins:
    - First pattern was rich in VLDL and IDL and poor in HDLs.
    - Second pattern was rich in HDL and poor in VLDL and IDL.

  These two groups were correlated with the protein concentration of the transudates and their underlying causative pathology. Based on the results, the authors suggested the following classification scheme and related suspected underlying causes:
    - Exudates: TNCC > 5000 cells/μl, regardless of the TP concentration.
    - Transudates: TNCC < 5000 cells/μl and:
        - TP < 15 g/l (1.5 g/dl): protein-losing enteropathy (PLE), chronic kidney disease (CKD) and acquired portosystemic shunt (PSS).
        - TP > 15 g/l (2.5 g/dl): heart disease, caudal vena cava syndrome and cavitary neoplasia.

Pearls and Pitfalls

- The classical fluid classification scheme currently used in veterinary medicine has its limitation, as different diseases may lead to effusions with overlapping TNCC and TP. Although total cell count and protein concentration provide an initial subclassification of the effusions, these should always be combined and interpreted in conjunction with the cytological findings, imaging results and clinical presentation, in order to achieve an accurate diagnosis of the underlying pathology (e.g. an effusion caused by neutrophilic peritonitis and one secondary to neoplastic exfoliation may have overlapping TNCC and TP).
- A less common classification method that has been investigated in veterinary medicine is an adaptation of the Light's criteria, widely used in human medicine. This scheme uses the concentration of pleural lactate dehydrogenase (LDH), $LDH_{pleural}$ fluid: LDH_{serum} ratio and total protein pleural fluid:total protein serum ratio to classify the effusions into transudates and exudates.

Table 3.1. Most commonly used parameters to classify effusions based on protein concentration and total cell count in veterinary medicine.

Type	Total protein (g/l)	Total cell count (cells/µl)
Raskin and Mayer		
Transudate	<25	<1000
Modified transudate	>25	>1000
Exudate	>30	>5000
Valenciano and Tyler		
Transudate	<25	<1500
Modified transudate	25–75	1000–7000
Exudate	>30	>7000
Stockham and Scott		
Transudate		
Protein-poor	<20	<1500
Protein-rich	≥20	<5000
Exudate	>20	>5000

Further reading

Alonso, F.H., Behling-Kelly, E. and Borjesson, D.L. (2022) Lipoprotein profile of pleural and peritoneal transudates in dogs and cats. *Journal of Internal Veterinary Medicine* 36(2), 464–472.
Zoia, A., Petini, M., Righetti, D., Caldin, M. and Drigo, M. (2020) Discriminating transudates and exudates in dogs with pleural effusion: diagnostic utility of simplified Light's criteria compared with traditional veterinary classification. *Veterinary Records* 187(1): e5.

3.5 Cell Types

Mesothelial cells

- They can exfoliate singly, in tessellating sheets or balls.
- When in clusters, a small clear gap may be seen in between contiguous cells (cell junctions).
- Mononucleated or occasionally bi- or multinucleated (especially when reactive).
- Anisokaryosis, anisocytosis and N:C ratio are variable.
- Nuclei are generally centrally placed, round to oval and have finely stippled to granular chromatin. Nucleoli can be single or multiple, round and variably visible.
- The cytoplasm is usually moderate in amount and pale to moderately basophilic. It can contain peripheral vacuoles (glycogen) or rarely a single medium-large vacuole, occasionally lightly pink in colour. Haematoidin crystals or haemosiderin granules may occasionally be seen in the cytoplasm, especially in haemorrhagic effusions.
- On the cell margins, small blebs may be seen (microvilli).

Macrophages

- Morphology is similar as observed in other locations.
- Cells have small-to-medium-sized, round-to-oval, central-to-paracentral nuclei.
- The cytoplasm is moderate to abundant and often vacuolated. It can contain amorphous phagosomes of variable nature.

Neutrophils

- Similar to those observed in the peripheral blood and in other locations.
- They can be variably degenerate showing karyolysis, pyknosis or karyorrhexis.
- In septic effusions, they may contain phagocytosed bacteria.

Lymphocytes

- Mostly small and medium sized.
- Similar to those observed in the peripheral blood.
- They have small round nuclei, indistinct nucleoli and a small cytoplasmic rim.
- Reactive lymphocytes may be found in inflammatory or reactive effusions. They are usually slightly larger with medium-large, round and eccentric nuclei, finely stippled chromatin and indistinct nucleoli. The cytoplasm is scant to moderate and moderately to deeply basophilic. Plasma cells may also be seen.

Eosinophils

- Similar to those observed in the peripheral blood and in other locations. They are polymorphonuclear leucocytes with lobulated nuclei. In dogs, they contain round, orange-pink granules. In cats, the granules are rod shaped.

Basophils

- Similar to those observed in the peripheral blood and in other locations. They are polymorphonuclear leucocytes with lobulated nuclei. In dogs granules appear purple and are not very numerous. Granules in cats are round or oval, light lavender or mauve in colour.
- Rarely observed in cavitary effusions.

Mast cells

- Morphology is similar as observed in other locations.
- Cells have medium-sized, round-to-oval nuclei variably positioned within the cell.
- The cytoplasm is moderate in amount and contains variable numbers of fine purple granules, which may obscure the nuclei.

Neoplastic cells

- Epithelial cells (carcinomatosis): the cell morphology reflects that of the cell of origin. Criteria of malignancy may be variable.
- Mesenchymal cells (sarcomatosis): the cell morphology reflects the lineage of the primary tumour. Criteria of malignancy may be variable.
- Round cells: e.g. lymphoma and mast cell tumour. The cell morphology mirrors that seen in other locations.
- Neoplastic mesothelial cells.

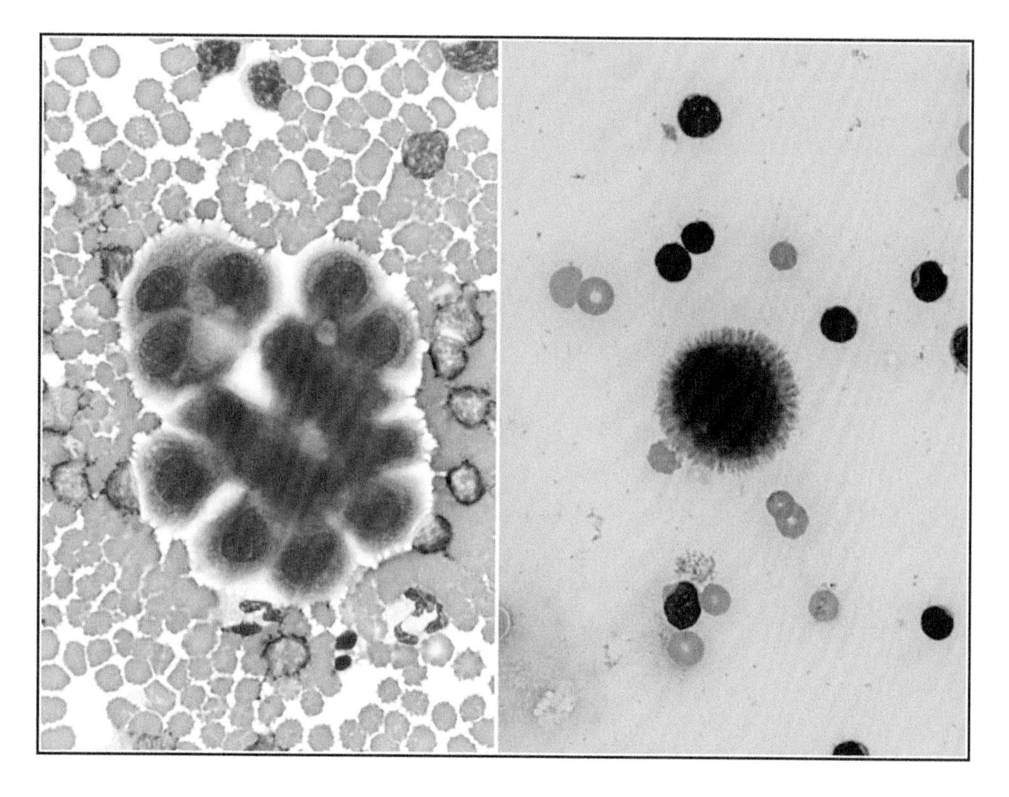

Fig. 3.2. Dog. Cavitary effusion. Left and right. Mesothelial cells. Wright-Giemsa.

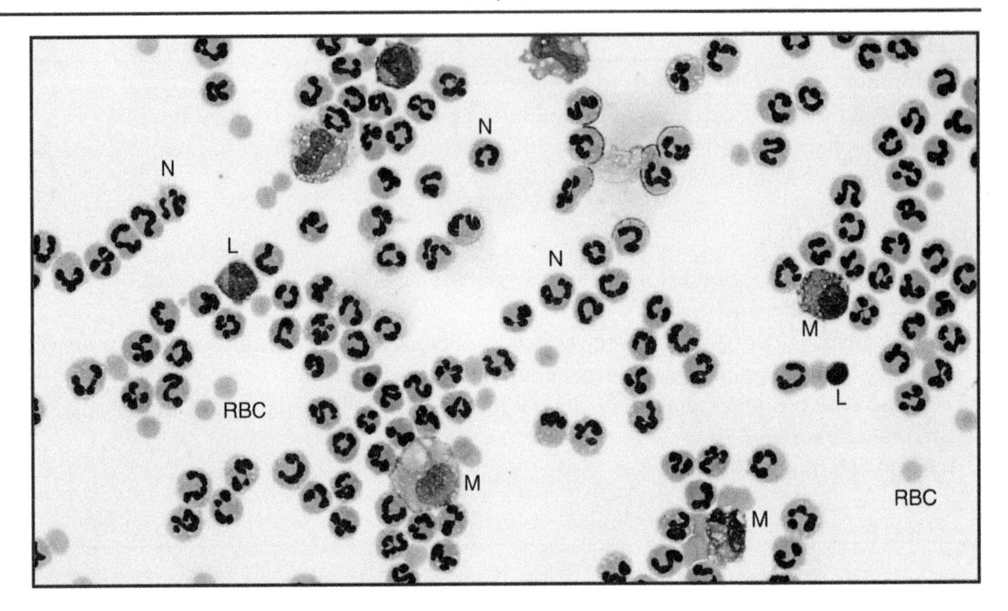

Fig. 3.3. Dog. Cavitary effusion. Mixed leucocytes in a haemodiluted background. N: neutrophils; L: lymphocytes; M: macrophages; RBC: red blood cells. Wright-Giemsa.

3.6 Pleural Effusions

Accumulation of fluid in the pleural space is caused by any process that alters the Starling forces, the lymphatic drainage and/or the vessel integrity.

In dogs and cats, pleural effusion usually accumulates bilaterally due to the fenestration of the mediastinum. Only in chronic processes, compartmentalization of the fluid may occur.

3.6.1 Pathophysiology

Pleural effusion occurs when the factors controlling the fluid dynamic are altered. This can be due to:

- Increased fluid formation.
- Reduced fluid absorption.
- Increased fluid formation and reduced fluid absorption.

Table 3.2. Causes of increased pleural fluid formation.

Increase of the hydrostatic pressure gradient, e.g.: – right-sided congestive heart failure (CHF) – pericardial tamponade – restrictive pericarditis – compression of a vessel by a neoplastic or inflammatory mass
Decreased colloid osmotic pressure secondary to hypoalbuminaemia, e.g.: – protein-losing nephropathy (PLN) – protein-losing enteropathy (PLE) – liver failure
Increased permeability of the capillary vessels, e.g.: – inflammation – infection – neoplasia
Disruption of the thoracic duct (chyle)
Disruption of the thoracic blood vessels (haemorrhage)

Table 3.3. Causes of reduced fluid reabsorption.

Left-sided CHF Obstruction of the venous or lymphatic drainage, e.g. – neoplasia – lung torsion Decreased pressure in the pleural space, e.g.: – bronchial obstruction – atelectasia

Pearls and Pitfalls

- In a recent retrospective study on 306 cats with pleural effusion, the most common causes were cardiac disease (35.3%), neoplasia (30.7%), pyothorax (8.8%), feline infectious peritonitis (FIP) (8.5%), chylothorax (4.6%) and others (12.2%). Of these, 8.5% has more than one aetiology.

Further reading

König, A., Hartmann, K., Mueller, R.S., Wess, G. and Schulz, B.S. (2019) Retrospective analysis of pleural effusion in cats. *Journal of Feline Medicine and Surgery* 21(12), 1102–1110.

3.6.2 Pleural Transudates

Pleural transudates are the accumulation of a low-cellular effusion in the pleural space. They can be classified as protein-poor and protein-rich transudates, depending on the protein concentration.

The primary cell types include non-degenerate neutrophils, monocytoid cells/macrophages, lymphocytes and mesothelial cells.

The aetiology of pleural transudates is wide and heterogeneous.

Clinical features

- Clinical signs relate to the mechanical interference with ventilation and reduced lung expansion caused by fluid accumulation in the pleural cavity.
  - They may include lethargy and exercise intolerance, cough, tachypnoea, dyspnoea and cyanosis.
  - The severity of the clinical signs is variable.

3.6.2.1 Non-infectious transudates

Hydrothorax

Accumulation of transudative fluid into the pleural space. It could be either protein-poor (pure transudate) or protein-rich.

Causes

This type of effusion is caused by a disturbance of the Starling forces:

- Protein-poor transudate:
  - Hypoproteinaemia:
    - Protein-losing nephropathy (PLN).
    - Protein-losing enteropathy (PLE).
    - Hepatic failure.
- Protein-rich transudate:
  - Right-sided CHF: it causes increased pleural fluid formation. It can also be associated with abdominal effusion.
  - Left-sided CHF: it decreases the pleural fluid absorption.
  - Pericardial disease.
  - Obstruction of venous and lymphatic drainage:
    - Lung lobe torsion (transudation of fluid through the lung capsule).
    - Diaphragmatic herniation of the liver into the thoracic cavity (transudation of fluid through the liver capsule).
    - Occlusion of caudal vena cava.
    - Neoplasia.

Cytological features

- Macroscopic appearance: clear and colourless. It can be variably haemodiluted due to iatrogenic haemorrhage during the sampling.
- Background: clear or pale basophilic with a variably small amount of blood (usually iatrogenic contamination).
- Cellularity is low. Total protein concentration can be low (protein-poor transudate) or high (protein-rich transudate).

- Nucleated cells usually consist of a mixture of segmented neutrophils, monocytoid cells or macrophages and small lymphocytes. Neutrophils are generally non-degenerate although *in vitro* swelling may occur.

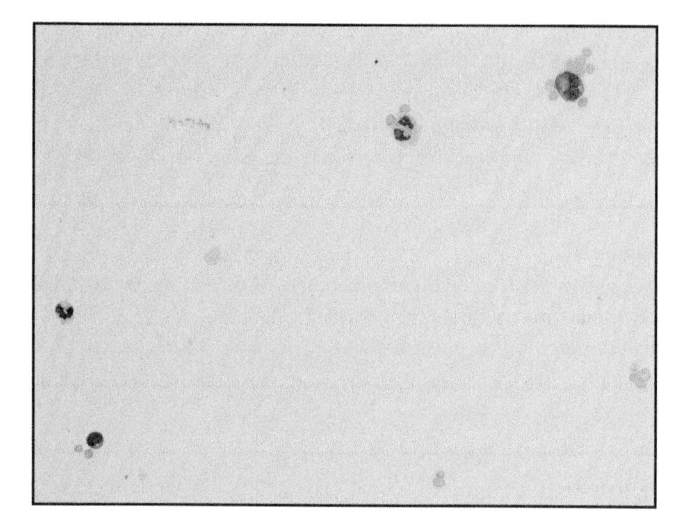

Fig. 3.4. Dog. Pleural effusion. Hydrothorax. Wright-Giemsa.

Lymphocyte-Rich Transudate (Cats)

Non-chylous lymphorrhagic pleural effusions characterized by a predominance of lymphocytes and absence of chylomicrons.

Clinical features

- Recently described in a cases series including 33 cats.
- Non-chylous lymphocyte-rich effusions are transudates that form due to the leakage of lymph, but that do not contain chylomicrons.
- Age: 6 months to 20 years.
- Clinical signs relate to the accumulation of fluid in the pleural space and to the underlying pathology causing the effusion.

Causes

In the study, the most common underlying causes associated with this type of effusion were:

- Cardiac disease (most common cause):
  - Restrictive cardiomyopathy.
  - Hypertrophic cardiomyopathy.
  - Dilatative cardiomyopathy.
  - Arrhythmia.
- Neoplasia:
  - Mediastinal lymphoma.
  - Carcinoma.
  - Thymoma.

Cytological features

- Macroscopic appearance: serous or serous-haemorrhagic.
- Cellularity: mean and median cell counts were 5051 cells/µl and 2400 cells/µl, respectively.
- Protein concentration: these transudates were often protein-rich (mean: 31.9 g/l).
- Triglycerides (TG) in the effusion were either < 100 mg/dl or $TG_{effusion} < TG_{serum}$.
- Background: clear to variably haemodiluted.
- Predominance of small lymphocytes: mean percentage of lymphocytes was 79%.

Differential diagnosis

- Chyle (especially in anorectic patients where the effusion may not have the typical *milky* appearance or may not contain chylomicrons)
- Lymphoma (although this is most frequently associated with large lymphoid cells)

Pearls and Pitfalls

While dogs with right-sided heart failure more commonly present with ascites, cats with heart disease more frequently develop pleural effusion. The cause for this difference is still poorly understood. It is postulated that feline visceral pleural veins and lymphatics drain into the pulmonary veins so, in case of increased pulmonary venous pressure, pleural exudation occurs.

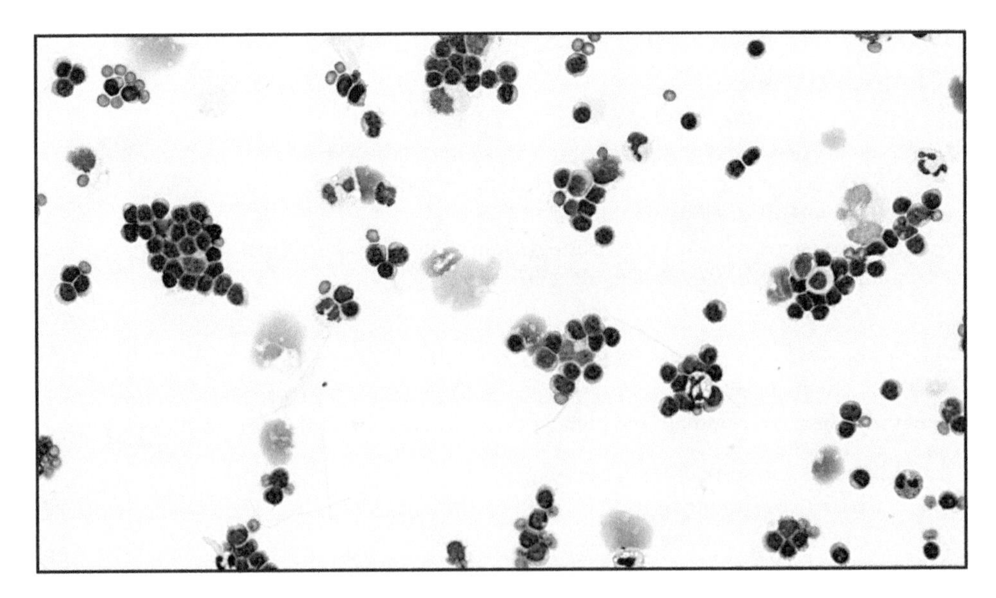

Fig. 3.5. Cat. Pleural effusion. Lymphocyte-rich effusion. Wright-Giemsa.

Further reading

Probo, M., Valenti, V., Venco, L., Paltrinieri, S., Lavergne, E. *et al.* (2018) Pleural lymphocyte-rich transudates in cats. *Journal of Feline Medicine and Surgery* 20(8), 767–771.

3.6.2.2 *Infectious transudates*

Feline Infectious Peritonitis

Feline infectious peritonitis is a fatal disease that occurs in domestic and wild felids worldwide. It is caused by the feline infectious peritonitis virus (FIPV), which derives from a mutation of the avirulent feline enteric coronavirus (FCoV).

Clinical features

- Most commonly occurs in young cats (<2 years old), but cats of all ages can be affected. A second peak in age-related risk is seen in cats over 10 years of age.
- Pedigree cats have been described as more susceptible than non-purebred cats. However, it seems that the predisposition to develop FIP occurs along familial lineages.
- Some studies report that males are more commonly affected.
- Patients living in multi-cats households are more at risk (e.g. breeders and rescue centres).
- Two forms exist:
  - Effusive (wet form): characterized by cavitary effusion (pleural and/or abdominal effusion). This is the most common form.
  - Non-effusive (dry form): characterized by granulomatous changes in different organs especially the CNS and eyes.
  - Mixed form.
- Clinical signs are often non-specific, especially in the dry form. They include anorexia, lethargy, weight loss, mild pyrexia, dyspnoea or tachypnoea, ocular and neurological signs, etc. Jaundice is possible.
- Abdominal masses may be found on physical examination due to omental and visceral adhesions. Mesenteric lymphadenomegaly can occur, especially in the dry form.
- Haematology: often non-specific changes are present, such as mild non-regenerative anaemia, neutrophilia and lymphopenia.
- Biochemistry: changes greatly depend on the organ/s that are involved. The most common abnormalities present in approximately 70% of cats with FIP are hyperproteinaemia and hyperglobulinaemia, with reduced albumin:globulin ratio (A:G). Although a low A:G ratio is relatively non-specific, values >0.6–0.8 have a high negative predictive value for FIP.
- Hypoalbuminaemia may also be present. This is often multifactorial due to protein-losing nephropathy and/or enteropathy and loss through extravasation secondary to vasculitis. On serum protein electrophoresis (SPE), a polyclonal gammopathy is often observed, often associated with an increase of the alpha2-globulins (mostly haptoglobin).
- Many cats with FIP also have hyperbilirubinaemia and bilirubinuria, mostly due to increased red blood cell destruction, rather than hepatic involvement.
- Alpha1-acid glycoprotein (A1GP) is often elevated at concentration ≥1.5 mg/ml in both serum and fluid.

Cytological features

- Fluid macroscopic appearance: often clear and yellow, sometimes viscous. It can be mildly haemodiluted due to iatrogenic haemorrhage during the sampling.
- Cellularity is variable (1000–30,000 cells/μl), but generally low. TP is high, often >35 g/l.
- A:G ratio: low. A:G values above 0.8 almost certainly exclude FIP. Effusions with TP > 35 g/l, A:G < 0.45 and low TCC are highly predictive of FIP.
- Background: pale to moderately basophilic, granular and often containing numerous protein crescents.
- Nucleated cells consist of a mixture of non-degenerate neutrophils, monocytoid cells/macrophages and small lymphocytes.
- Additional testing:
  - Immunostaining for FCoV antigen: detection of a large amount of viral antigen within macrophages (cytology or histopathology samples) indicates high viral replication in these cells. This is highly specific and is considered the gold standard for the diagnosis of FIP. Negative results do not exclude the disease. In particular, the sensitivity of FCoV immunostaining in the effusions is reported to vary between 57% and 100%.
  - Fluid FCoV PCR: this may be used to confirm FCoV as the underlying cause of the clinical signs. However, less virulent FCoV can occasionally spread systemically in cats without FIP. Therefore, this test is not necessarily specific for a diagnosis of FIP, although it is highly sensitive. Detection of higher viral loads by real time RT-qPCR increases the probability of FIP.
  - Alpha-1 acid glycoprotein: It has been identified as the best acute phase protein to distinguish between cats with and without FIP. One study reported that the AGP level was high in FIP effusions (>1.55 mg/ml), with a sensitivity and specificity of 93%.
  - Rivalta test: not so commonly used any more. This test is highly sensitive but poorly specific.
  - Usually, an antemortem diagnosis requires a combination of multiple test results that support the diagnosis of FIP.
  - Histopathology: this is considered the gold standard to confirm FIP, often in association with immunohistochemistry to confirm the presence of the virus in the lesion.

Differential diagnoses

- Non-exfoliating neoplasia.
- Cardiac heart failure.

Pearls and Pitfalls

Feline infectious peritonitis is an inaccurate terminology because affected patients do not have peritonitis. The common presence of abdominal effusion is a consequence of a pyogranulomatous vasculitis that leads to fluid exudation.

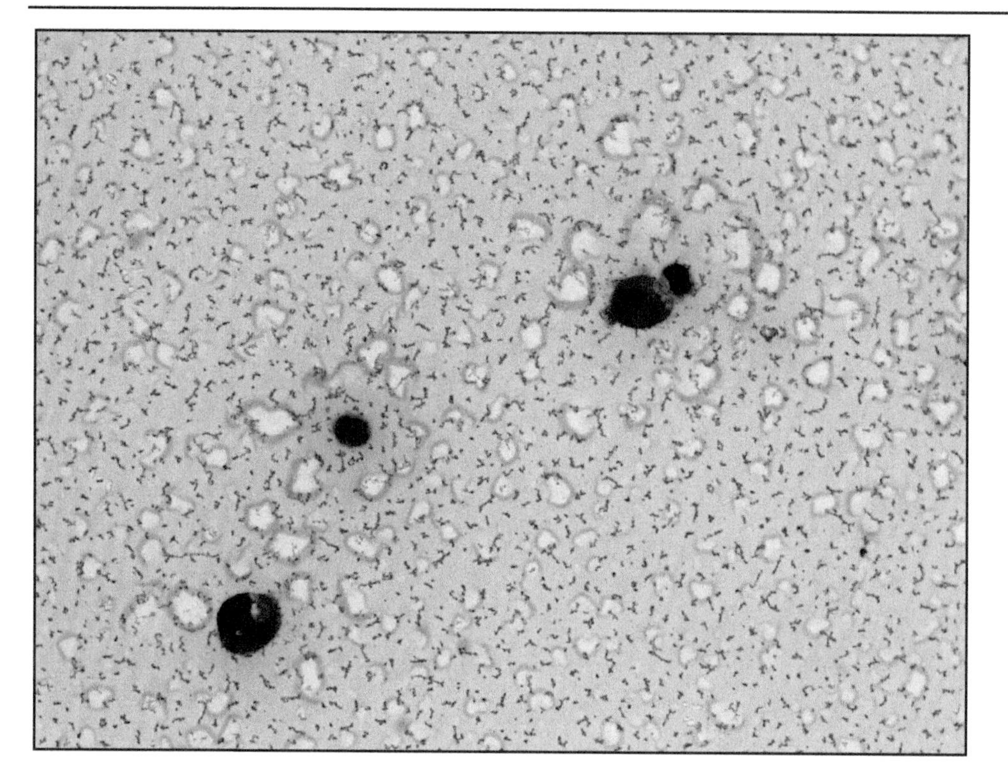

Fig. 3.6. Cat. Pleural effusion. Feline infectious peritonitis. Wright Giemsa (*Courtesy of Ugo Bonfanti.*)

Further reading

Kennedy, M. (2020) Feline infectious peritonitis update on pathogenesis, diagnostics, and treatment. *Veterinary Clinics of North America: Small Animal Practice* 50, 1001–1011.
Taske, S. (2018) Diagnosis of feline infectious peritonitis: update on evidence supporting available tests. *Journal of Feline Medicine and Surgery* 20, 228–243.
Thayer, V., Gogolski, S., Felten, S., Hartmann, K., Kennedy, M. *et al.* (2022) 2022 AAFP/EveryCat feline infectious peritonitis diagnosis guidelines. *Journal of Feline Medicine and Surgery* 24(9), 905–933.

Protozoal Disease

- *Toxoplasma gondii* is the most common protozoa that can be associated with pleural effusion.
- Effusions secondary to protozoal infection can be transudates (protein-poor and protein-rich) or exudates.
- Nucleated cells that may be more often seen include neutrophils, macrophages and lymphocytes.
- *Toxoplasma* spp. is characterized by banana-shape morphology with a pale basophilic cytoplasm and a small, round, purple nucleus.

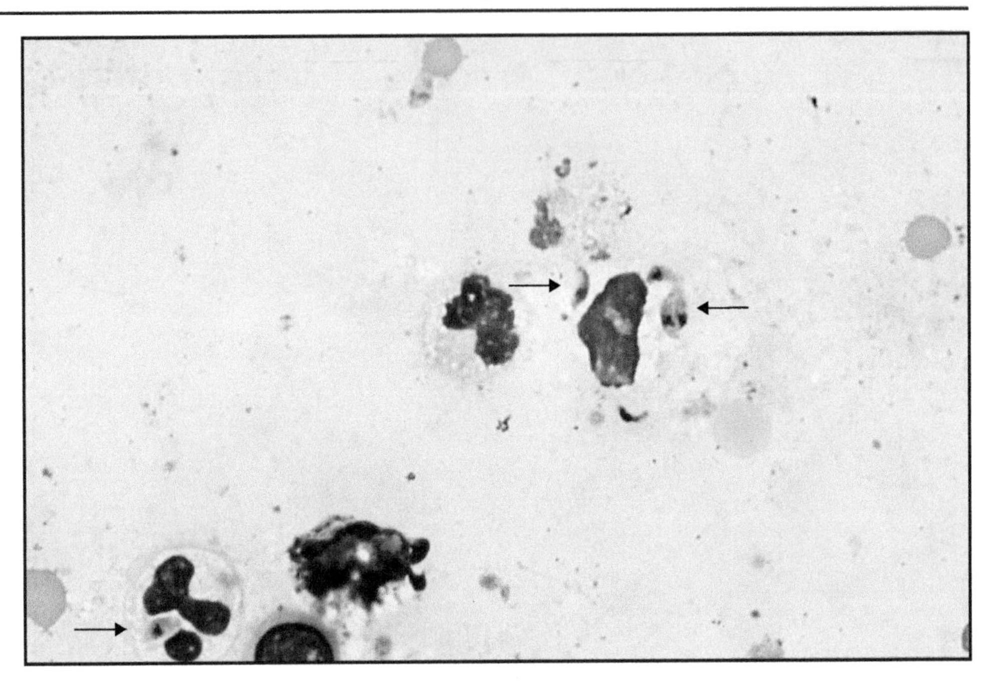

Fig. 3.7. Cat. Pleural effusion. Toxoplasmosis. Wright-Giemsa.

3.6.3 Pleural Exudates

Exudative effusions are caused by an inflammation within the pleural space. The triggers that can induce inflammation in the pleural cavity could be:

- Exogenous: e.g. bacteria, fungi and foreign bodies/material.
- Endogenous: e.g. bile, chyle and urine.

It is important to remember that the absence of infectious agents in cytological examination does not exclude an underlying infection.

Pathophysiology

- Increased capillary wall permeability due to the effect of cytokines and vasoactive amines released during inflammation and endothelial damage. This allows proteins, cells and macromolecules to enter the pleural space.
- Increased hydrostatic pressure secondary to hyperaemia (increased blood flow) in the pleural capillaries and due to inflammation.
- Reduced lymphatic drainage secondary to the thickening of the parietal pleura.
- Increased oncotic pressure within the pleural space secondary to the accumulation of proteins within the pleural fluid.
- Exudates can be broadly subdivided in septic and non-septic.

3.6.3.1 Non-infectious exudates

Neutrophilic and Mixed Exudates

Causes

- Extension of an inflammatory process from inflamed organs or structures in the pleural cavity.
- Neoplasia.
- Sterile irritants, such as bile and urine (Section 3.6.4) and foreign bodies.

Cytological features

- The cellularity is variably high and TP is usually increased.
- Background: variably haemodiluted and clear to pale basophilic. Exogenous or endogenous material can be found, depending on the underlying cause.
- Predominance of non-degenerate neutrophils. Occasionally, karyorrhexis and pyknosis are observed (age-related degenerative changes).
- Other leucocytes such as macrophages, lymphocytes, plasma cells and eosinophils can be observed in variable percentages. Mesothelial cells may be present in variable numbers.

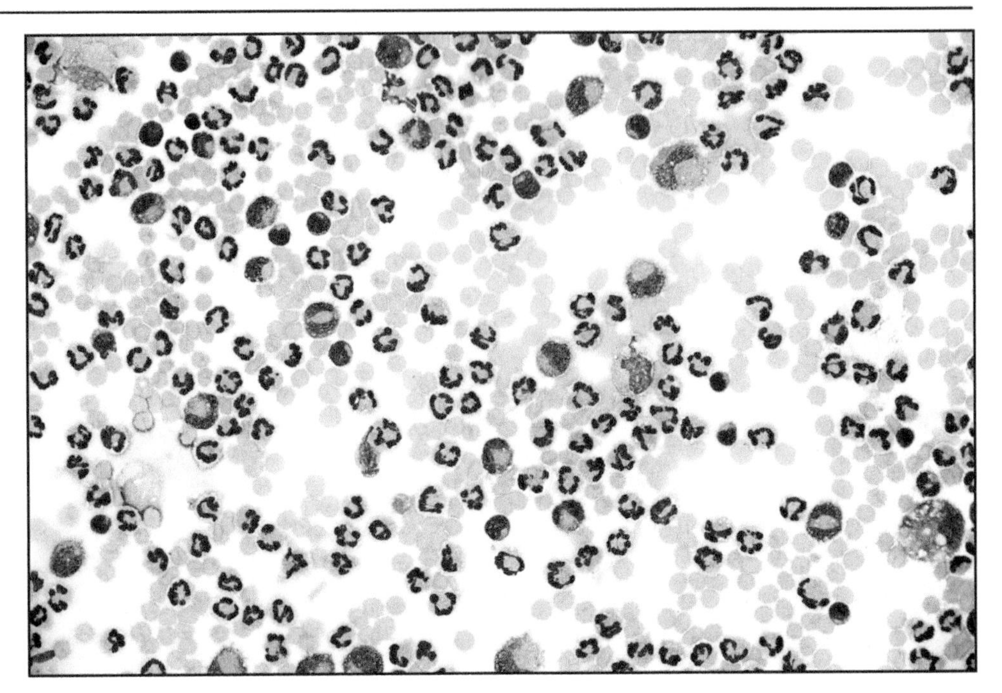

Fig. 3.8. Dog. Pleural effusion. Neutrophilic exudate. In a mildly haemodiluted background, there are non-degenerate neutrophils, low numbers of macrophages and occasional small lymphocytes. Wright-Giemsa. (*Courtesy of Melissa White.*)

Eosinophilic Exudates

Causes

- Neoplasia: e.g. mast cell tumour and T-cell lymphoma.
- Idiopathic hypereosinophilic syndrome.
- Allergy.
- Pneumothorax.

Cytological features

- The cellularity is variable to high, and TP is also often raised.
- Background: variably haemodiluted and clear to pale basophilic.
- An increased proportion of eosinophils (>10%) is observed. Other nucleated cells may include variable percentages of non-degenerate neutrophils, monocytoid cells/macrophages, small lymphocytes and reactive mesothelial cells.

Pearls and Pitfalls

- Pleural eosinophilic effusions can be either exudates or transudates, but the differential diagnoses are the same.

Further reading

Fossum, T.W., Wellman, M., Relford, R.L. and Slater, M.R. (1993) Eosinophilic pleural or peritoneal effusions in dogs and cats: 14 cases (1986–1992). *Journal of American Veterinary Medical Association* 202(11), 1873–1876.

Sykes, J.E., Weiss, D.J., Buoen, L.C., Blauvelt, M.M., and Hayden, D.W. (2001) Idiopathic hypereosinophilic syndrome in 3 Rottweilers. *Journal of Veterinary Internal Medicine* 15(2), 162–166.

3.6.3.2 Infectious exudates

Infectious agents that penetrate the pleural space often cause an inflammatory process leading to accumulation of an exudative fluid. Infectious agents that may cause pleural exudate include bacteria, fungi/yeasts, protozoa, algae and parasites and can reach the thoracic cavity by different routes, such as:

- Migrating foreign body.
- Penetrating wound.
- Oesophageal perforation.
- Parasitic migration.
- Haematogenous, lymphatic or parapneumonic bacterial spread.
- Previous thoracic surgery or thoracocentesis.
- Ruptured lung abscess.
- Parasitic migration (cats), e.g. *Aelurostrongylus abstrusus*, *Toxocara cati* and *Cuterebra*.

Bacteria

- Cocci: they are round and can be found in chains (e.g. *Streptococcus* spp.) or in groups (e.g. *Staphylococcus* spp.). They are most frequently Gram-positive bacteria. An uncommon septic pyothorax described in cats and rarely in dogs is that caused by *Rhodococcus equi*. These are facultative intracellular bacteria that preferentially infect histiocytic cells. This aetiology should be suspected when the bacteria are seen more frequently in macrophages rather than in neutrophils, as more typically observed in other septic infections.
- Rods/bacilli: they are elongated and vary in size from small to relatively large. They are usually Gram-negative. They can be found singly or in chains.
- Filamentous: they are very thin elongated bacteria often forming long chains in bundles. Typical examples are *Nocardia* and *Actinomyces* spp.
- Helicoidal: they are very thin elongated bacteria with a spiral morphology. The most common spiral bacterium that can be found in pyothorax following bite-penetrating wounds is *Treponema* spp. (e.g. *Treponema denticola*). This is a commensal of the oral cavity. Conventional culture fails to grow this bacterium.
- Negatively stained bacilli: this characteristic appearance is often associated with mycobacterial infection. The bacteria are usually found either in the macrophages or free in the background. Acid-fast stain may facilitate their identification.
- In pyothorax from dogs, obligate anaerobic bacteria (*Bacteroides* spp., *Fusobacterium* spp.) and Gram-positive filamentous organisms, such as *Nocardia* and *Actinomyces* spp., are most commonly isolated. In cats, *Pasteurella multocida* and anaerobes are the most frequent isolates.

Fungi and Yeasts

Examples of fungi/yeasts that can cause pleural exudates include:

- *Histoplasma* spp.: small, round-to-oval organisms measuring approximately 2–5 µm. They are pale basophilic yeasts surrounded by a thin clear capsule. Usually found within macrophages.
- *Cryptococcus neoformans*: round organisms measuring approximately 2–20 µm. They usually have a thick, negatively staining capsule of mucopolysaccharides. Narrow-based buddings are characteristic.
- *Blastomyces dermatitidis*: the yeasts are round, basophilic and measure between 6 µm and 15 µm. They have a thick, clear and distinct capsule and show broad-based buddings.

- *Candida albicans*: round to oval basophilic structures of approximately 3–8 μm. They may show narrow-base budding. They can also form hyphae and pseudohyphae. These are chains of fungal cells that show various degrees of elongation, with a constriction between adjacent cellular compartments. True hyphae consist of long tubes with parallel sides and no visible constrictions.
- Partial identification can be attempted on morphology, but ultimately culture and/or PCR would be required for definitive diagnosis.

Parasites

Parasitic infestations are rare but have been reported. Examples include:

- *Spirocerca lupi*.
- *Aelurostrongylus abstrusus*.
- *Angiostrongylus vasorum*.
- *Mesocestodides* spp.

Protozoa

Most commonly *Toxoplasma gondii*, although rare.

Neutrophilic exudate (pyothorax)

This is defined as an accumulation of purulent fluid within the pleural space. Infectious agents that can cause a neutrophilic exudate include bacteria, fungi/yeast and parasites. Most common causes are listed in Section 3.6.3.2.

Clinical features

- Commonly seen in both dogs and cats.
- Usually bilateral, but unilateral pyothorax is not uncommon.
- Age: younger animals seem to be more commonly affected (3–6 years old).
- Males of both species are over-represented in multiple studies.
- Common clinical signs: tachypnoea, dyspnoea, lethargy, weight loss, anorexia/hyperoxia and cough. Pyrexia is also possible. Only 50% or less of cats with pyothorax are hyperthermic.
- Haematological abnormalities are common and include mild anaemia of chronic disease and leucocytosis with variable toxic changes and left shift seen in the neutrophils.

Cytological features

- Cellularity and TP are high, in the range of an exudate.
- Background: clear to pale basophilic and finely granular (proteinaceous) and variably haemodiluted. Protein crescents might be observed, especially in direct smears.
- The majority of the cells consist of neutrophils (>50%). These are often degenerate displaying variable degree of karyolysis. Nuclear swelling can also be an *in vitro* change due to cellular suspension in fluid. In some cases, neutrophils may not show signs of degeneration.

- Other inflammatory cells may be seen including macrophages and fewer lymphocytes and plasma cells. Macrophages often have abundant and foamy cytoplasm, may contain amorphous phagosomes and can display leucophagia. In chronic processes, the inflammation may become pyogranulomatous.
- Bacteria, foreign body material, fungi, etc. may be found on cytology, depending on the underlying cause of the effusion.
- Bacteria usually trigger a neutrophilic inflammation. Chronic forms may become pyogranulomatous. Bacteria can be found free in the background or phagocytosed by the neutrophils. When free in the background, they can be observed individually, in pairs, chains or forming variably sized groups.
- Yeast and fungal elements can be found free in the background or within the macrophages. They are more commonly found in thick areas of the smears, hidden within dense aggregates of inflammatory cells.
- Parasites usually trigger a neutrophilic to pyogranulomatous inflammation. Variable numbers of eosinophils may also be present.
- The protozoal tachyzoites can be found in the background or within the macrophages. The type of effusion associated with this type of infection is variable from transudates to exudates.

Pearls and Pitfalls

- In septic pyothorax, the infectious agents may not always be found, especially if the patient had already been treated with antimicrobials at time of sampling (for bacterial infections).
- Although pyothorax is a relatively common condition in dogs and cats, in a review of the veterinary literature it emerged that in only 2–22% of cases the underlying cause was found.

Further reading

Stillion, J.R. and Letendre, J.A. (2015) A clinical review of the pathophysiology, diagnosis, and treatment of pyothorax in dogs and cats. *Journal of Veterinary Emergency and Critical Care* 25(1), 113–129.

Epstein, S.E. and Balsa, I.M. (2020) Canine and feline exudative pleural diseases. *Veterinary Clinics of North America: Small Animal Practice* 50, 467–487.

Mixed and Macrophagic Exudate

- These types of effusions have similar underlying causes and clinical features as neutrophilic exudates, but they are characterized by a higher percentage of macrophages.
- They could represent the evolution of a pyothorax to a more chronic form (resolving of an acute effusion).
- While bacteria tend to be more irritant and elicit a more selective neutrophilic inflammatory response, other infectious agents, such as fungi/yeasts and protozoa, tend to trigger a more mixed inflammation.

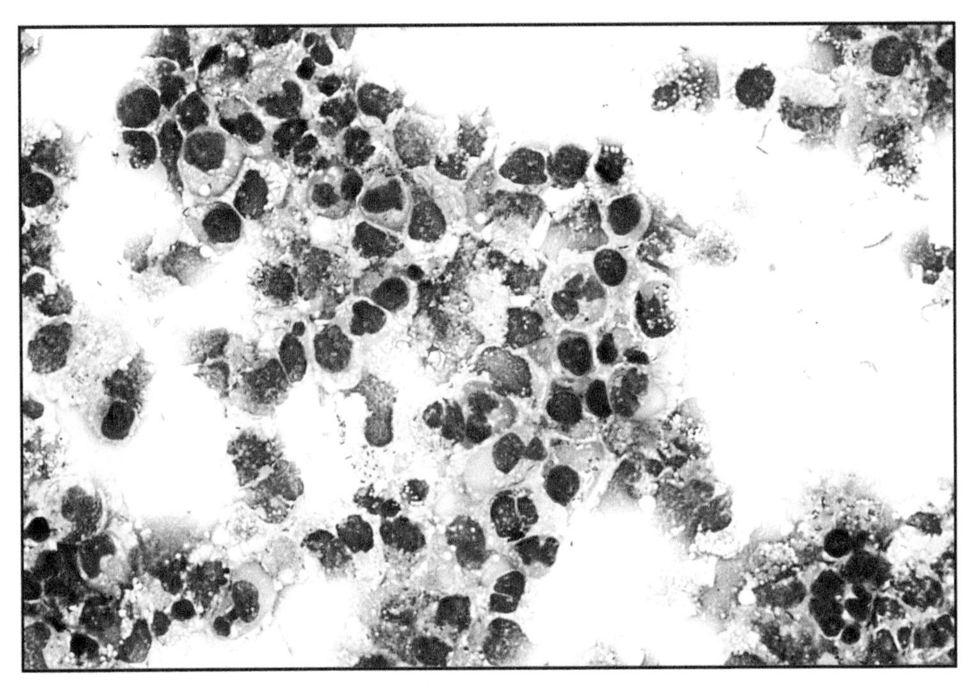

Fig. 3.9. Dog. Pleural effusion. Septic neutrophilic exudate. Degenerate neutrophils and rod bacteria. Wright-Giemsa. (*Courtesy of Nic Ilchyshyn.*)

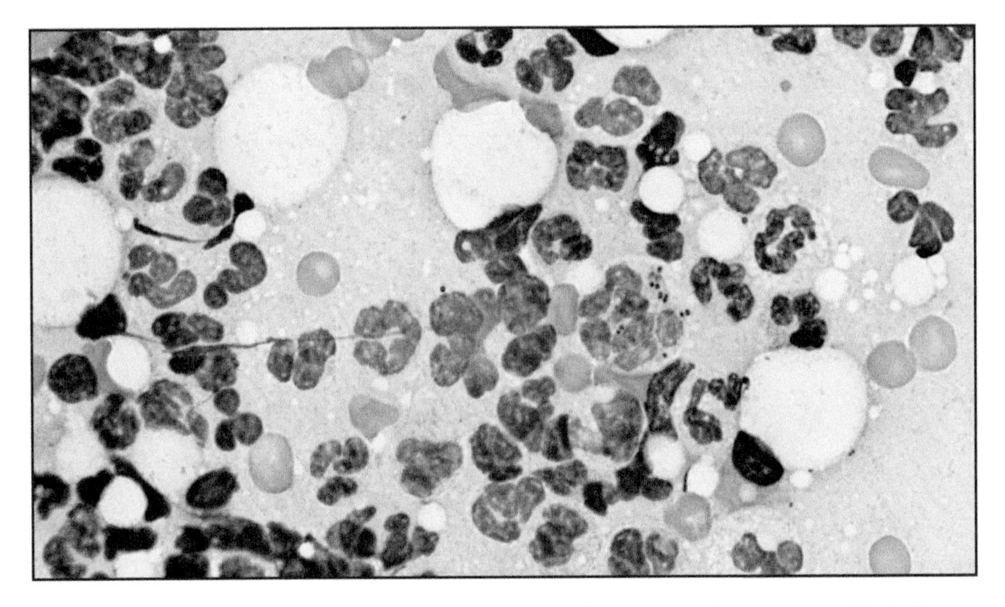

Fig. 3.10. Dog. Pleural effusion. Septic neutrophilic exudate, neutrophil containing phagocytes cocci. Wright-Giemsa.

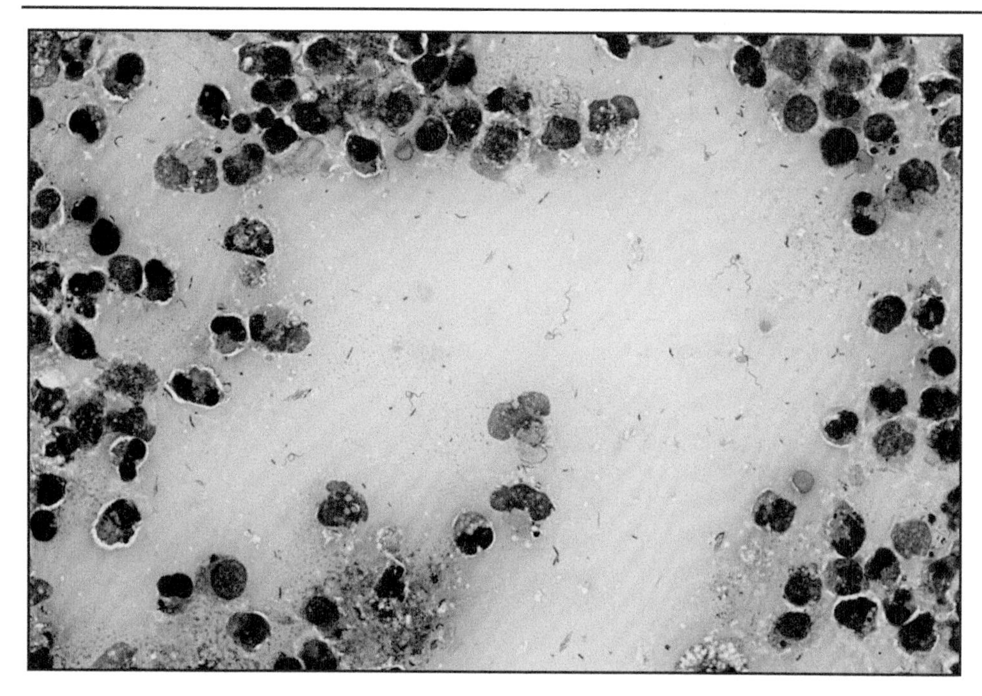

Fig. 3.11. Cat. Pleural effusion. Septic neutrophilic exudate with mixed bacteria including spiral bacteria compatible with *Treponema* spp. Wright-Giemsa. (*Courtesy of Nic Ilchyshyn.*)

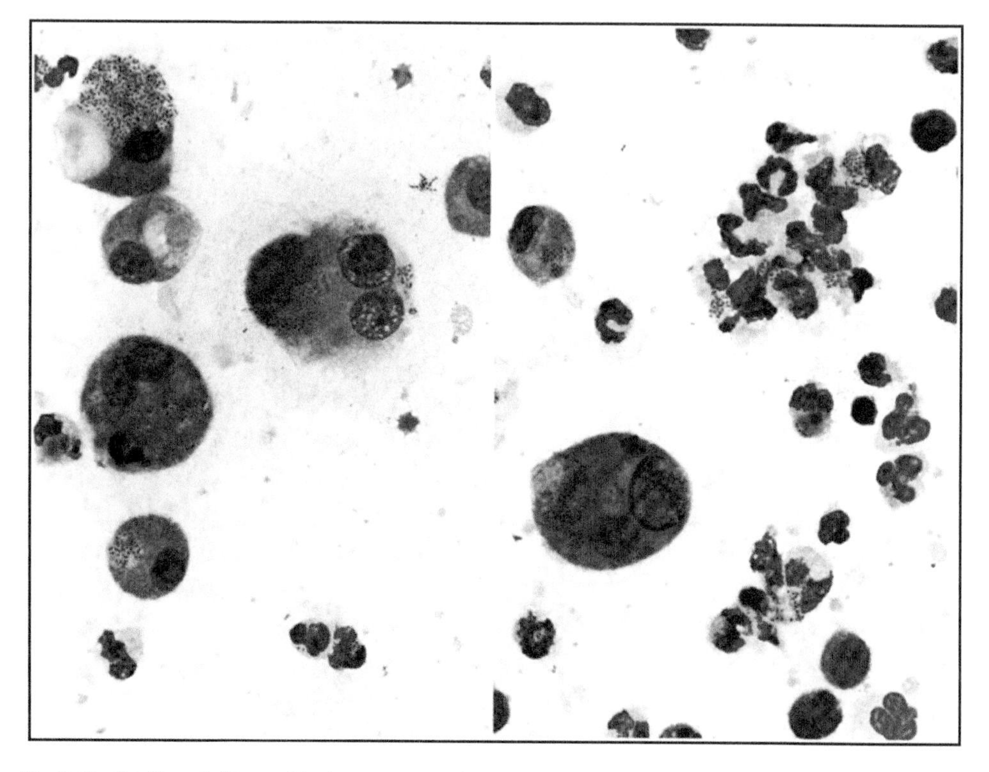

Fig. 3.12. Cat. Pleural effusion. *Rhodococcus equi* infection. Bacteria are seen within both neutrophils and macrophages. (*Courtesy of Gary Lee, case from Eric Morissette.*)

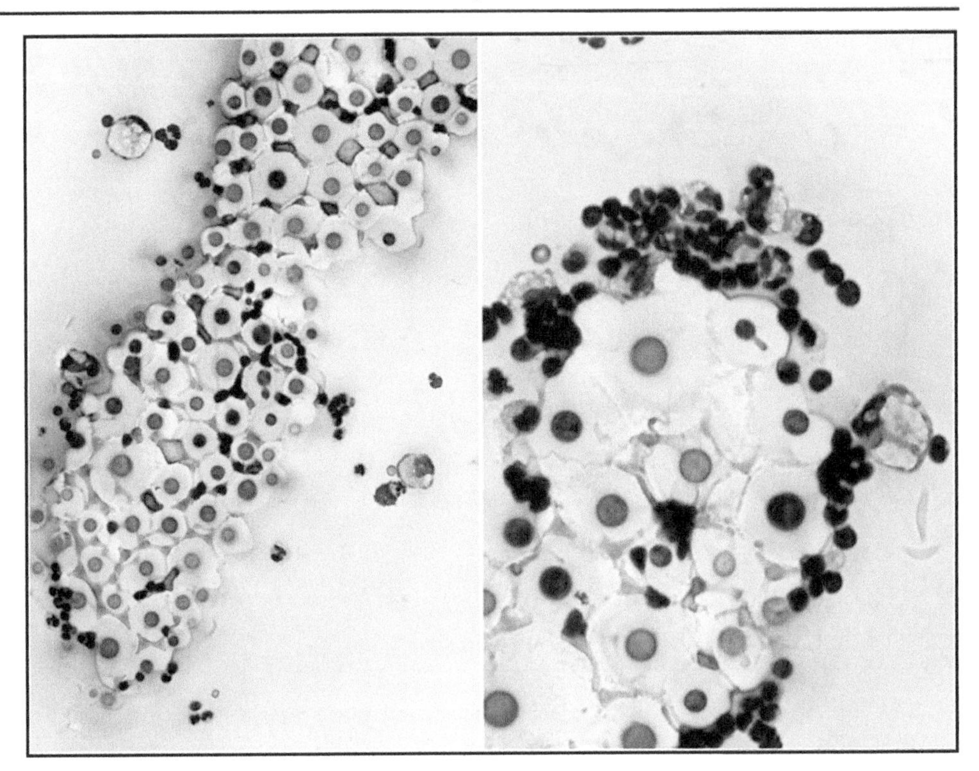

Fig. 3.13. Cat. Pleural effusion. Cryptococcosis. Wright-Giemsa.

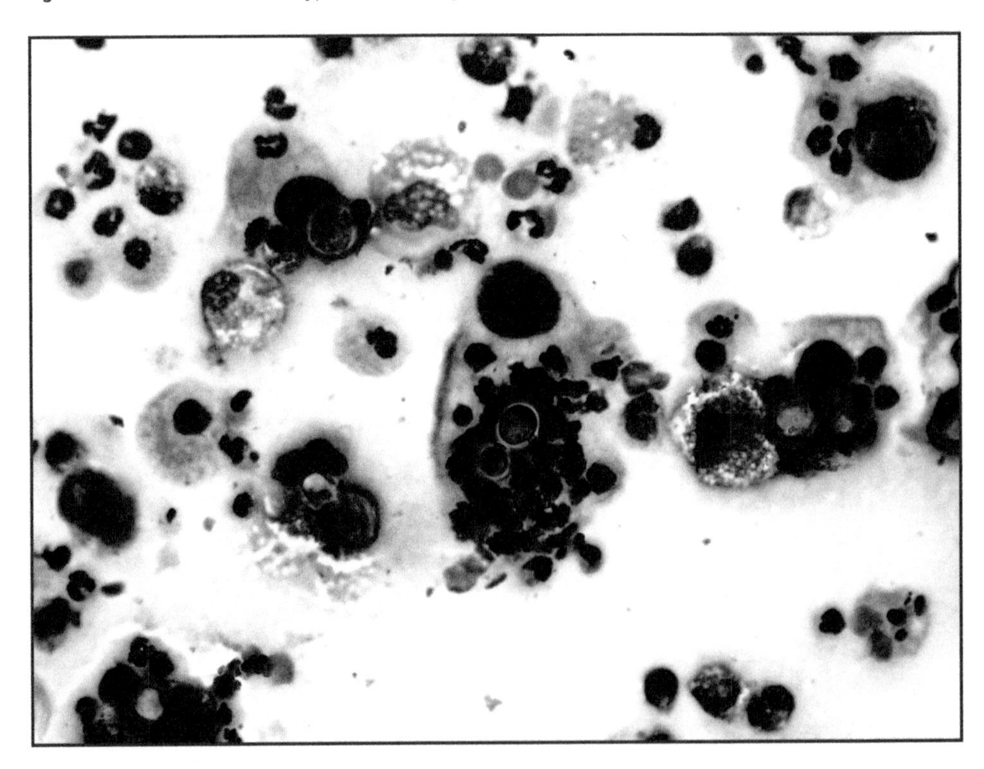

Fig. 3.14. Dog. Pleural effusion. Blastomycosis. Wright-Giemsa. (*Courtesy of Reema Patel.*)

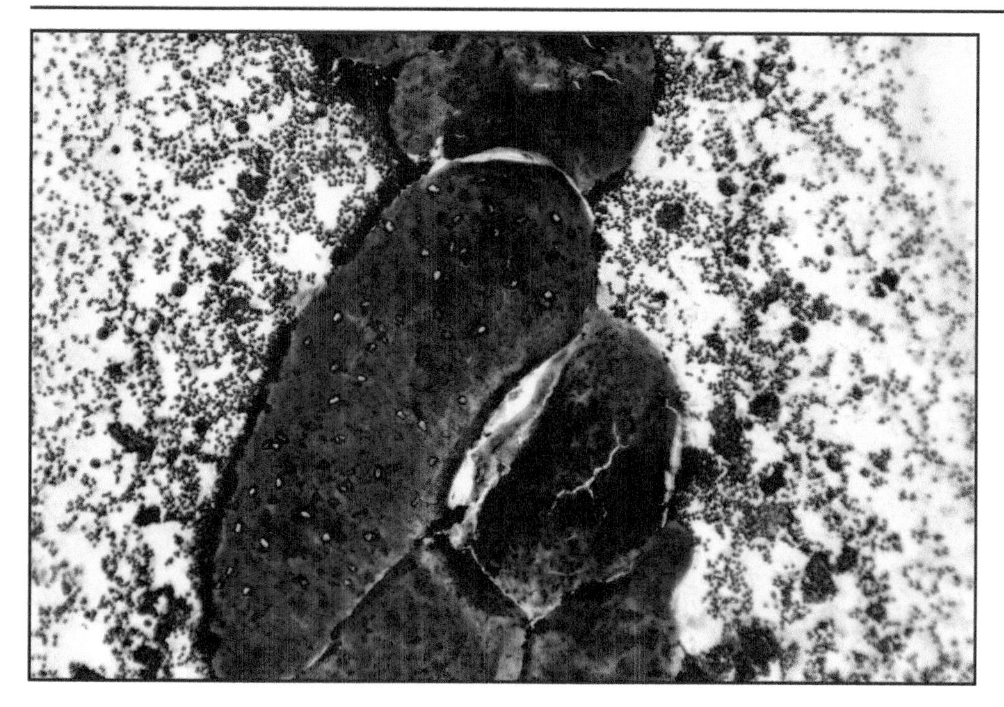

Fig. 3.15. Dog. Pleural effusion. Mesocestoidiasis. Wright-Giemsa. (*Courtesy of Walter Bertazzolo.*)

Eosinophilic Exudate

- Infectious eosinophilic pleural exudates in dogs and cats are rare. A case report of a dog with systemic coccidioidomycosis and eosinophilic exudate is reported in literature. *Angiostrongylus* sp. has been identified as the cause of eosinophilic pleural effusion in a cat.

Cytological features

- The cellularity and protein concentrations are in the range of an exudate.
- By definition, an exudate is defined eosinophilic when at least 6–10% of the TNCC are eosinophils (depending on the source).
- Numerous neutrophils and macrophages are also present, with fewer numbers of lymphocytes and plasma cells. Neutrophils may or may not be degenerate.
- The underlying infectious agent might not be found in the effusion.

3.6.4 Pleural effusions from ruptured or leaky vessels or organs

Chylothorax

Accumulation of chyle (lymph) within the pleural cavity. *Chylos* derives from the Greek word that means juice.

Pathophysiology

- Chyle drains from the thoracic duct (TD) into the venous system. The TD is the largest lymphoid vessel in the body that runs dorsal to the aorta and ventral to the thoracic vertebrae. One of its functions is to maintain the fluid balance and to prevent tissue oedema by returning the interstitial fluid to the vascular system.
- It is made up of lymphatic fluid and chylomicrons. The chylomicrons are a mixture of long-chain triglycerides (TG), cholesterol esters and phospholipids and derive from dietary lipids processed in the gastrointestinal tract.

Causes

- Obstruction of the lymphatic flow into the TD:
  - Mechanical:
    - Mediastinal and pulmonary neoplasia: e.g. thymoma, lymphoma and lymphangiosarcoma. These can impair the flow from the outside by compressing the TD or from the inside with neoplastic emboli.
    - Thoracic fungal granuloma.
    - Inflammatory foci.
    - Lung lobe torsion.
    - Cranial vena cava thrombosis.
    - Congenital abnormalities of the TD.
    - Diaphragmatic hernia.
  - Functional:
    - Cardiovascular disease: e.g. cardiomyopathy, pericardial effusion, restrictive pericarditis and heartworm disease.
    - Increased lymphatic flow due to increased lymph production.
- Idiopathic.
- Rupture of the TD.

Clinical features

- More frequent in cats than in dogs.
- Clinical signs relate to the accumulation of fluid in the pleural space and to the underlying cause of the chylothorax. They may include cough, laboured breathing, dyspnoea, etc.
- Over-represented canine breeds: in one study, Afghan Hounds had a higher incidence compared with other breeds. This may be due to their predisposition to lung torsion.

Cytological features

- Macroscopic appearance: chyle is often described as a *milky* fluid. This reflects the typical high content of fat and, in particular, of chylomicrons. However, this depends on the diet of the patient and, in anorectic patients, a clear effusion might be observed instead. A pink-red discolouration suggests blood contamination.
- Cellularity and protein concentration: usually in the range of a protein-rich transudate. In chronic forms, both TNCC and TP may increase in the range of an exudate. Protein measurement might be inaccurate due to the lipaemia of the sample.
- Background: pale basophilic, finely granular and variably haemodiluted.
- The majority of the nucleated cells are small lymphocytes. Macrophages can also be seen in established effusions. They typically contain characteristic punctate clear vacuoles of lipids. In more chronic forms, the irritant effect of the chyle on tissues causes a neutrophilic inflammatory response and neutrophils may replace the lymphocytic component.
- The final diagnosis of chylothorax is made by confirming the high TG content in the fluid as follow:
  - $TG_{effusion} > TG_{serum}$. This ratio is generally >3:1.
  - $TG_{effusion} > 100$ mg/dl (1.1 mmol/1). This criterion should be used carefully in anorectic patients.
  - C:T < 1 (mg/dl) (cholesterol to triglyceride ratio). This method can lead to false-positive results. In a study on 23 dogs and 25 cats, all the patients with chylothorax had a C:T < 1. However, 12% of the dogs with non-chylous effusion and 50% of the cats also had a ratio <1.

Differential diagnoses

- Lymphocyte-rich effusion.
- Lymphoma (although this is most frequently associated with large lymphoid cells).

Pearls and Pitfalls

- The 'milky' appearance of a pleural effusion does not *per se* define a chylothorax. For a definitive diagnosis of chylous effusion, the demonstration of a high triglyceride concentration is required.
- Similarly, a non-milky appearance does not rule out chylothorax. In anorectic patients, the chyle might be clear and triglyceride content may be low.
- Although numerous causes of chylothorax have been described in dogs and cats, the underlying cause is often not found (idiopathic).

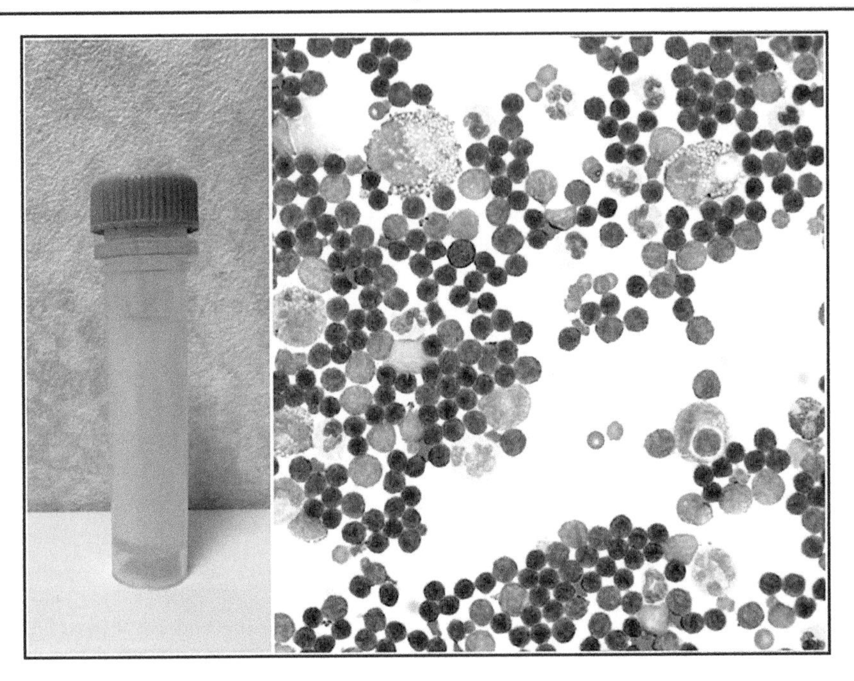

Fig. 3.16. Cat. Pleural effusion. Chyle. (Left) Macroscopic milky appearance. (Right) Prevalence of small lymphocytes with low numbers of macrophages containing clear punctate vacuoles. Wright-Giemsa.

Further reading

Singh, A., Brisson, B. and Nykamp, S. (2012) Idiopathic chylothorax: pathophysiology, diagnosis, and thoracic duct imaging. *Compendium: Continuing Education for Veterinarians* 34(8), E2.

Waddle, J.R. and Giger, U. (1990) Lipoprotein electrophoresis differentiation of chylous and non-chylous pleural effusions in dogs and cats and its correlation with pleural effusion triglyceride concentration. *Veterinary Clinical Pathology* 19(3), 80–85.

Haemothorax

Haemorrhagic extravasation into the pleural space.

Clinical features

- Clinical signs relate to the accumulation of fluid in the pleural space and to the loss of blood. They include pale mucus membranes and prolonged capillary refill time, weak peripheral pulse, tachypnea and dyspnoea, hypotension, hypothermia, tachycardia, hypovolemic shock, collapse, etc.

Causes

- Dogs: trauma, iatrogenic, congenital or acquired coagulopathy, neoplasia, and/or lung lobe torsion, *Angiostrongylus vasorum* (dog). Of the acquired coagulopathies, rodenticide intoxication is a relatively common cause.
- Cats: trauma, coagulopathy secondary to rodenticide intoxication, traumatic fat embolism, underlying neoplasia, lung lobe torsion, etc.
- Examples of tumours reported to cause haemorrhagic pleural effusion include mediastinal fibrosarcoma (dog), osteosarcoma (dog), thymoma and thoracic haemangiosarcoma.

Cytological features

- Macroscopically, the effusion appears as frank blood or as a serosanguineous fluid, depending on the duration of the effusion.
- In acute forms, the cellularity and protein are very similar to the peripheral WBC count and TP. In more chronic forms, these decrease secondary to a dilutional effect.
- In veterinary literature, there are no standardized criteria to classify an effusion as haemothorax. Generally, a haematocrit (HCT) >25% of the peripheral haematocrit is considered consistent with a haemothorax. In some texts, a PCV of pleural fluid >20% is also used as a criterion for the diagnosis. The same sources suggest that a PCV <20% still reflects haemorrhage although, in this case, the effusion is often associated with another concurrent pathology.
- In acute/per-acute forms, most of the cells consist of mixed blood-derived leucocytes in haemic proportion and a few mesothelial cells, in a heavily haemodiluted background. Platelets can sometimes be seen. Low numbers of macrophages displaying erythrophagia might be encountered.
- In more dated effusions, macrophages and mesothelial cells tend to increase in numbers. Macrophages may contain products of the RBC degradation, such as haemosiderin and haematoidin crystals. Mesothelial cells might be hyperplastic and reactive and sometimes can contain haematoidin crystals. Platelets, if present, usually represent concurrent iatrogenic haemorrhage.

Bilothorax (bilious pleural effusion)

This is a rare type of inflammatory effusion secondary to extravasation of bile into the pleural space.

Clinical features

- Described in both dogs and cats, but rare.
- Clinical signs are non-specific and include lethargy, depression, hypothermia or hyperthermia, dyspnoea and jaundice.

Causes

- Dogs: gunshot injuries with diaphragmatic tears, traumatic bile duct rupture (but intact diaphragm), penetrating thoracic injuries, post-cholecystectomy (but intact diaphragm).
- Cats: pleuro-biliary fistula secondary to thoracostomy tube placement and bite wounds.

Cytological features

- The fluid is usually dark brown in colour and turbid.
- The cellularity of the effusion can be variable, but usually moderate to high and the protein concentration increased, in the order of a typical exudate.
- The background is pale basophilic and variably haemodiluted. Lakes of eosinophilic mucinous material can be observed.
- Cells consist of a mixture of neutrophils and macrophages, with fewer lymphocytes. Neutrophils are often non-degenerate, and macrophages are activated with abundant and foamy cytoplasm. They can contain phagocytosed dark-black-green amorphous granules corresponding to bile pigment. Reactive mesothelial cells are also frequently present.
- Infectious agents are usually not found (unless a pre-existing biliary infection was present).
- Bilirubin concentration is usually higher in the fluid than in blood, and this can be used as a diagnostic tool. A $\text{bilirubin}_{\text{fluid}}$: $\text{bilirubin}_{\text{serum}} > 1$ is usually diagnostic.

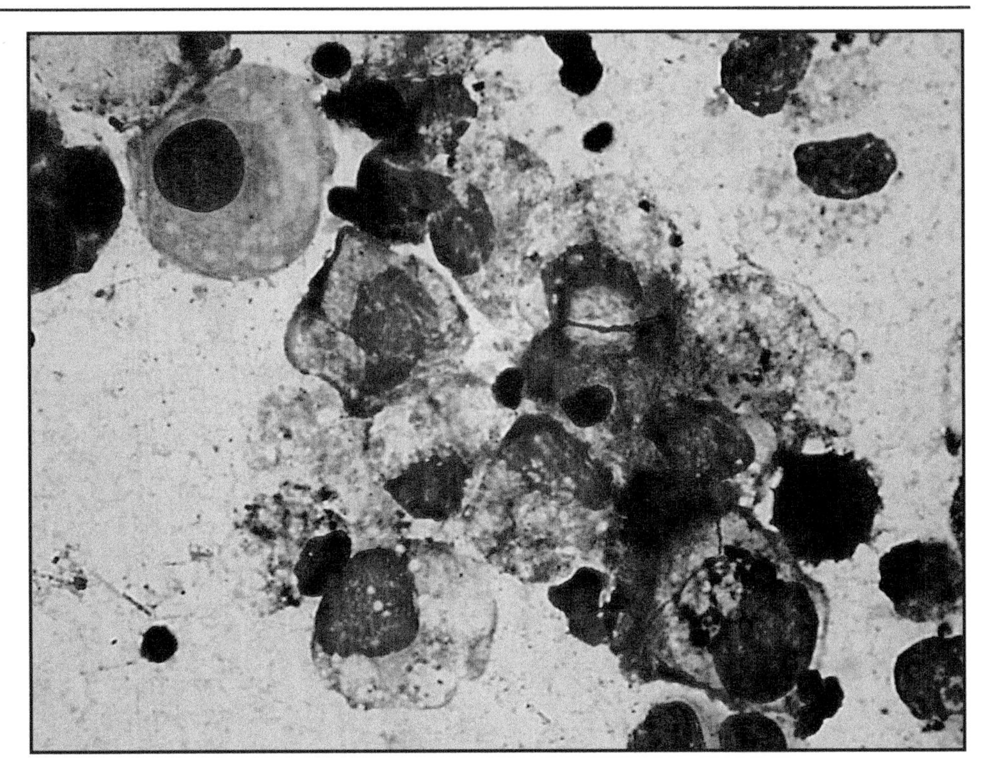

Fig. 3.17. Dog. Pleural effusion. Bilothorax. Macrophages contain dark bile pigment. Needle-like bilirubin crystals are seen in the background. Wright-Giemsa. (*Courtesy of Walter Bertazzolo.*)

Further reading

Bartolini, F., Didier, M., Iudica, B., Torti, E. and Bertazzolo, W. (2015) What is your diagnosis? Pleural effusion in a dog with a gunshot wound. *Veterinary Clinical Pathology* 44(2), 333–334.

Charcoal-induced pleural exudate (lung rupture)

Charcoal extravasation into the pleural cavity is a rare trigger of pleuritis and secondary pleural effusion. It has been described in a dog with inadvertent inhalation of charcoal and subsequent lung rupture.

Clinical features

- Clinical signs are non-specific and relate to the accumulation of fluid in the pleural cavity and inflammation.

Cytological features

- The fluid is variably haemodiluted and turbid.
- The cellularity of the effusion is moderate to high and TP is increased.
- A variable amount of black amorphous material can be found (charcoal).

- Cells are predominantly non-degenerate neutrophils with fewer activated macrophages. Both can contain phagosomes of black-dark amorphous material. A few lymphocytes can also be present. Mesothelial cells can be reactive.

Further reading

Caudill, M.N., Stilwell, J.M., Howerth, E.W. and Garner, B. (2019) Chronic granulomatous pneumonia and lung rupture secondary to aspiration of activated charcoal in a French Bulldog. *Veterinary Clinical Pathology* 48(1), 67–70.

Urothorax

Rare type of inflammatory effusion secondary to accumulation of urine in the pleural space, secondary to the presence of uroabdomen.

Clinical features

- Described in both dogs and cats, but rare.
- Clinical signs relate to the accumulation of fluid in the thoracic cavity and to the electrolyte and acid-base imbalances caused by the extravasation of the urine from the urinary tract.
- In two dogs, the urothorax was caused by blunt trauma leading to bladder rupture. In one of these dogs, the diaphragm appeared intact.
- In one of the two cats reported in literature, the urothorax was secondary to trauma-induced kidney avulsion and rupture of the diaphragm. In the second cat, the urothorax was secondary to bladder rupture, in the absence of trauma or compromised diaphragmatic integrity.
- The pathophysiology of urothorax in patients without diaphragm defects is likely secondary to migration of urine from the abdomen into the pleural space through the pleural lymphatics.

Cytological features

- In three of the cases reported in literature where the type of pleural effusion was classified, it was defined as pure transudate or modified transudate with a variable degree of haemorrhage.
- The effusion contained a high concentration of creatinine, which was higher than the plasma concentration.
- The cellular elements present in the effusions were not described.

Pearls and Pitfalls

A creatinine ratio ($[\text{Creatinine}]_{\text{pleural fluid}}/[\text{Creatinine}]_{\text{plasma}}$) cutoff for urothorax is not reported in veterinary literature. In people, a cutoff >1 is used.

Oesophageal Rupture

Typically caused by ingestion of foreign bodies that penetrate and lacerate the oesophageal wall or could be iatrogenic during endoscopic procedures.

Clinical features

- Depending on the case, pneumothorax, haemothorax or an exudate may develop.
- Clinical signs are non-specific and mostly relate to the accumulation of fluid in the pleural space. They include tachycardia, tachypnea and increased respiratory effort.
- The diagnosis is reached by combining the history, imaging findings and fluid analysis.

Cytological features

- The cytological findings are also non-specific and may include:
  - Septic pyothorax: characterized by high TNCC and TP; prevalence of variably degenerate neutrophils. Intracellular and/or extracellular bacteria may be found. Squamous epithelial cells from the oesophageal mucosa can also exfoliate in the effusion and can be found in the cytological preparations.
  - Haemothorax: heavily haemodiluted sample containing low numbers of macrophages showing erythrophagia, haemosiderophagia and/or containing haematoidin crystals.

3.6.5 Neoplastic pleural effusions (effusions from cell exfoliation)

- Neoplastic effusions can present as either transudates or exudates. There are no specific numerical parameters for neoplastic effusions.
- The absence of tumour cells in the fluid does not exclude an underlying neoplastic process. In literature, a sensitivity of 64% in dogs and 61% in cats is reported for fluid cytology in patients with neoplasia (high numbers of false-negative results). The same study reports a specificity for the diagnosis of neoplasia of 99% and 100%, respectively.
- The tumour cells in thoracic effusions may exfoliate from a local primary or metastatic solid tumour or from multiple small nodular metastases (miliary carcinomatosis).
- In dogs and cats, tumours that most commonly cause neoplastic effusions are carcinoma (dogs) and lymphoma (cats). Sarcomas rarely exfoliate into fluids.
- In this section, only the tumours that have been reported to have exfoliated in the pleural effusions of dogs and cats are described.

Pathophysiology

Intrathoracic neoplasia can cause pleural fluid accumulation following different mechanisms:

- Increased hydrostatic pressure: the tumour may cause venous compression leading to a transudative effusion.
- Compression of the lymphatics: this usually leads to the accumulation of chyle.
- Increased vascular permeability: secondary to the effects of cytokines and vasoactive amines released by the tumour.
- Inflammation associated with the tumour: this usually leads to the formation of an exudate.

Pearls and Pitfalls

- The term 'neoplastic effusion' should only be used to describe effusions when a neoplastic cell population has been identified on fluid cytology.

Further reading

Hirschberger, J., DeNicola, D.B., Hermanns, W. and Kraft, W. (1999) Sensitivity and specificity of cytologic evaluation in the diagnosis of neoplasia in body fluids from dogs and cats. *Veterinary Clinical Pathology* 28(4), 142–146.

Epithelial Tumours

Clinical features

- Effusion caused by carcinomas may be the result of intra-cavitary or extra-cavitary neoplasms.
- Primary epithelial tumours of the thoracic cavity: pulmonary adenocarcinoma, thymoma and ectopic thyroid carcinoma.
- Metastatic epithelial tumours: examples include mammary carcinoma, urothelial carcinoma and prostatic carcinoma.
- Cytologically, it is often difficult to confirm the tissue of origin, although the clinical history and imaging findings may help.

Cytological features

- Cellularity and protein concentration: variable.
- Background: clear to pale basophilic and variably haemodiluted.
- Neoplastic epithelial cells usually exfoliate in cohesive clusters or rafts of cells.
- Acinoid formations may be seen in adenocarcinoma, while squamous differentiation is observed in metastatic squamous cells carcinoma or in primary pulmonary adenosquamous carcinoma.
- The cell morphology depends on the tissue of origin. Cells can be cuboidal, columnar, angular or polygonal.
- Variable degree of anisokaryosis and anisocytosis may be observed and multi-nucleated cells might be present.
- Nuclei are round, variably positioned in the cell and may contain one to multiple, variably sized and shaped prominent nucleoli. The chromatin pattern may be variable.
- The cytoplasm also varies in amount and is often moderately to deeply basophilic. It may contain clear vacuoles.
- Mixed leucocytes are also often present including neutrophils, macrophages and fewer small lymphocytes.

Differential diagnoses

- Mesothelioma
- Reactive and hyperplastic mesothelial cells

Pearls and Pitfalls

- The differentiation between epithelial cells, reactive mesothelial cells and neoplastic mesothelial cells is often challenging. The combination of the morphological findings with the clinical presentation and imaging results may sometimes help in the diagnosis.
- Some sources suggest that at least five strong criteria of malignancy should be present to suspect a malignant process (epithelial or mesothelial), as opposed to a reactive/hyperplastic mesothelial population.
- When neoplasia is suspected but the morphology of the cells is non-specific, immunocytochemistry can be attempted, although has its limitations. Although dual expression of cytokeratin and vimentin has often been used to confirm a mesothelial origin, some epithelial tumours may express the same immunohistochemical pattern (e.g. pulmonary epithelial neoplasms).

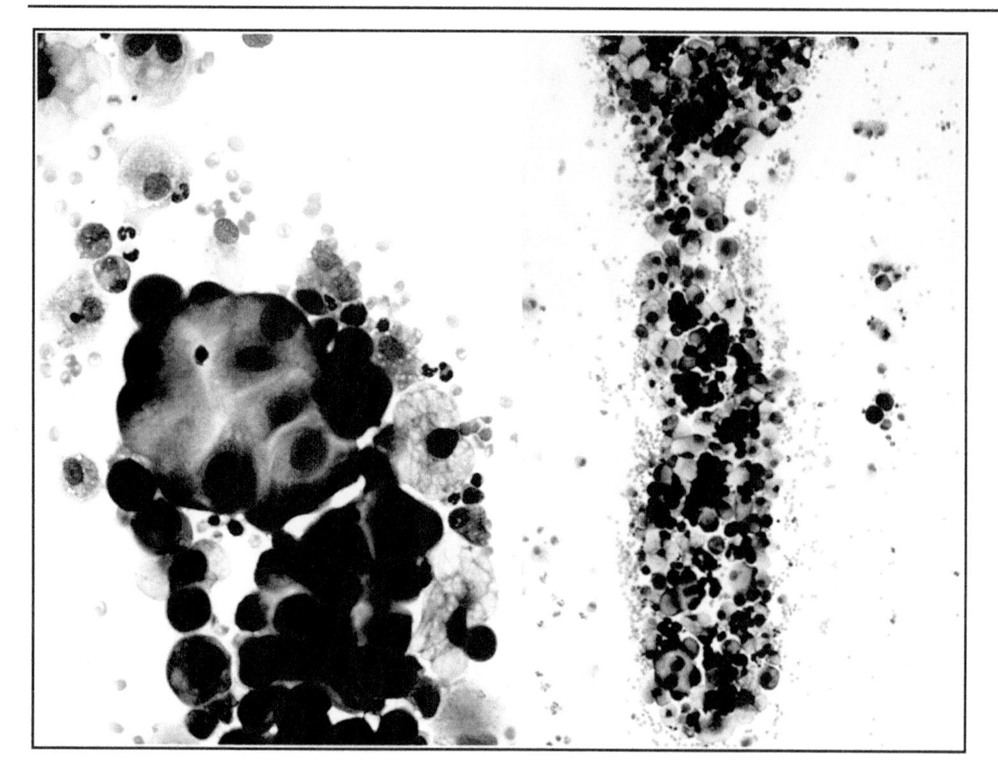

Fig. 3.18. Dog. Pleural effusion. Pulmonary adenocarcinioma. Neoplastic cells have exfoliated in cohesive clusters, low numbers of inflammatory cells are also present. Wright-Giemsa. (*Courtesy Giulia Mangiagalli.*)

Further reading

Stewart, J., Holloway, A., Rasotto, R. and Bowlt, K. (2016) Characterization of primary pulmonary adenosquamous carcinoma-associated pleural effusion. *Veterinary Clinical Pathology* 45(1), 179–183.

Round-Cell Tumours

Lymphoma

Clinical features

- Lymphoma is the most common cause of neoplastic effusion in cats and is often associated with mediastinal (thymic) lymphoma. Lymphomatous pleural effusions caused by mediastinal lymphoma have also been reported in dogs. The most common clinical signs in patients with mediastinal lymphoma include:
    - Dogs: lethargy, anorexia, coughing, dyspnoea/tachypnoea, polyuria/polydipsia (PU/PD) and vomiting. The PU/PD is usually secondary to paraneoplastic hypercalcaemia.
    - Cats: dyspnoea, inappetence, regurgitation, cough and pyrexia.
- Based on data in the literature, pleural effusion is present at time of diagnosis in 45% of dogs with mediastinal lymphoma and in 51% of cats.

Continued

- Age:
  - Dogs: median age of 7.8 years old (range 2.5–12.1 years).
  - Cats: patients with mediastinal lymphoma are usually young (median age: 3 years old, range: 6 months to 12 years). A smaller peak of incidence is noted at 8 years.
- Over-represented breeds:
  - Dogs: medium-large breeds and mixed-breed dogs are more commonly affected.
  - Cats: Domestic Shorthairs and Siamese.
- Cats might be feline leukaemia virus (FeLV) positive.

Cytological features

- Cellularity and protein concentration: variable.
- Background: variably haemodiluted.
- The neoplastic lymphoid cells appear monomorphic.
  - Dogs:
    - Lymphoblastic lymphoma: mediastinal lymphoma in dogs is usually a T-cell lymphoblastic lymphoma. The cells are medium sized with round and eccentric nuclei and often exhibit nuclear membrane irregularities. The chromatin is immature with a smooth/open texture. Nucleoli are often indistinct. The cytoplasm is scant and moderately basophilic. Mitoses are frequent.
    - Large cell lymphoma: mediastinal large cell lymphoma is also more frequently of T-cell origin. Lymphoid cells are large, monomorphic and characterized by having large, round and eccentric nuclei, finely stippled chromatin and often multiple small nucleoli are observed. The cytoplasm is scant to moderate and moderately basophilic. Occasionally, the neoplastic cells could be of the granular cell type. Mitoses are frequent.
  - Cats: in a recent study on flow cytometry of mediastinal masses in cats, the most common immunophenotype of lymphoma was the double positive CD4+ CD8+ T cell lymphoma. In the same study, the neoplastic cells were either small to medium sized or large.

Differential diagnoses

- Lymphocyte-rich effusion (cat) (although in this case cells are small mature lymphocytes).
- Chyle (although in this case cells are mostly small mature lymphocytes).

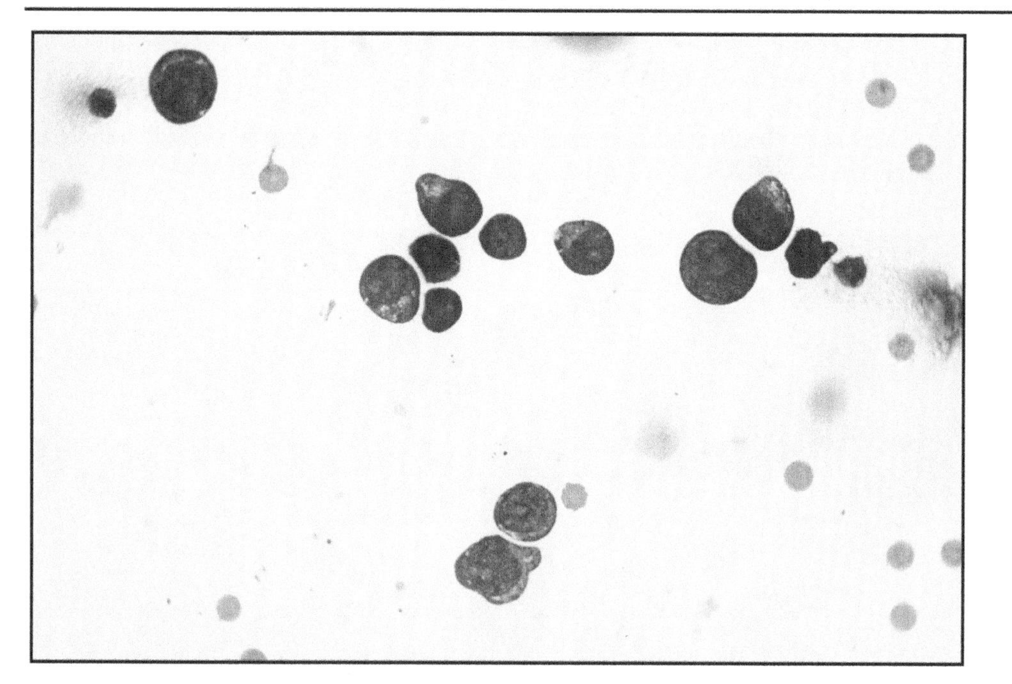

Fig. 3.19. Cat. Pleural effusion. Mediastinal lymphoma with pleural effusion. Predominance of large lymphoid cells. Wright-Giemsa.

Further reading

Bernardi, S., Martini, V., Perfetto, S., Cozzi, M. and Comazzi, S. (2020) Flow cytometric analysis of mediastinal masses in cats: a retrospective study. *Frontiers in Veterinary Science* 7, 444.
Fabrizio, F., Calam, A.E., Dobson, J.M., Middleton, S.A., Murphy, S. *et al.* (2014) Feline mediastinal lymphoma: a retrospective study of signalment, retroviral status, response to chemotherapy and prognostic indicators. *Journal of Feline Medicine and Surgery* 16(8), 637–644.
Moore, E.L., Vernau, W., Rebhun, R.B., Skorupski, K.A. and Burton, J.H. (2018) Patient characteristics, prognostic factors and outcome of dogs with high-grade primary mediastinal lymphoma. *Veterinary Comparative Oncology* 16(1), E45–E51.

Mast cell tumour

Clinical features

- Thoracic mast cell tumours are uncommon but have been reported in dogs and rarely in cats.
- They are most frequently metastases from cutaneous mast cell tumours. Rare forms of visceral mastocytosis have also been described.
- Presumptive primary pulmonary mast cell tumour has been described in two dogs.

Cytological features

- Cellularity and protein concentration: variable.
- Background: variably haemodiluted. It may contain free purple granules.
- The neoplastic mast cells are similar to those observed in other locations. Anisokaryosis and anisocytosis may be variable and multi-nucleated cells may be present or absent. The degree

of granulation is also variable. Cells have round-to-oval nuclei and a moderate amount of cytoplasm containing variable numbers of purple granules.

- Variable numbers of eosinophils may also be present.
- In some cases, the neoplastic mast cell may not be found in the pleural fluid but only an eosinophilic effusion might be present.

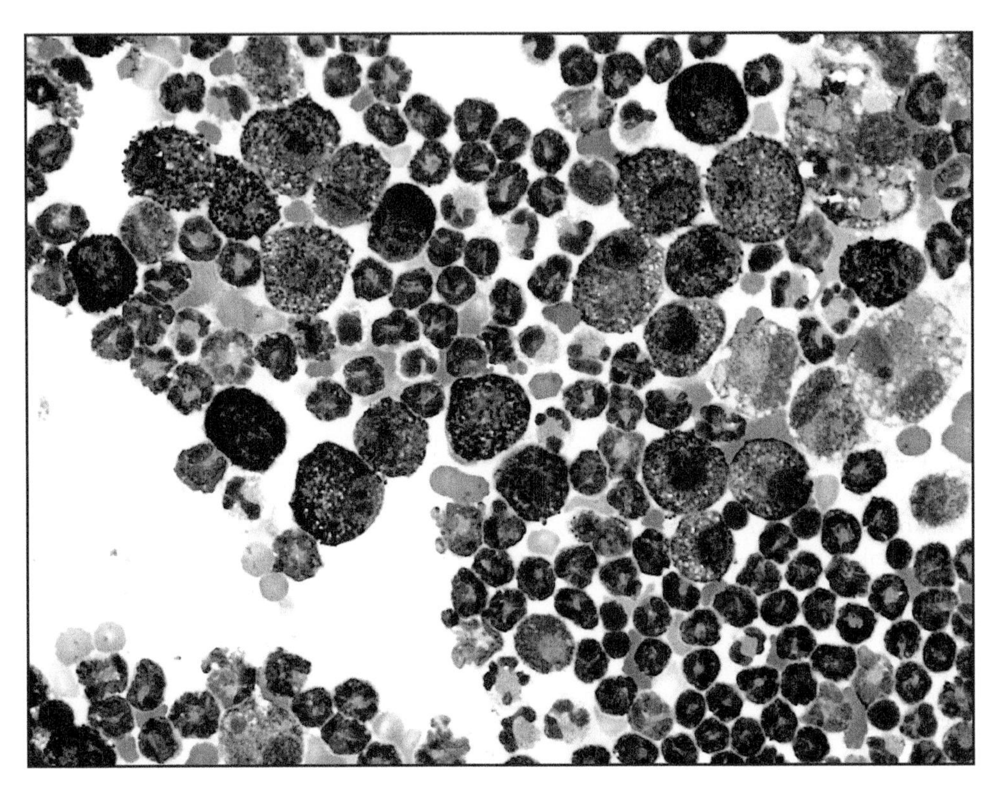

Fig. 3.20. Dog. Pleural effusion. Mast cell tumour. Numerous eosinophils and mast cells are present. Wright-Giemsa.

Further reading

Campbell, O., de Lorimier, L.P., Beauregard, G., Overvelde, S. and Johnson, S. (2017) Presumptive primary pulmonary mast cell tumor in 2 dogs. *Canadian Veterinary Journal* 58(6), 591–596.
Cowgill, E. and Neel, J. (2003) Pleural fluid from a dog with marked eosinophilia. *Veterinary Clinical Pathology* 32(3), 147–149.

Mesenchymal tumours

- Mesenchymal tumours of the thoracic cavity can be primary or metastatic and are rare.
- They can originate from the pulmonary connective tissue. They include osteosarcoma, chondrosarcoma, fibrosarcoma, undifferentiated sarcoma and mesothelioma.
- They can also arise in the mediastinum and reported cases include fibrosarcoma and haemangiosarcoma. In these cases, it is often difficult to understand the exact site and tissue of origin.
- Histiocytic sarcoma in the thoracic cavity can be primary or metastatic. Primary HS arises from the interstitial dendritic cells present in this location.
- Sarcomas in the thoracic cavity may sometimes cause pleural effusion, but the neoplastic cells rarely exfoliate in the fluid.

Cytological features

- Neoplastic cells, if present, are found in low numbers.
- Background: variably haemodiluted.
- Cells can exfoliate individually or in aggregates. Morphological features may be similar to those observed in sarcomas arising in other anatomical locations. Features of atypia vary from mild to prominent. Neoplastic cells can occasionally be associated with a small amount of pink amorphous material.

Melanoma

Thoracic melanomas are uncommon and usually reflect the metastasis of a distant primary mass. They can cause pleural effusion and neoplastic cells can exfoliate in the fluid. In literature, only a few case reports have been published in dogs and cats.

Cytological features

- Cellularity and protein concentration: variable.
- Background: variably haemodiluted. Free melanin granules may be found.
- Neoplastic cells are round to spindle-shaped and can exfoliate singly or in small clusters. They have round-to-oval nuclei with fine chromatin and prominent large nucleoli. The cytoplasm is abundant, basophilic and contains grey-green intracytoplasmic granules of melanin.
- Binucleated cells can be observed, and anisokaryosis and anisocytosis can be prominent.
- Low numbers of neutrophils and macrophages can also present in the effusion. Macrophages can contain phagocytosed melanin pigment (melanophages).

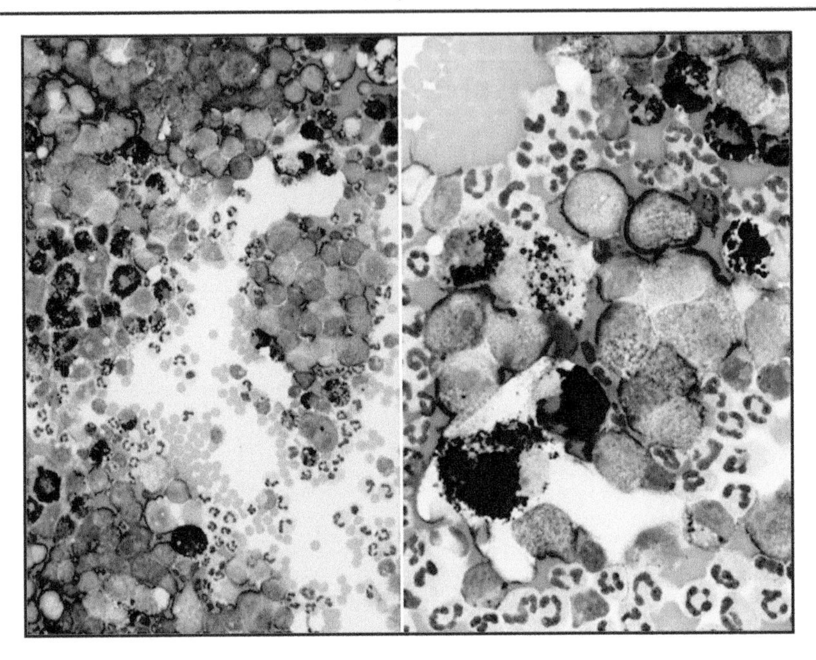

Fig. 3.21. Dog. Pleural effusion. Melanoma, neoplastic cells contain a variable amount of melanin pigment. Wright-Giemsa. (*Courtesy of Erica Corda.*)

Further reading

Corda, E., Vilar Saavedra, P., Berghoff, N., Smedley, R.C. and Thomas, J.S. (2020) Neoplastic melanocytic pleural effusion in a Portuguese water dog. *Veterinary Clinical Pathology* 49(4), 652–654.

Morges, M.A. and Zaks, K. (2011) Malignant melanoma in pleural effusion in a 14-year-old cat. *Journal of Feline Medicine and Surgery* 13(7), 532–535.

Mesothelioma

Mesothelioma is an aggressive neoplasm that arises from the mesothelial cells that line the serosal surface of the body cavities.

Clinical features

- Rare neoplasm more frequently seen in dogs than cats.
- It can present as diffuse or localized thickening of the mesothelium, plaques or discrete nodules.
- The majority of mesotheliomas in the thoracic cavity cause effusion, which could be in the form of haemorrhagic effusion, transudate, exudate or chyle.
- Dogs: effusions can be monocavitary, bicavitary or tricavitary. In a recent study that included 34 dogs, 16 patients had a monocavitary effusion (mostly pleural), 12 dogs had a bicavitary effusion (mostly pleural and pericardial) and 5 dogs had a tricavitary effusion.
- Cats: the majority of the reported feline mesotheliomas affected the thoracic cavity.
- Mesothelial cells can differentiate either into the epithelial-like cells that line the serosal membrane or into the mesenchymal-like cells that form the underlying connective tissue stroma. Similarly, neoplastic mesothelial cells can either have an epithelial-like or mesenchymal-like differentiation. Due to this, mesotheliomas are subclassified as:
  - Epithelioid.
  - Sarcomatous (fibrous).
  - Biphasic (or mixed).

Cytological features

- Cellularity and protein concentration: variable.
- Background: variably haemodiluted.
- Cells can be individualized or in cohesive clusters, often forming variably sized balls. Cell crowding and nuclear moulding may be noticed.
- Cells are most frequently round to slightly polygonal. Occasionally, they can be spindle-shaped, probably reflecting the sarcomatous/fibrous variant.
- Nuclei are generally large, round to oval and often central to paracentral. They can be hyperchromatic, and the chromatin is finely to coarsely stippled. One to multiple, small-to-large, round or irregular shaped, prominent nucleoli may be present.
- The cytoplasm is variable in amount. In some of the cells, it is scant, in others is abundant and may contain one to multiple, small-to-large vacuoles. Fringed margins may be observed.
- Anisokaryosis and anisocytosis are usually prominent and multi-nucleated cells are frequent.

Differential diagnoses

- Carcinoma
- Reactive mesothelial hyperplasia
- Sarcoma (for sarcomatous/fibrous variant)

Pearls and Pitfalls

- Mesotheliomas are challenging to diagnose on cytology (and small biopsies) due to the inherent difficulty in differentiating a neoplastic mesothelial population from an epithelial neoplastic population and reactive mesothelial hyperplasia.
- In people, the presence of non-neoplastic reactive mesothelial cells in lymph nodes has been described in a few patients (defined as nodal mesothelial cell inclusion). All cases had large volumes of cavitary effusion. Also in these patients, the diagnostic dilemma exists.

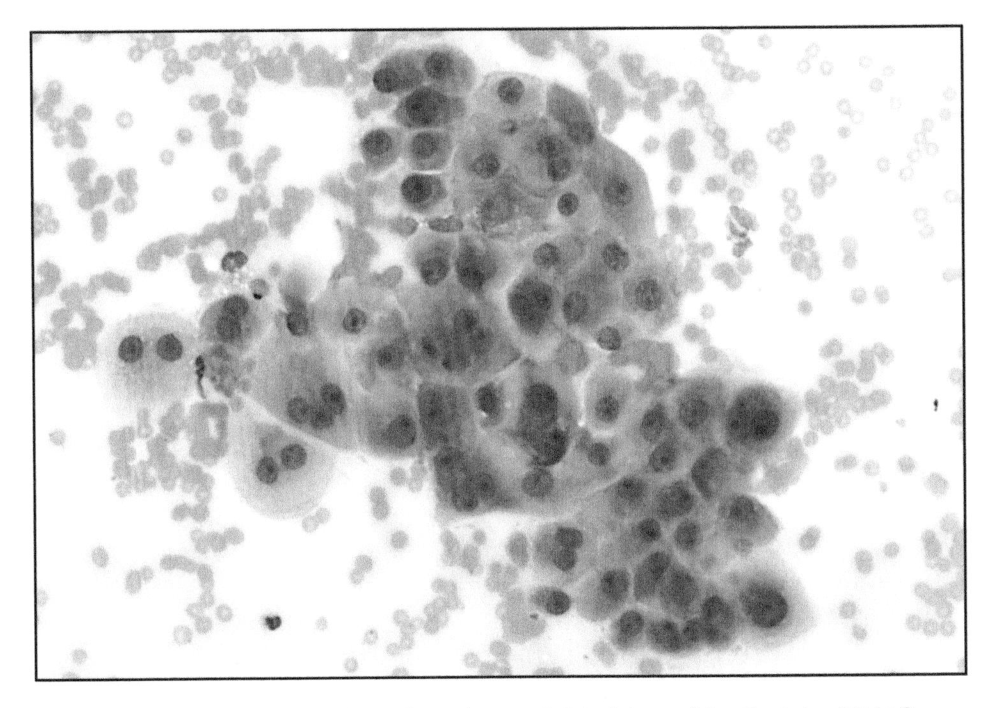

Fig. 3.22. Cat, pleural effusion, mesothelioma. Plemorphic mesothelial cells have exfoliated in clusters. Wright-Giemsa.

Further reading

Bacci, B., Morandi, F., De Meo, M. and Marcato, P.S. (2006) Ten cases of feline mesothelioma: an immunohistochemical and ultrastructural study. *Journal of Comparative Pathology* 134, 347–354.

Moberg, H.L., Gramer, I., Schofield, I., Blackwood, L., Killick, D. *et al.* (2022) Clinical presentation, treatment and outcome of canine malignant mesothelioma: a retrospective study of 34 cases. *Veterinary Comparative Oncology* 20(1), 304–312.

3.6.6 Microbiology testing of pleural fluids (Marta Costa)

Pleural fluids suspected of septic pyothorax should be submitted for aerobic and anaerobic culture. Gram staining could also be considered.

Information regarding the presumed organism(s) inferred from cytology should be provided to the microbiology laboratory because:

- Some organisms may require additional diagnostic tests (e.g. antigen testing or PCR for *Cryptococcus* spp.).
- Special media (e.g. *Mycoplasma* spp.) might be needed.
- Some organisms require prolonged incubation times (e.g. *Actinomyces* spp. or *Nocardia* spp.).

3.6.6.1 Bacteriology

- Septic pyothorax cases are often polymicrobial.
- Dogs and cats: most common organisms recovered from septic pyothorax include mixed anaerobes such as *Prevotella* spp., *Peptostreptococcus* spp., *Propionibacterium acnes*, *Clostridium* spp., *Bacteroides* spp., and *Fusobacterium* spp.
- Dogs: aerobic or facultative anaerobic organisms frequently isolated in dogs include Gram negatives, such as enterobacterales, *Pasteurella* spp., and Gram positive such as *Staphylococcus* spp. and *Streptococcus canis*.
- Cats: *Pasteurella* spp., *Streptococcus* spp. and *Staphylococcus* spp. are the most common organisms recovered from aerobic culture, with other Gram-negative organisms also isolated. Mycoplasmas have also been rarely reported in feline pyothorax.
- *Nocardia* spp., *Actinomyces* spp. and *Rhodocococcus equi* are less commonly recovered. Several other bacteria have been described in few cases.

Actinomyces spp.

- *Actinomyces* spp. infections can be suspected based on cytological findings. However, some morphological overlap can occur with other organisms.
- In some cases, there are large aggregates of organism colonies that can be visible microscopically or even grossly forming white to tan to yellow granules – 'sulfur granules'. Microscopically the organisms are seen as filamentous rods, thin, with varied length and irregular staining leading to a beaded appearance. They are occasionally branched. Other organisms including *Nocardia* spp., some *Corynebacterium* spp. and anaerobes can be confused with *Actinomyces* spp. Actinomycetes are Gram-positive and non-acid-fast filamentous organisms.
- Actinomycosis may be challenging to diagnose and treat, as organisms can be difficult to culture. Short courses of antimicrobials are not effective.
- Most Actinomycetes are facultative anaerobes, but some are obligate anaerobes, so both aerobic and anaerobic cultures are recommended. Some growth can be seen quickly at 48 h, but it may require prolonged incubation (5–7 days or longer). For this reason, if *Actinomyces* spp. are suspected on cytology, it is useful to inform the microbiology laboratory to allow for extended culture. Identification of *Actinomyces* spp. to the species level may be challenging, and some have recently been assigned to a new genus (e.g. *Actinomyces canis* is now *Schaalia canis*). Overgrowth with concurrent bacteria that are less fastidious to grow is also possible.

Nocardia spp.

- *Nocardia* spp. are similar to *Actinomyces* spp. in morphology, with a beaded appearance and branching filamentous bacilli.

- They are also Gram-positive, but contrary to *Actinomyces* spp., have some degree of acid-fast resistance (partially or weak acid-fast bacteria) and may stain positive with modified Ziehl-Neelsen staining (not all strains are acid-fast).
- They are less frequently associated with sulfur granules or other bacteria.
- *Nocardia* spp. infections are less common than *Actinomyces* spp. In humans, they are associated with immunosuppression (e.g. AIDS, autoimmune diseases on long-term treatment with immunosuppressants, transplant patients and haemic neoplasia). Less data are available for dogs and cats but underlying immunosuppression (from disease or therapeutic drugs) also appears to be a predisposing factor.
- Like *Actinomyces* spp., some cases can grow quickly and easily in standard culture, while others may require longer incubation times (weeks), so alerting the microbiology laboratory to allow for longer incubation times is recommended. Definitive differentiation between *Nocardia* spp. and *Actinomyces* spp. requires culture, particularly for the non-acid-fast strains.

Antimicrobial susceptibility testing

- Antimicrobial susceptibility testing (AST) should be used to help guiding the antimicrobial therapy.
- Some organisms have growth characteristics that interfere with routine AST and, in such cases, predicted susceptibilities may be considered (e.g. mixed anaerobes, Mycoplasmas, Actinomyces and Nocardia).
- The use of an antimicrobial drug with activity against anaerobes in the treatment regime of septic pleural effusions should be considered independently of the culture results because of the possibility of:
    - False negatives.
    - Presence of fastidious anaerobic bacteria.
    - High frequency of anaerobic involvement in pyothorax cases either associated with bite wounds and normal oral flora or related to penetrating wounds and foreign bodies.

3.6.6.2 Mycology

- Fungal organisms have been infrequently recovered from pyothorax cases associated with systemic mycosis including *Candida* spp., *Cryptococcus* spp., *Histoplasma* spp., *Aspergillus* spp. and *Blastomyces* spp. but are considered rare.
- If cytologically there is suspicion for *Cryptococcus* spp., *Histoplasma* spp. or *Blastomyces* spp., PCR or antigen testing rather than culture is recommended given the zoonotic risk of culturing these organisms. *Candida* spp. and *Aspergillus* spp. can be grown easily in fungal/yeast culture.

3.7 Peritoneal Effusions

Peritoneal/Abdominal effusions also known as ascites, arise when the net transfer of fluid from the peritoneal capillary bed to the peritoneal cavity occurs at a rate higher than the fluid re-absorption and lymphatic drainage, leading to accumulation of peritoneal fluid.

3.7.1 Pathophysiology

As for pleural effusion, accumulation of peritoneal fluid may occur due to:

- Increased hydrostatic pressure gradient (most commonly portal hypertension [PH]).
- Decreased colloid osmotic pressure (hypoalbuminaemia).
- Increased permeability of the peritoneal capillaries (inflammation).
- Decreased fluid removal by the lymphatic system.

The mechanisms involved in fluid accumulation secondary to reduced oncotic pressure, lymphatic drainage and increased permeability of the vessels are similar to those described in the section on pleural effusions. The pathophysiology of fluid accumulation associated to PH is unique to abdominal cavity and requires further description.

Portal hypertension

The liver receives its blood supply from:

- Portal vein: approximately 75%. This is rich in nutrients and poor in oxygen. This is a low-pressure system.
- Hepatic artery: approximately 25%. This is rich in oxygen and poor in nutrients.

The portal vein and the hepatic artery enter in the liver at the level of the portal triad and mix together in the hepatic sinusoids. After the hepatic cords, the sinusoidal blood drains into the hepatic central vein and exits the liver through the hepatic veins to empty into the caudal vena cava.

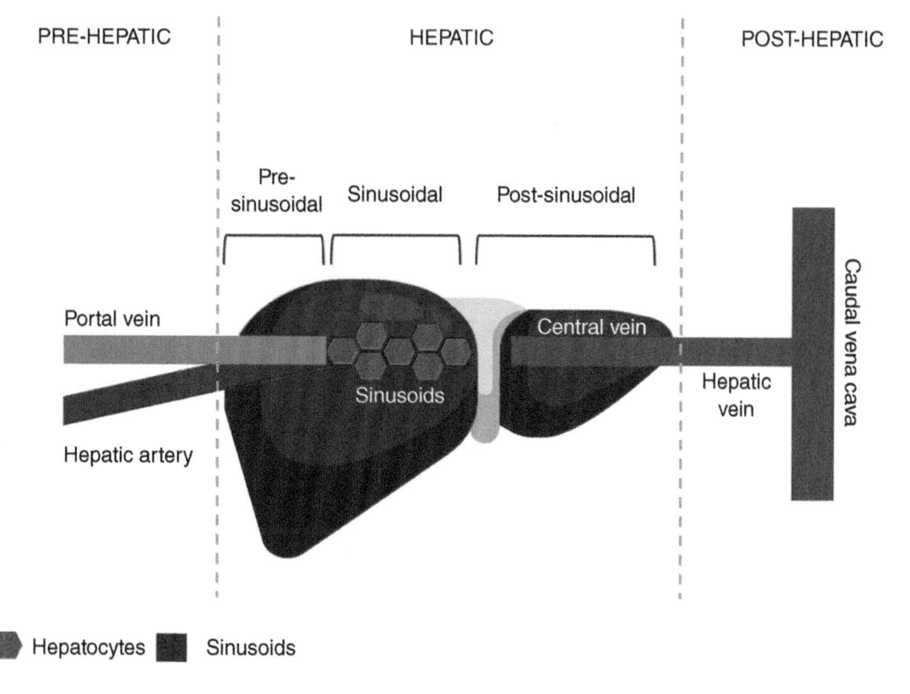

Fig. 3.23. Liver anatomy.

Portal hypertension can be classified into:

- Pre-hepatic: caused by increased resistance in the extra-hepatic portal vein.
- Hepatic: caused by increased resistance in the microscopic portal vein tributaries, sinusoids or small hepatic veins. This can be further subdivided into:
  - Pre-sinusoidal.
  - Sinusoidal.
  - Post-sinusoidal.
- Post-hepatic: caused by increased resistance in the larger hepatic veins, post-hepatic caudal vena cava and right atrium.

Table 3.4. Causes of pre-hepatic PH (Portal vein).

Causes
Congenital portal vein atresia
Intraluminal portal vein obstruction – thrombus – neoplasia – stenosis
Extraluminal obstruction caused by mass effect, e.g.: – neoplasia – mesenteric lymphomegaly – granuloma/abscess

Table 3.5. Causes of intra-hepatic PH (Liver).

Causes
Pre-sinusoidal – primary hypoplasia of portal vein – chronic cholangitis – hepatic arteriovenous fistula – nodular hyperplasia (PH is an uncommon consequence) – schistosomiasis – idiopathic hepatic fibrosis (dog) – canine chronic hepatitis
Sinusoidal – canine chronic hepatitis/cirrhosis – chronic cholangiohepatitis – lobular dissecting hepatitis
Post-sinusoidal – veno-occlusive disease

Table 3.6. Causes of post-hepatic PH (Hepatic veins, caudal vena cava, heart).

Hepatic veins and caudal vena cava intraluminal obstruction
– thrombosis
– vena cava syndrome
– neoplasia
Hepatic veins and caudal vena cava extraluminal obstruction
– Neoplasia
– Kinking of caudal vena cava
Right heart failure
– CHF
– Pericardial tamponade
– Constrictive pericarditis
– Intracardiac neoplasia

During PH, the increased pressure in the portal vein drives fluid in the interstitial space, following the Starling law. When the capacity of lymphatic drainage is overwhelmed, fluid accumulates and ascites forms. Additionally, PH is also associated with splanchnic vasodilation. This causes pooling of blood in the abdomen and subsequent systemic hypovolaemia and hypotension. This triggers compensatory mechanisms, such as increased cardiac output, that are initially able to compensate these haemodynamic imbalances. As the disease progresses, the compensatory mechanisms fail, with eventual activation of the renin-angiotensin-aldosterone system (RAAS), with resultant fluid retention, volume expansion and further increase of the hydrostatic pressure.

Further reading

Buob, S., Johnston, A.N. and Webster, C.R. (2011) Portal hypertension: pathophysiology, diagnosis, and treatment. *Journal of Veterinary Internal Medicine* 25(2), 169–186.

3.7.2 Peritoneal transudates

Peritoneal transudates are a consequence of altered fluid dynamics. They are usually subclassified into protein-poor and protein-rich transudates, depending on the protein concentration of the effusion (refer to Section 3.4).

3.7.2.1 Non-infectious transudates

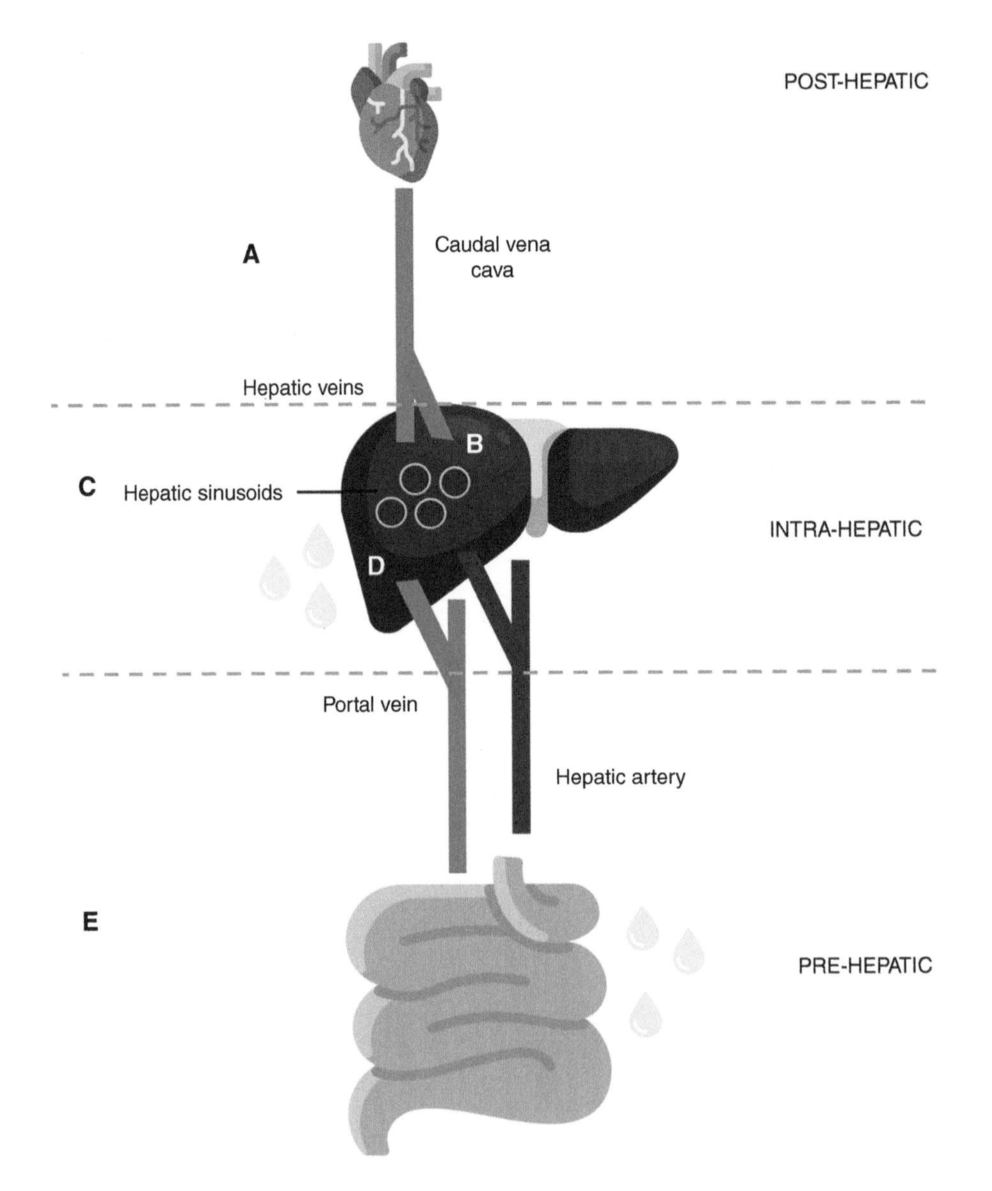

Fig. 3.24. (A, B, C) Post-hepatic, post-sinusoidal and sinusoidal PH. These cause leakage of fluid from the sinusoidal endothelium. The effusion will be poorly cellular and high in protein (protein-rich transudate). However, sinusoidal PH caused by chronic liver disease is often associated with capilarization of the sinusoids and hepatic failure (with hypoalbuminaemia) and the ascites is more commonly poor in protein. (D, E). Pre-sinusoidal and pre-hepatic PH. These will increase intestinal lymph formation but, due to the large absorptive capacity of the intestinal lymphatic system and the tight capillary beds, the ascites will be a protein-poor transudate.

Protein-poor transudate

Also known as *pure transudate*, it is characterized by low cellularity and low-protein concentration.

Clinical features

- It can be associated with a similar pleural effusion.
- Most frequently observed in dogs, less common in cats.

Causes

- Severe hypoalbuminaemia (usually <15 g/l): since there is no change in the endothelial or mesothelial permeability, there is no concurrent cell leakage. Usually associated to:
    - Protein-losing nephropathy (PLN).
    - Protein-losing enteropathy (PLE).
    - Hepatic failure/cirrhosis.
- Increased hydraulic pressure gradient: in patients with PLN and hepatic cirrhosis, there is an altered regulation of the blood volume causing activation of the renin-angiotensin-aldosterone axis. This results in sodium and water retention, leading to increased hydrostatic pressure and consequent transudation.
- Portal hypertension:
    - Pre-hepatic and pre-sinusoidal PH increase the formation of intestinal lymph. Because the intestinal lymphatic system has a large absorptive capacity and tight capillary beds, the effusion typically has a low-protein concentration. This also depends on the fact that portal blood contains lower protein than hepatic sinusoidal blood. Causes of pre-hepatic and pre-sinusoidal PH are illustrated in tables 3.4 and 3.5.
    - In some patients with sinusoidal PH, the transudate could be protein-poor, if a concurrent liver insufficiency and secondary severe hypoalbuminaemia develops.

Cytological features

- Macroscopic appearance: clear and colourless. It can be variably haemodiluted due to iatrogenic haemorrhage during the sampling.
- Background: clear with a variable (usually small) amount of blood.
- Cellularity and TP concentration are low.
- Nucleated cells usually consist of a mixture of segmented neutrophils, monocytoid cells/macrophages and small lymphocytes. Neutrophils are generally non-degenerate although *in vitro* swelling may occur. Low numbers of mesothelial cells may also be present.

Protein-rich transudate

Accumulation in the peritoneal cavity of a hypocellular fluid with high-protein concentration.

Causes

- Sinusoidal, post-sinusoidal and post-hepatic PH: they increase hepatic lymph formation, resulting in loss of a high-protein fluid through the leaky sinusoidal endothelium (sinusoids are more permeable to proteins). They can be secondary to:
    - Cardiovascular disease (post-hepatic PH):
        - CHF.
        - Pericardial tamponade.

        - Constrictive pericarditis.
        - Cardiac neoplasia.
    - Extraluminal obstruction of hepatic veins and vena cava (post-hepatic PH):
        - Neoplasia.
        - Kinking of caudal vena cava.
    - Intraluminal obstruction of hepatic veins and vena cava (post-hepatic PH):
        - Thrombosis.
        - Vena cava syndrome.
        - Neoplasia.
    - Veno-occlusive disease (post-sinusoidal PH).
    - Liver disease (sinusoidal PH): e.g. chronic hepatitis/cholangiohepatitis.

Cytological features

- Macroscopic appearance: clear and colourless. It can be variably haemodiluted due to iatrogenic haemorrhage during the sampling.
- Background: pale basophilic and finely granular. Protein crescents might be observed. It might contain a small amount of blood.
- Cellularity is low, and TP concentration is greater than 20-25 g/l.
- Nucleated cells usually consist of a mixture of segmented neutrophils, monocytoid cells or macrophages and small lymphocytes. Neutrophils are generally non-degenerate although *in vitro* swelling may occur. A few mesothelial cells might be present.

Pearls and Pitfalls

The percentage of neutrophils in an effusion as well as an absolute neutrophil cutoff has a limited diagnostic value in discriminating between transudates and exudates.

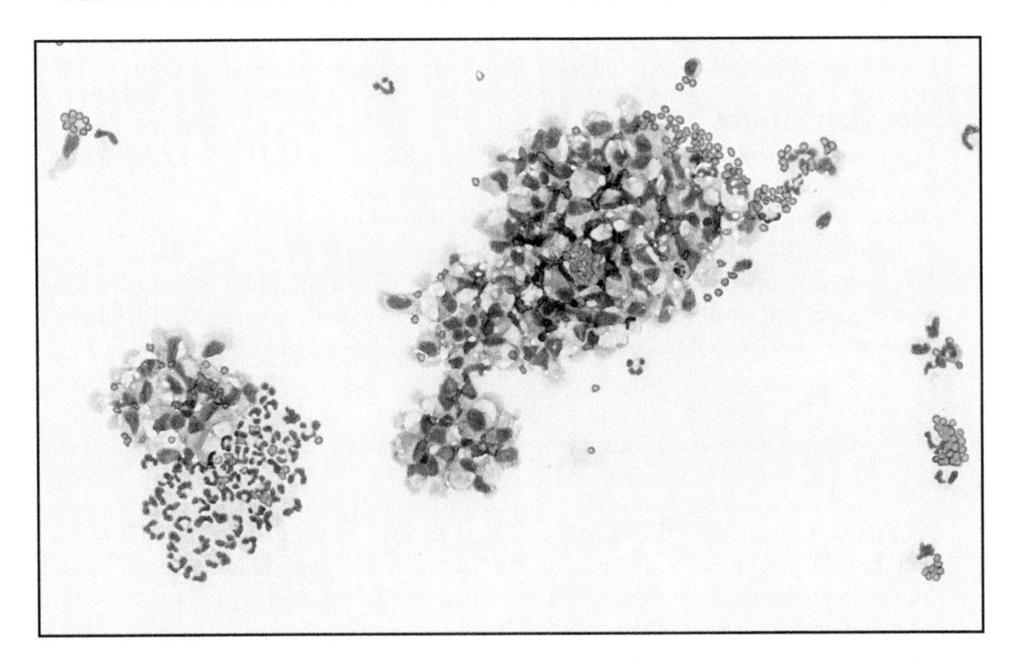

Fig. 3.25. Cat. Abdominal effusion. Protein-rich transudate. Mixture of non-degenerate neutrophils and macrophages. Wright-Giemsa.

Further reading

Buob, S., Johnston, A.N. and Webster, C.R. (2011) Portal hypertension: pathophysiology, diagnosis, and treatment. *Journal of Veterinary Internal Medicine* 25(2), 169–186.

3.7.2.2 Infectious transudates

Feline infectious peritonitis

Fatal disease that occurs in domestic and wild felids worldwide. It is caused by the FIPV, which derives from a mutation of the avirulent feline enteric coronavirus (FCoV).

Clinical features

- Described in Section 3.6.2.2.

Cytological features

- Fluid macroscopic appearance: often clear and yellow, sometimes viscous. It can be mildly haemodiluted due to iatrogenic haemorrhage during the sampling.
- Cellularity is variable (1000–30,000 cells/μl) but generally low. TP is high, often >45 g/l.
- Albumin:globulin ratio (A:G): low. A:G values above 0.8 almost certainly exclude FIP. Effusions with TP > 35 g/l, A:G < 0.45 and low TCC are highly predictive of FIP.
- Background: pale to moderately basophilic and granular and often containing numerous protein crescents.
- Nucleated cells consist of a mixture of non-degenerate, neutrophils, monocytes/macrophages and small lymphocytes.
- Additional testing:
  - Immunostaining of FCoV antigen: detection of a large amount of viral antigen within macrophages (cytology or histopathology samples) indicates high viral replication in these cells and is highly specific and is considered the gold standard for the diagnosis of FIP. Negative results do not exclude the disease. In particular, the sensitivity of FCoV immunostaining in the effusions is reported to vary between 57% and 100%.
  - Fluid FCoV PCR: this may be used to confirm FCoV as the underlying cause of the clinical signs. However, less virulent FCoV can occasionally spread systemically in cats without FIP. Therefore, this test is not necessarily specific for a diagnosis of FIP, although it is highly sensitive. Detection of higher viral loads by real time RT-qPCR increases the probability of FIP.
  - Alpha-1 acid glycoprotein: it has been identified as the best acute phase protein to distinguish between cats with and without FIP. One study reported that the AGP level was high in FIP effusions (>1.55 mg/ml), with a sensitivity and specificity of 93%.
  - Rivalta test: not so commonly used any more. This test is highly sensitive but poorly specific.
  - Usually, an antemortem diagnosis requires a combination of multiple test results that support the diagnosis of FIP.
  - Histopathology: this is considered the gold standard to confirm FIP, often in association with immunohistochemistry to confirm the presence of the virus in the lesion.

Differential diagnoses

- Cardiovascular disease.
- Non-exfoliating neoplasia.

Further reading

Kennedy, M. (2020) Feline infectious peritonitis update on pathogenesis, diagnostics, and treatment. *Veterinary Clinics of North America: Small Animal Practice* 50, 1001–1011.
Taske, S. (2018) Diagnosis of feline infectious peritonitis: update on evidence supporting available tests. *Journal of Feline Medicine and Surgery* 20, 228–243.
Thayer, V., Gogolski, S., Felten, S., Hartmann, K., Kennedy, M. *et al.* (2022) 2022 AAFP/EveryCat feline infectious peritonitis diagnosis guidelines. *Journal of Feline Medicine and Surgery* 24(9), 905–933.

Bacterial peritonitis

- Most typically, bacterial peritonitis is associated with an exudative effusion. However, in a few cases of primary and secondary bacterial peritonitis, the cellularity of the ascites can be low, in the range of a transudate.
- In a study on bacterial peritonitis in dogs and cats, some of the effusions had a TNCC as low as 1570 cell/µl in primary peritonitis and 800 cells/µl in secondary peritonitis.
- The mean protein concentration was high (31 g/l and 35 g/l, respectively).

Cytological features

- The cellularity is low, and the protein concentration can be variable.
- Low numbers of neutrophils and macrophages are seen. Neutrophils may be non-degenerate or display karyolysis.
- Bacteria are usually seen in low numbers within the neutrophils.

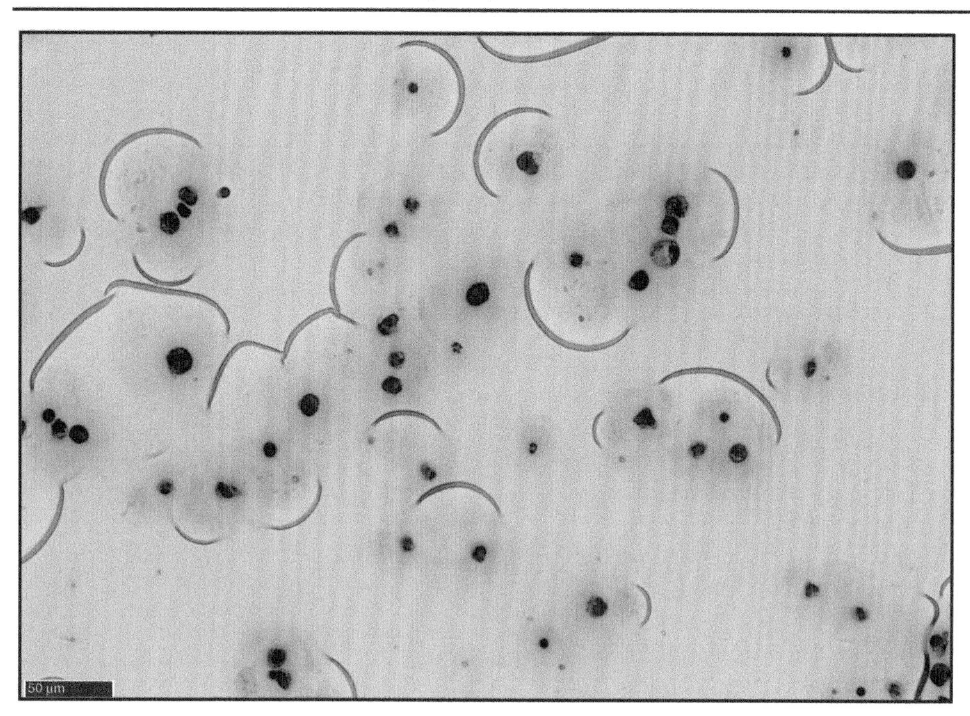

Fig. 3.26. Cat. Abdominal effusion. FIP. The background is basophilic and contains protein crescents. Mixed, often condensed leucocytes are present. Wright-Giemsa.

Further reading

Culp, W.T., Zeldis, T.E., Reese, M.S. and Drobatz, K.J. (2009) Primary bacterial peritonitis in dogs and cats: 24 cases (1990–2006). *Journal of American Veterinary Medical Association* 234(7), 906–913.

3.7.3 Peritoneal exudates

Exudates are the result of increased vascular permeability and inflammation. As for the pleural cavity, abdominal exudative effusions can be caused by:

- Exogenous substances: e.g. bacteria, fungi and foreign bodies.
- Endogenous substances: e.g. urine, bile and cystic content. Peritonitis caused by endogenous irritants is also called *chemical* peritonitis.

It is important to remember that the absence of infectious agents on cytological examination does not exclude an underlying infection.

Pathophysiology

- Increased capillary permeability secondary to endothelial cell contraction and injury. This allows proteins, cells and macromolecules to exit into the peritoneal space.
- Increased hydrostatic pressure secondary to hyperaemia (increased blood flow).
- Reduced lymphatic drainage.
- Increased oncotic pressure within the peritoneal space secondary to the accumulation of proteins within the ascitic fluid.

3.7.3.1 Non-infectious exudates

Neutrophilic and mixed exudates

Causes

- Sterile irritants such as urine, bile and cystic content (see Section 3.7.4).
- Extension of an inflammatory process from inflamed intraabdominal organs or structures.
- Pancreatic secretions.
- Uncomplicated intra-abdominal surgery: in a study performed in dogs subject to experimental celiotomy, the highest TNCC of the peritoneal fluid was observed on days 3 and 4 post-surgery.
- Neoplasia.
- Long-standing protein-rich transudates.

Cytological features

- The cellularity is variably high, and TP is increased.
- Background: variably haemodiluted and clear to pale basophilic. Exogenous or endogenous material can be found, depending on the underlying cause.
- The majority of the cells are non-degenerate neutrophils. Lower numbers of monocytoid cells/macrophages, small lymphocytes and reactive mesothelial cells are seen.

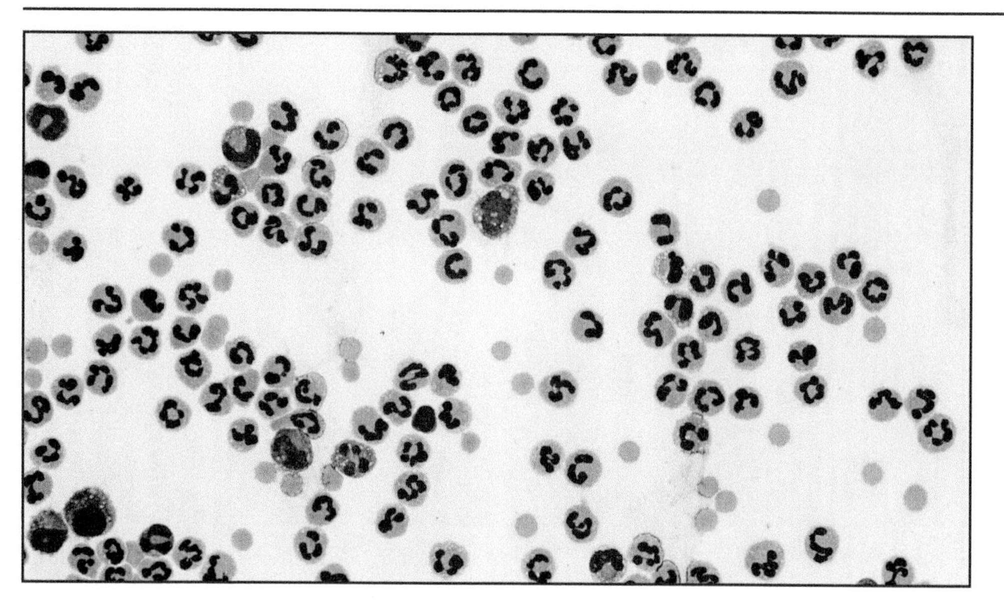

Fig. 3.27. Dog. Abdominal effusion. Non septic neutrophilic exudate. Predominance of non-degenerate neutrophils. Wright-Giemsa.

Eosinophilic exudates

Causes

- Systemic mastocytosis and mast cell tumour.
- T-cell lymphoma.
- Feline eosinophilic gastrointestinal sclerosing fibroplasia (FGESF).

Cytological features

- The cellularity is variably high. TP may be either low or high.
- Background: variably haemodiluted.
- A percentage of eosinophils ≥10% is usually required to define an exudate as eosinophilic or mixed eosinophilic. Other inflammatory cells such as neutrophils, monocytoid cells/ macrophages and lymphocytes may be found in variable numbers.

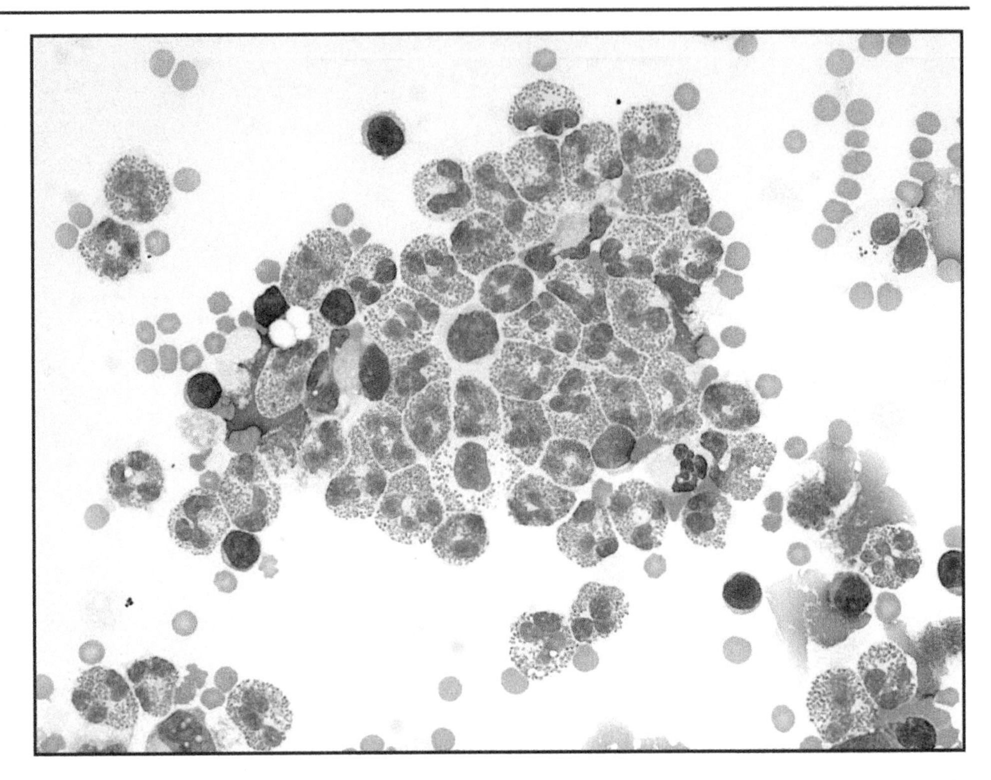

Fig. 3.28. Cat. Abdominal effusion. Feline eosinophilic gastrointestinal sclerosing fibroplasia. The majority of the nucleated cells are eosinophils. Wright-Giemsa.

Pancreatitis-associated effusions

Cytological features

- Effusions caused by acute pancreatitis could fall in the category of either a protein-rich transudate or an exudate.
- The cellularity is variable, and the protein concentration is usually increased.
- The background could be clear to pale basophilic and mildly haemodiluted.
- The majority of the cells are generally non degenerate neutrophils with variable numbers of monocytoid cells/macrophages. Low numbers of small lymphocytes might be present.
- Infectious agents are usually not present, and the effusion is sterile.
- Measurement of the fluid lipase can be used to help in the diagnosis of pancreatitis, alongside the clinical presentation, imaging results and haematology and biochemistry findings.
- In dogs, peritoneal fluid lipase measured by pancreas-specific lipase immunoreactivity (cPLI) assay showed a sensitivity of 100% and specificity of 94.7% for the diagnosis of acute pancreatitis when a cutoff value of 500 μg/l was used.

Further reading

Chartier, M.A., Hill, S.L., Sunico, S., Suchodolski, J.S., Robertson, J.E. *et al.* (2014) Pancreas-specific lipase concentrations and amylase and lipase activities in the peritoneal fluid of dogs with suspected pancreatitis. *Veterinary Journal* 201(3), 385–389.

3.7.3.2 Infectious exudates

Infectious agents that can cause peritoneal exudate include bacteria, fungi/yeasts, protozoa and parasites.

Bacterial peritonitis (septic neutrophilic peritonitis)

This is an inflammation of the peritoneal cavity caused by bacteria and is usually characterized by a marked neutrophilic inflammatory response.

Clinical features

- Commonly seen in both dogs and cats.
- It can be generalized or localized. In localized forms, only a small portion of the peritoneum is involved.
- Bacterial peritonitis can be classified as:
  - Primary: infection of the peritoneal cavity with no identifiable intraperitoneal source of infection or history of a penetrating wound in the abdominal cavity. The term 'spontaneous bacterial peritonitis' is sometime used as a synonym. Primary bacterial peritonitis is uncommon but reported in both dogs and cats.
  - Secondary: most common form of septic peritonitis. It can be caused by leakage into the peritoneal cavity of bacteria, most frequently from the gastroenteric tract.
  - Tertiary: persistent or recurrent peritonitis after previous treatment of a primary or secondary peritonitis.
- Clinical signs are non-specific and may include lethargy, vomiting, anorexia, diarrhoea, tachypnoea, depression, abdominal discomfort, dehydration and fever.

Causes of secondary septic peritonitis

- Leakage from the GI tract
  - Bacterial translocation through the intestinal wall (e.g. during GI lymphoma).
  - Perforating foreign body.
  - Perforating ulcer.
  - Intestinal ischaemia.
  - Rupture of the gastric wall (e.g. gastric dilation-volvulus).
  - Iatrogenic.
- Urogenital
  - Ruptured prostatic abscess.
  - Ruptured pyometra.
  - Ruptured bladder with urinary tract infection.
- Pancreatic abscess.
- Splenic abscess, torsion.
- Liver abscess, hepatitis or ruptured gallbladder with biliary infection.
- Iatrogenic.

Cytological features

- The cellularity and protein concentration are usually high. One study found that a TNCC > 13,000 cells/μL was 100% specific for septic peritonitis (as opposed to non-septic peritonitis) in 18 dogs and 12 cats.
- Background: often pale basophilic and finely granular. Variably haemodiluted.
- The majority of the cells are neutrophils, which often show variable degree of degeneration (karyolysis). Absence of signs of degeneration does not exclude an underlying bacterial infection. Low numbers of macrophages and a few lymphocytes and reactive mesothelial cells may also be found.

- Bacteria can be seen either free in the background or phagocytosed by the neutrophils. When deriving from the GI tract, they are often mixed and most frequently bacilli. Absence of bacteria does not exclude septic peritonitis.
- Further testing:
  - Culture and sensitivity.
  - Blood and peritoneal fluid glucose: in a study performed on 18 dogs and 12 cats, $glucose_{blood}$ > 20 mg/l more than $glucose_{fluid}$ resulted 100% specificity for a septic process in dogs and cats and 100% and 86% sensitivity in dogs and cats, respectively.
  - Peritoneal fluid lactate: in a study, all dogs with septic effusions had a peritoneal fluid lactate concentration >2.5 mmol/l, a peritoneal fluid lactate concentration higher than blood lactate and a negative blood to fluid lactate difference. In the same study, the peritoneal fluid lactate concentration and blood to fluid lactate difference were not accurate tests for detecting septic peritoneal effusions in cats.

Pearls and Pitfalls

- The use of a glucometer is not indicated for the measurement of glucose in pleural or peritoneal fluids. Glucometeres are usually validated for whole blood, serum and/or plasma and results of whole blood analysis are affected by the haematocrit of the sample.

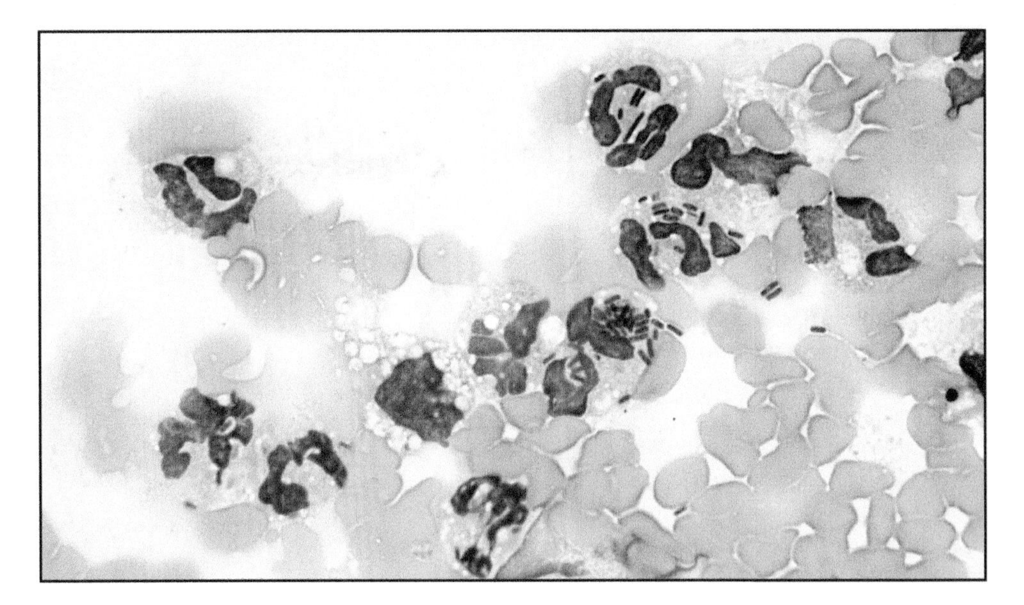

Fig. 3.29. Dog. Abdominal effusion. Septic neutrophilic peritonitis. Neutrophils contain phagocytosed rods. Wright-Giemsa.

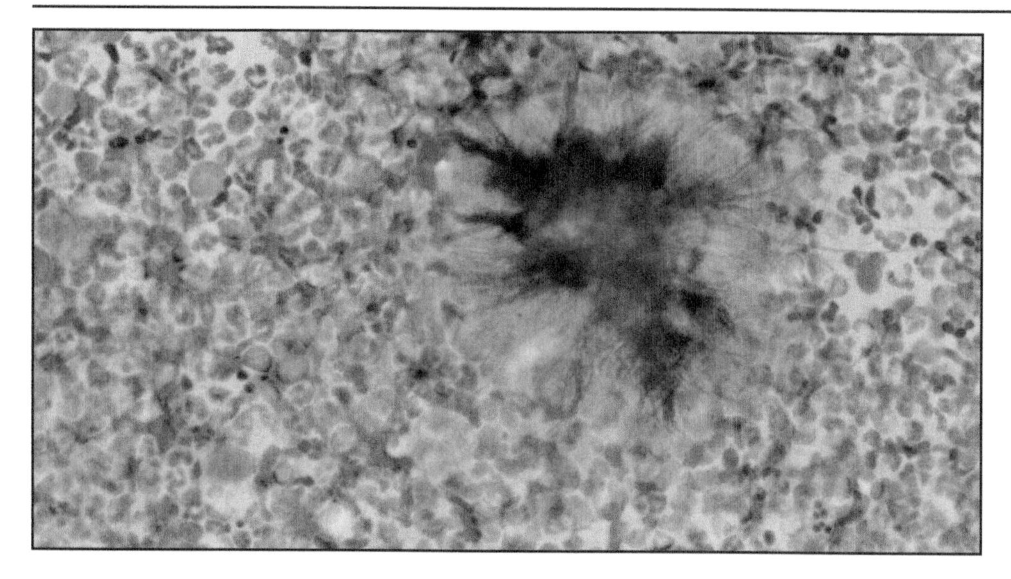

Fig. 3.30. Dog. Abdominal effusion. Septic neutrophilic peritonitis caused by *Actinomyces* spp. Wright-Giemsa. (*Courtesy of Marta Costa.*)

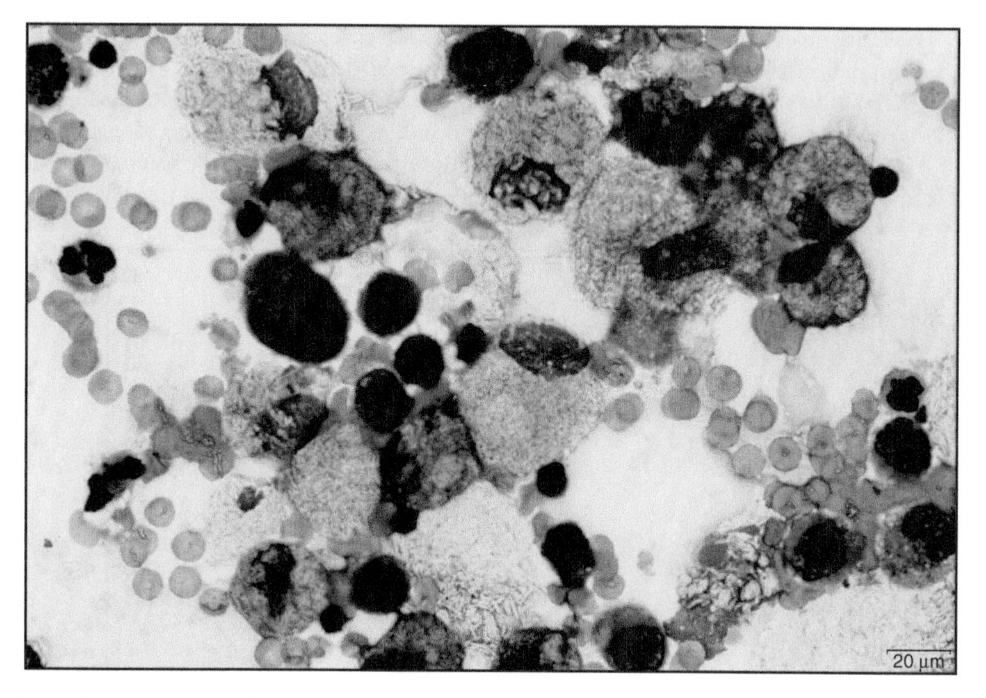

Fig. 3.31. Cat. Abdominal effusion. Macrophagic inflammation caused by *Mycobacterium* spp. The macrophages contain numerous negatively stained bacilli. Wright-Giemsa. (*Courtesy of Candice Pei-Hua Chu, University of Pennsylvania.*)

Further reading

Bonczynski, J.J., Ludwig, L.L., Barton, L.J., Loar, A. and Peterson, M.E. (2003) Comparison of peritoneal fluid and peripheral blood pH, bicarbonate, glucose, and lactate concentration as a diagnostic tool for septic peritonitis in dogs and cats. *Veterinary Surgery* 32(2), 161–166.

Levin, G.M., Bonczynski, J.J., Ludwig, L.L., Barton, L.J. and Loar, A.S. (2004) Lactate as a diagnostic test for septic peritoneal effusions in dogs and cats. *Journal or American Animal Hospital Association* 40(5), 364–371.

Peritoneal larval cestodiasis

Parasitic infestation of the canine peritoneal cavity caused by *Mesocestoides* spp. and *Echinococcus* spp.

Clinical presentation

Clinical features

- The adult tapeworms usually reside in the small intestinal lumen, but the larvae can occasionally penetrate the intestinal wall and invade the abdominal cavity causing peritonitis. The clinical signs are non-specific and can vary from asymptomatic to very severe and life threatening. They include abdominal distension, lethargy, anorexia, vomiting, PU/PD, etc.

Cytological features

- Fluid macroscopic appearance: often serous-haemorrhagic. It may contain small white particles. It has sometimes been described as similar to a cream of wheat or tapioca pudding.
- The cellularity and protein concentration are usually high.
- Background: clear or pale basophilic and haemodiluted and can contain the organism, intact or in fragments.
- Cells are predominantly neutrophils with lower numbers of macrophages, small lymphocytes and eosinophils. Neutrophils are generally are non-degenerate.
- The parasites stain homogenously pink to deeply basophilic and can contain variable numbers of clear to yellow, round, irregularly shaped or ovoid, refractile structures, occasionally with concentric rings. These represent calcareous corpuscles, which are specifically found in cestode stromal tissue. When the organisms are intact, four suckers may be observed (tetrathyridia).

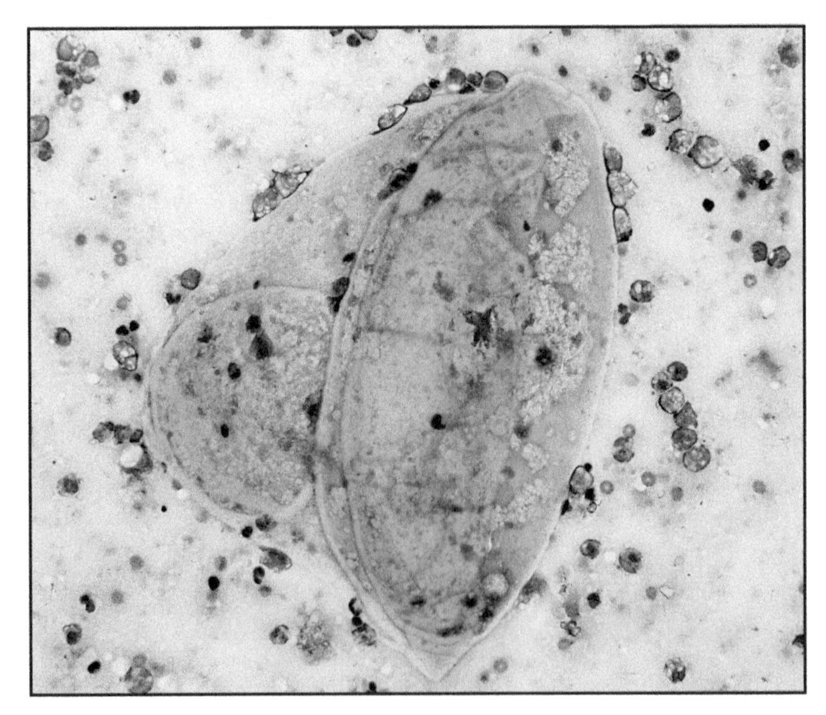

Fig. 3.32. Dog. Abdominal effusion. Cestodiasis caused by *Echinococcus* spp. Basophilic membrane-like folded structures are seen among mixed inflammatory cells. Wright-Giemsa. (*Courtesy of Erica Corda.*)

Further reading

Carta, S., Corda, A., Tamponi, C., Dessì, G., Nonnis, F. *et al.* (2021) Clinical forms of peritoneal larval cestodiasis by *Mesocestoides* spp. in dogs: diagnosis, treatment and long term follow-up. *Parasitology Research* 120(5), 1727–1735.

Caruso, K.J., James, M.P., Fisher, D., Paulson, R.L. and Christopher, M.M. (2003) Cytologic diagnosis of peritoneal cestodiasis in dogs caused by *Mesocestoides* sp. *Veterinary Clinical Pathology* 32(2), 50–60.

Yeast and fungi peritonitis

Different fungi and yeasts are reported to occasionally cause-peritonitis in dogs and cats.

Cytological features

- Depending on the infectious agent involved and the host response, the effusion could fall in the category of a transudate (protein-rich or protein-poor) or exudate. Most frequently, the effusion is an exudate.
- Cellularity and protein concentration can be variable.
- Background: clear or pale basophilic and variably haemodiluted. It may contain free organisms.
- In most of the cases, a mixed neutrophilic inflammation is observed. Neutrophils could be non-degenerate or show signs of degeneration with variable degree of karyolysis. Macrophages are also often present. They may have abundant and vacuolated cytoplasm and contain small phagosomes. They can also contain phagocytosed infectious agents.
- The cytomorphology of the organisms depends on the type of yeast and fungal infection:
    - *Histoplasma* spp.: small, round-to-oval organisms measuring approximately 2–5 µm. They are pale basophilic yeasts surrounded by a thin clear capsule. Usually found within macrophages.
    - *Blastomyces dermatitidis*: the yeasts are round, basophilic and measure between 6 µm and 15 µm. They have a thick, clear and distinct capsule and show broad-based buddings.
    - *Coccidioides immitis*: the organisms are large, from 20 µm to 200 µm. They are spherules with a thick refractile wall and granular basophilic protoplasm or multiple internal endospores (approximately 2–5 µm).
    - *Candida albicans*: round-to-oval basophilic structures of approximately 3–8 µm. They may show narrow-base budding. They can also form hyphae and pseudohyphae.
- Initial identification can be attempted on morphology, but ultimately culture and/or PCR would be required for definitive diagnosis.

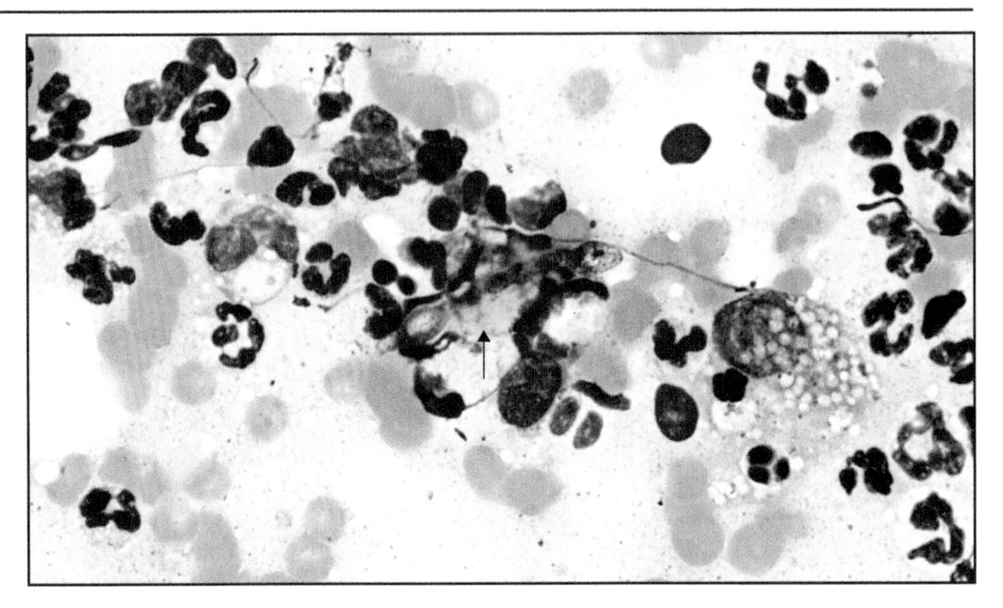

Fig. 3.33. Dog, abdominal effusion, fungal peritonitis. Hyphae present in between mixed inflammatory cells. Wright-Giemsa.

Pearls and Pitfalls

Candida spp. is a commensal of the GI tract in dogs and cats. Peritonitis secondary to this yeast has only occasionally been reported and, in a recent study, all dogs had a history of antimicrobial administration coupled with either intestinal or biliary surgery or intestinal ulceration and perforation secondary to the administration of non-steroidal anti-inflammatory drugs.

Further reading

Bradford, K., Meinkoth, J., McKeirnen, K. and Love, B. (2013) Candida peritonitis in dogs: report of 5 cases. *Veterinary Clinical Pathology* 42(2), 227–233.

Protozoa peritonitis

Rarely, protozoal infections (*Toxoplasma* spp., *Neospora* spp. and *Sarcocystis* spp.) can cause peritoneal exudates.

Cytological features

- The cellularity and protein concentration are variably high.
- Inflammatory cells include neutrophils and macrophages mostly. In some cases, an eosinophilic response may be elicited.
- The organisms are usually crescent- or banana-shaped with a small purple nucleus and clear or pale basophilic cytoplasm. They can be found free in the background or phagocytosed by the macrophages.
- Accurate speciation requires PCR.

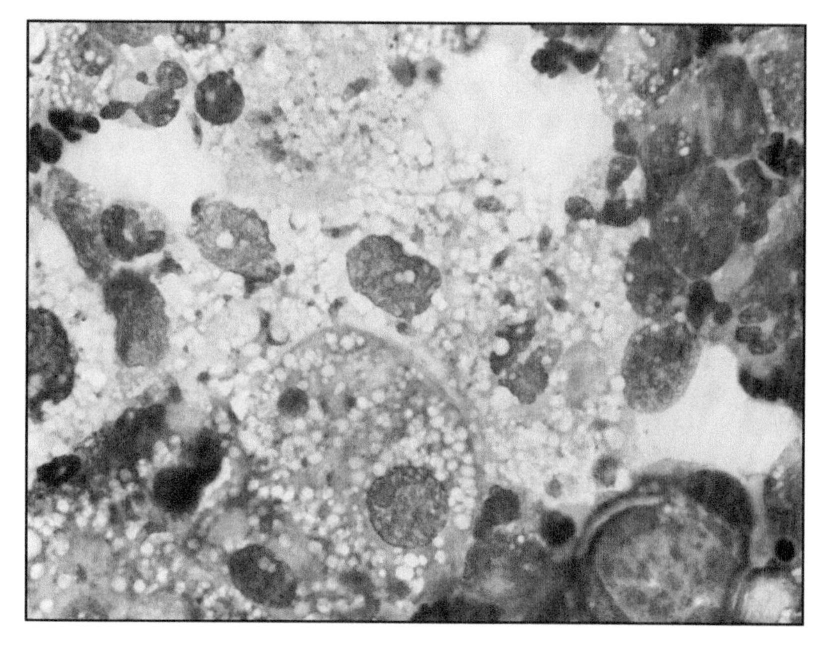

Fig. 3.34 Cat. Peritoneal effusion. Numerous tachyzoites are seen in the background and within macrophages. Wright-Giemsa. (*Courtesy of Lucia Sanchini.*)

3.7.4 Peritoneal Effusions from ruptured or leaky vessels or organs

Haemoabdomen

Haemorrhagic extravasation into the peritoneal space due to ruptured blood vessels.

Clinical features

- Clinical signs are non-specific and of varying severity. They may vary from mild signs of episodic weakness to severe signs of unconsciousness and shock.
- In case of compensated hypovolemic shock, mild tachycardia might be observed. In uncompensated and more severe cases, significant tachycardia, hypotension, pallor, prolonged capillary refill time and hypotension can be seen. Abdominal distension and abdominal thrill may be present.

Causes

In dogs and cats, haemoperitoneum can be classified as:

- Traumatic: e.g. motor vehicle accident, high-rise falls, penetrating wounds and gunshots.
- Non-traumatic:
  - Haemorrhagic neoplasia: up to 87% in dogs and 60% in cats. Examples of tumours that have been associated with haemoperitoneum include:
    - Haemangiosarcoma (up to 76% in dogs and 60% in cats)
    - Adrenal neoplasia
    - Lymphoma
    - Hepato-biliary tumours (cats)
    - Myelolipoma (cats)
  - Rupture of non-neoplastic masses: e.g. splenic haematoma.
  - Liver rupture due to amyloidosis.
  - Coagulopathy: e.g. ingestion of rodenticides and inherited factor deficiency.
  - Torsion of an organ: e.g. gastric dilation-volvulus, splenic torsion, liver torsion.
  - Anaphylaxis: haemoperitoneum has been described in some patients with anaphylactic reactions. However, the exact mechanism remains to be fully understood.

Cytological features

- Macroscopic appearance of the fluid: frank blood to serosanguineous fluid. Depending on the duration of the effusion, the supernatant can be clear (acute) or xanthochromatic (chronic).
- In acute forms, the cellularity and protein concentration are very similar to the peripheral WBC count and TP. In more chronic effusions, these decrease secondary to a dilutional effect.
- In veterinary literature, there are no standardized criteria to classify an effusion as haemoabdomen. As a guideline, a haematocrit (HCT) >25% of the peripheral haematocrit is considered consistent with haemoperitoneum. In several books, a cutoff >3% is indicated to suggest that a haemorrhagic process has occurred. However, in cases with such a low HCT, the haemorrhage often is not the primary cause of the effusion.
- Cytology samples contain numerous erythrocytes and mixed blood-derived leucocytes. In very early stages, platelets may also be observed (usually in sample collected not later than 1 h from the blood extravasation). In acute forms, signs of active red blood cell degradation are not found.

- In more chronic forms, macrophages and reactive mesothelial cells are frequently present. Macrophages usually have abundant and foamy cytoplasm and may contain products of red blood cell degradation (haemosiderin and haematoidin crystals) or display erythrophagia. Mesothelial cells can be found singly or in clusters, can be mononucleated to bi-/multi-nucleated and often have the characteristic fringed outlines.
- In haemoabdomen caused by haemorrhagic neoplasia, tumour cells are infrequently encountered on cytology.

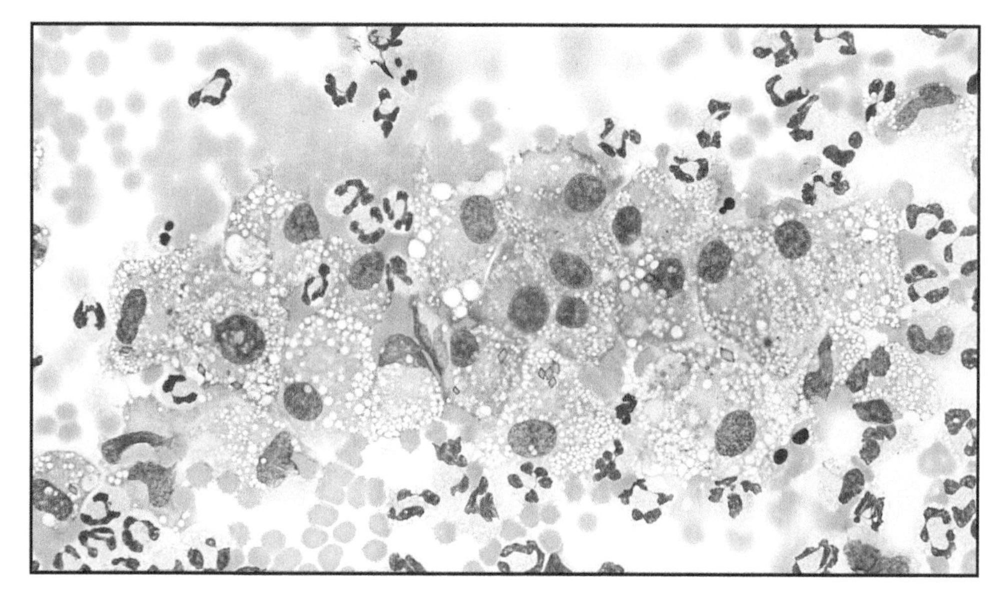

Fig. 3.35. Dog. Abdominal effusion. Haemoabdomen. In a haemic background, neutrophils containing haematoidin crystals are seen. Wright-Giemsa.

Further reading

Brockman, D.J., Mongil, C.M., Aronson, L.R. and Brown, D.C. (2000) A practical approach to hemoperitoneum in the dog and cat. *Veterinary Clinics of North America: Small Animal Practice* 30(3), 657–668.
Culp, W.T., Weisse, C., Kellogg, M.E., Gordon, I.K., Clarke, D.L. *et al.* (2010) Spontaneous hemoperitoneum in cats: 65 cases (1994–2006). *Journal of American Veterinary Medical Association* 236(9), 978–982.
Hnatusko, A.L., Gicking, J.C. and Lisciandro, G.R. (2021) Anaphylaxis-related hemoperitoneum in 11 dogs. *Journal of Veterinary Emergency and Critical Care (San Antonio)* 31(1), 80–85.

Bile peritonitis

Inflammation of the peritoneum caused by generalized or localized extravasation of bile in the abdominal cavity.

Clinical features

- More common in dogs than in cats.
- Clinical signs can be acute or chronic and depend if the peritonitis is septic or sterile.
- Most common signs include abdominal pain, weakness, anorexia, vomiting, diarrhoea, weight loss, distended abdomen, jaundice and pyrexia.

Causes

- Blunt or penetrating abdominal trauma.
- Biliary obstruction.
- Iatrogenic rupture of the common bile duct or gallbladder.
- Necrotizing choledochitis or cholecystitis. In dogs, necrotizing cholecystitis is frequently a result of a mature gallbladder mucocele that stretches the gallbladder wall to the extent of causing ischaemic necrosis.
- Cholelithiasis.
- Neoplasia.

Cytological features

- Macroscopic appearance of the fluid: yellow-green and turbid.
- Cellularity is high in the range of an exudate. The protein concentration is variable.
- The background is pale basophilic and may contain either bile pigment or pale basophilic mucinous material.
- Cells are predominantly neutrophils. These are usually non-degenerate in sterile effusions or can show variable degrees of degeneration in septic cases. Macrophages are usually found in lower numbers. They may contain phagocytosed bile pigment. Reactive mesothelial cells may also be seen.
- In the majority of the cases, bile pigment is found free in the background or phagocytosed by the inflammatory cells. It is usually present as a yellow, green or black granular material. Occasionally, crystals of bile pigment are also found. They resemble haematoidin crystals. They are rhomboid or needle-like, orange-golden and variably sized.
- In other cases, the typical bile pigment is not observed but instead a variable amount of pale basophilic mucinous to fibrillar amorphous material is found. This is usually defined as 'white bile' and has more frequently been associated with the rupture of the common bile duct and mucocele.
- The diagnosis of bile peritonitis may be aided by the measurement of the bilirubin in the fluid that is usually 2.0–2.5 times greater than the serum bilirubin and patients are often icteric with hyperbilirubinaemia.
- Recently, a few canine cases of anicteric gallbladder rupture and secondary peritonitis have been described. Anicteric gallbladder rupture is reported more commonly in patients with gallbladder mucoceles. In these patients, the bilirubin concentration in the serum and abdominal fluid is low. However, fluid bile acid concentration is greater than in serum. Although this finding requires further studies, when a mucocele is suspected on abdominal imaging and free abdominal fluid is present, a comparison of serum to peritoneal fluid bile acid concentrations may provide additional support for a diagnosis of gallbladder rupture.
- In septic bile peritonitis, bacteria (rods and cocci) can be found either free in the background or phagocytosed by the neutrophils.

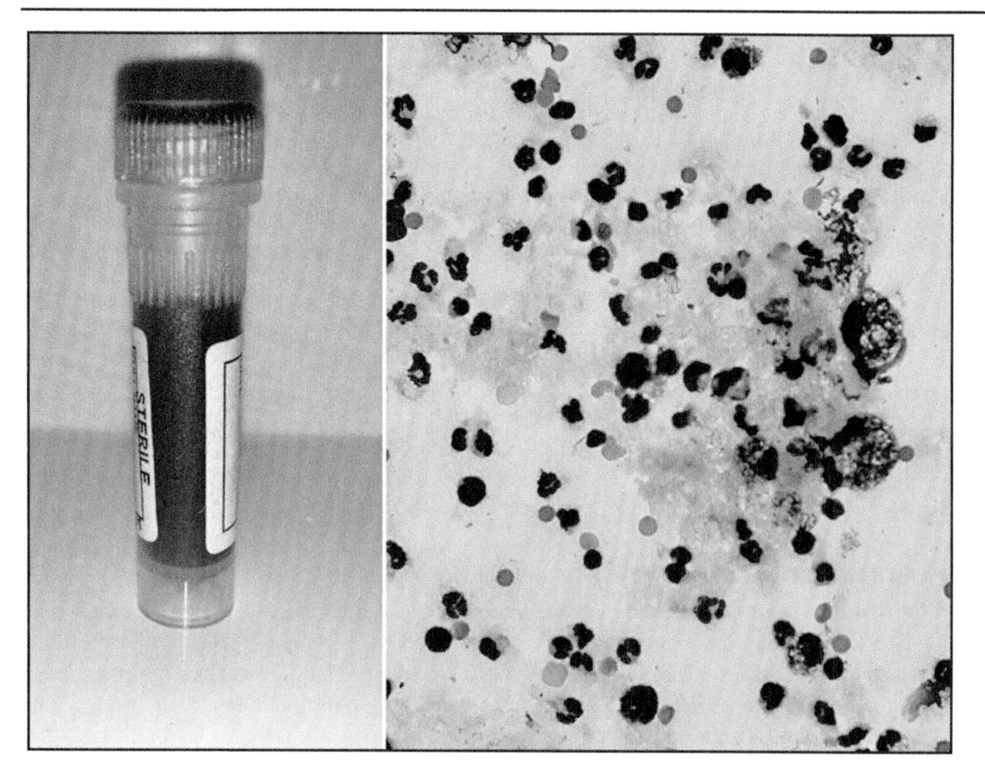

Fig. 3.36. Dog. Abdominal effusion. Bile peritonitis. (Left) Macroscopic appearance of the effusion. (Right) Large amount of biliary pigment present in the background and within the macrophages. Wright-Giemsa.

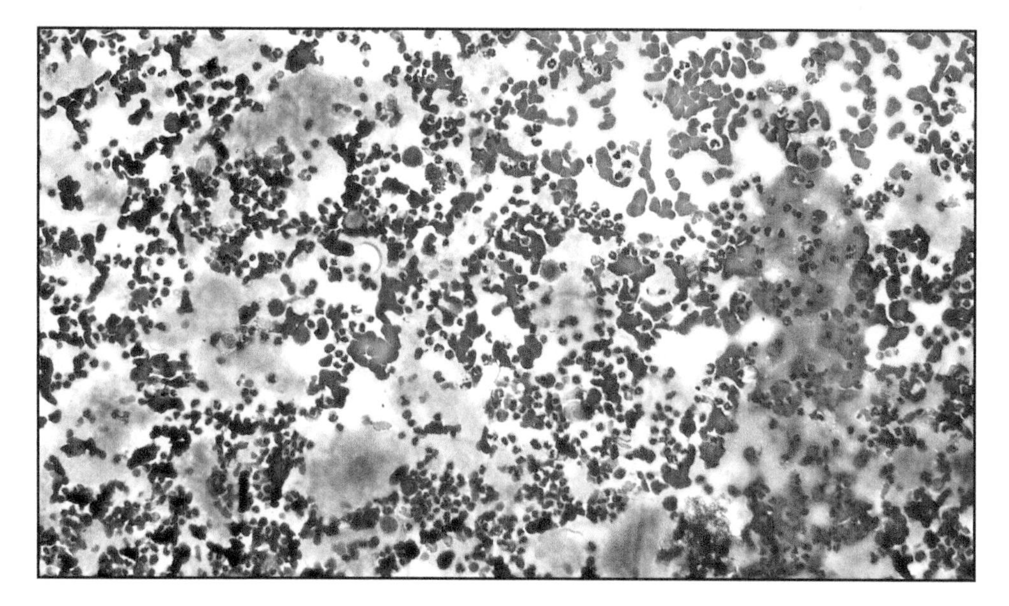

Fig. 3.37. Dog. Abdominal effusion. White bile peritonitis, large amount of mucoid amorphous material seen. Wright-Giemsa.

Further reading

Guess, S.C., Harkin, K.R. and Biller, D.S. (2015) Anicteric gallbladder rupture in dogs: 5 cases (2007–2013). *Journal of American Veterinary Medical Association* 247(12), 1412–1414.
Ludwig, L.L., McLoughlin, M.A., Graves, T.K. and Crisp, M.S. (1997) Surgical treatment of bile peritonitis in 24 dogs and 2 cats: a retrospective study (1987–1994). *Veterinary Surgery* 26(2), 90–98.
Owens, S.D., Gossett, R., McElhaney, M.R., Christopher, M.M. and Shelly, S.M. (2003) Three cases of canine bile peritonitis with mucinous material in abdominal fluid as the prominent cytologic finding. *Veterinary Clinical Pathology* 32(3), 114–120.
Pascual, M., Fauchon, E., Monti, P. and Valls, F. (2022) Anicteric gallbladder rupture with elevated bile acids in abdominal effusion in a dog with cholecystitis. *Journal of American Veterinary Medical Association* 58(3), 146–151.

Uroabdomen

Accumulation of urine in the peritoneal cavity. Urine causes chemical irritation leading to inflammation.

Clinical features

- Clinical signs can relate either to the cause that lead to the rupture of the urinary bladder and to the accumulation in the abdomen and secondary absorption of urine.
- Motor vehicle accident is a common cause of urinary bladder rupture, and patients can present concurrent signs of organ contusion, brain injury, fractures, etc.
- Other clinical signs may reveal lethargy, altered mentation, tachycardia, bradycardia or other arrhythmias, abdominal pain, palpable abdominal fluid wave and bruising of the inguinal region or perineum.
- The urinary bladder may not be palpable and patients can be anuric or dysuric.
- On blood analysis, the most common abnormalities associated with uroabdomen are azotaemia, metabolic acidosis and electrolyte imbalances including mild hyponatremia, hyperphosphatemia and hyperkalemia. Azotaemia and hyponatremia often develop within the 24 h following the onset of uroabdomen; hyperkalemia may not develop for 48 h or more.

Causes

Uroperitoneum occurs secondary to rupture of urinary bladder or of other urinary tract structures that are located within the peritoneal cavity. Causes are:

- Traumatic: blunt trauma (e.g. motor vehicle accident) or penetrating wounds.
- Non-traumatic: spontaneous bladder rupture secondary to neoplasia or urethral obstruction.
- Iatrogenic: e.g. during catheterization or bladder expression.
- Urine leakage: e.g. following cystotomy or cystoscopy if the bladder wall is affected by inflammation or neoplasia.

Cytological features

- Macroscopically, the fluid could be colourless or blood tinged, clear or turbid.
- The cellularity and protein concentration are variable. Abdominal effusions secondary to uroabdomen can fall in the category of a transudate (protein-poor or protein-rich) in the early phases or of an exudate in the later stages following the irritant effect of the urine.

- Urine is a chemical irritant and causes inflammation. In the early phases, mononuclear cells predominate but these are replaced by neutrophils in the later stages. Neutrophils can show karyorrhexis and pyknosis in sterile effusions or can display variable degree of karyolysis in septic infections. Bacteria, when present, may be found phagocytosed by the neutrophils.
- Measurement of fluid creatinine and potassium and comparison with the serum values help in the diagnosis of uroperitoneum.
- A retrospective study investigating the creatinine and potassium concentration ratios of peritoneal fluid to peripheral blood in dogs with uroperitoneum found that:
  - $Creatinine_{fluid}$: $creatinine_{serum}$ > 2:1 was predictive of uroabdomen with a specificity of 100% and sensitivity of 86%.
  - $Potassium_{fluid}$: $potassium_{serum}$ > 1.4:1 was also consistent with uroabdomen with both the specificity and sensitivity being 100%.
- A retrospective study in cats evaluating the creatinine and potassium concentration ratios of peritoneal fluid to peripheral blood in patients with uroabdomen found the following ratios:
  - The mean $creatinine_{serum}$: $creatinine_{fluid}$ was 1:2 (range, 1:1.1–1:4.1).
  - The mean $potassium_{serum}$: $potassium_{fluid}$ was 1:1.9 (range, 1:1.2–1:2.4).

Further reading

Stafford, J.R. and Bartges, J.W. (2013) A clinical review of pathophysiology, diagnosis, and treatment of uroabdomen in the dog and cat. *Journal of Veterinary Emergency and Critical Care (San Antonio)* 23(2), 216–229.

Peritonitis secondary to gastroenteric leakage

Common cause of septic peritonitis in dogs and cats, secondary to GI leakage and secondary intraperitoneal infection by commensal intestinal bacteria.

Clinical features

- GI diseases account for 38–75% of all cases of secondary septic peritonitis.
- A study on 44 dogs and 11 cats found that the most common sites of preformation were the pylorus (38%), other areas of the stomach (11%) and the intestine (51%) (predominantly small intestine and less frequently the colon).
- Peritonitis caused by GI rupture is often septic. The bacterial species involved in peritonitis reflect the normal flora of the gastrointestinal tract. Infections are often mixed anaerobic-aerobic. *Escherichia coli* is the most common isolate from both dogs and cats, followed by *Enterococcus* and *Clostridium* spp.
- Clinical signs are non-specific and include anorexia, vomiting and diarrhoea, abdominal distension and pain, weakness and collapse.

Causes

- Gastrointestinal surgical site dehiscence (e.g. resection and anastomosis).
- Penetrating abdominal trauma (e.g. gunshot).
- Non-steroidal or steroidal anti-inflammatory drug toxicity.
- Ingested foreign bodies.
- Gastrointestinal neoplasia: most common tumours associated with GI leakage are lymphoma and adenocarcinoma.

- Eosinophilic gastroenteritis.
- Torsion, intussusception, intestinal entrapment, gastric-dilatation volvulus: these usually cause bacterial translocation secondary to splanchnic hypoperfusion and secondary ischaemia-reperfusion injury.
- Gastric ulcer.
- Uremic gastropathy.

Cytological features

- Macroscopic appearance of the fluid: often turbid and of variable colour.
- Cellularity and protein concentration are high, often in the range of an exudate.
- The background can be pale basophilic, variably haemodiluted and can contain ingesta and brown amorphous material.
- Inflammatory cells are predominantly degenerate neutrophils, which display variable degree of karyolysis. Macrophages and reactive mesothelial cells are often seen in lower numbers. Macrophages usually have abundant and foamy cytoplasm and may contain phagocytosed amorphous material.
- Infectious agents may include bacteria and yeasts. Bacteria are frequently mixed (often thin and thick rods, but also cocci). They can be found phagocytosed by the inflammatory cells or free in the background.
- Exogenous material other than ingesta may be seen in the background or within the inflammatory cells (e.g. barium used during the clinical workup).

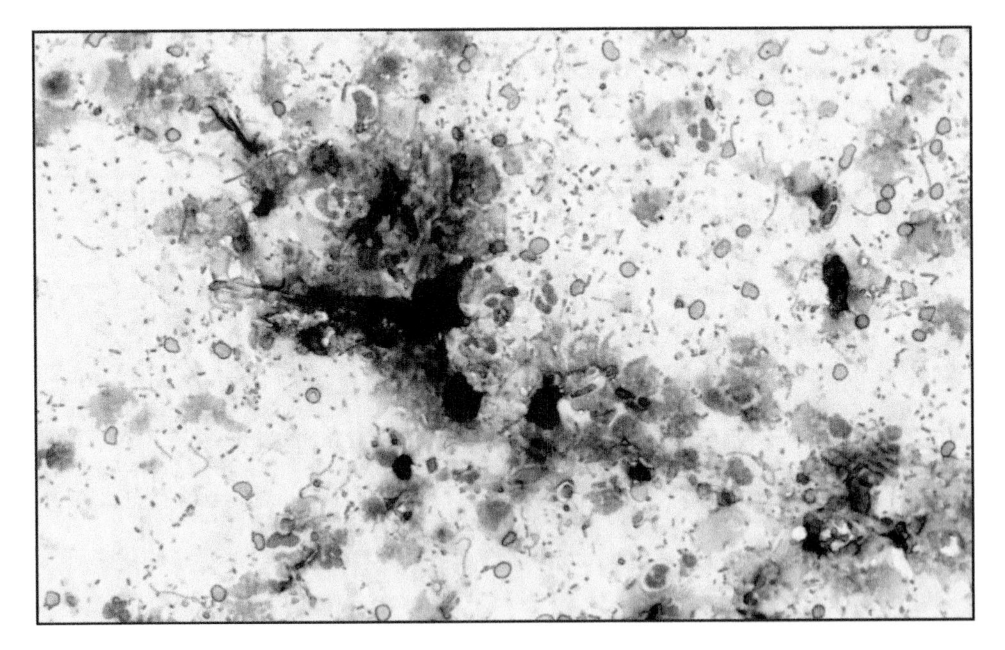

Fig. 3.38. Dog. Abdominal effusion. Septic peritonitis secondary to GI rupture. Numerous mixed extracellular bacteria and amorphous ingesta are present in the background. Wright-Giemsa.

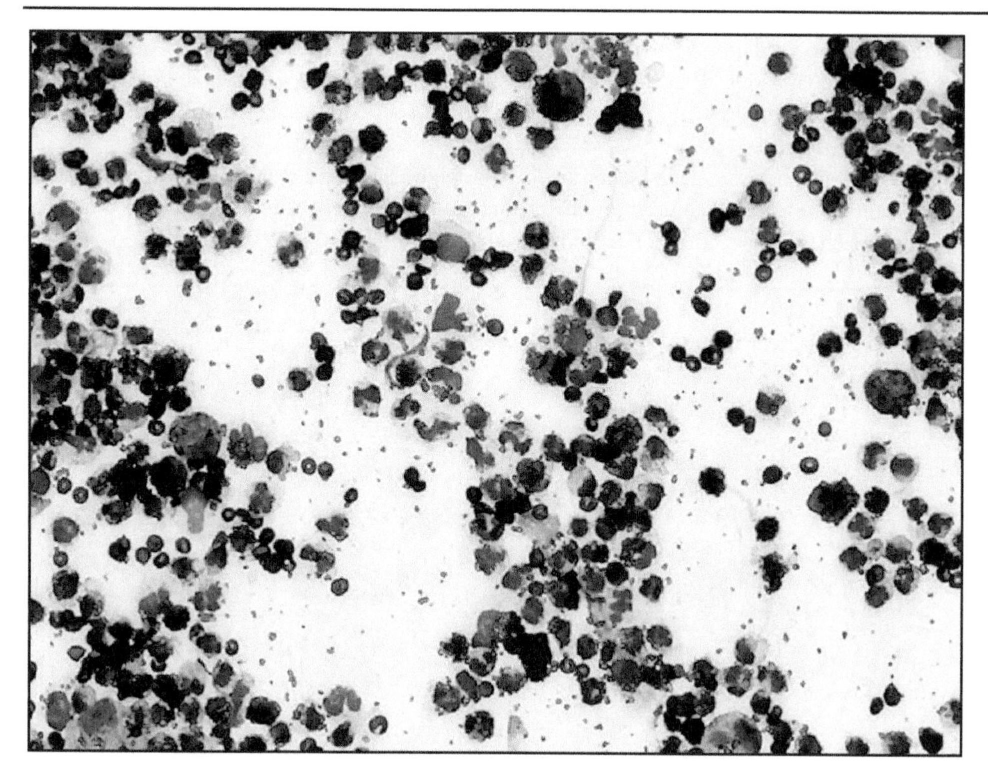

Fig. 3.39. Cat. Abdominal effusion. GI rupture with extravasation of contrast medium. Numerous small refractile structures (barium) are seen among the inflammatory cells. Wright-Giemsa.

Chyloabdomen

Rare condition that results from leakage of lipid-rich lymph into the peritoneal cavity secondary to blockage or impaired lymphatic drainage.

Clinical features

- Most common clinical signs include anorexia, lethargy and vomiting. Some patients may present with abdominal distension.
- Chylothorax is a common comorbidity (47%).
- Malignant neoplasia is the most common underlying cause (45%).

Causes

- Cardiac disease.
- Thromboembolic disease.
- Trauma.
- Neoplasia.
- Infectious diseases: e.g. FIP (cat).
- Iatrogenic causes: e.g. surgical complications.

Cytological features

- Macroscopic appearance of the fluid: usually milky due to the high content of chylomicrons. In anorectic patients, it can be clear.
- Cellularity and protein concentration: variable.

- The majority of the nucleated cells are small lymphocytes. Macrophages can also be seen in established effusions. They usually contain small clear, punctate vacuoles of lipids.
- As chyle acts as an irritant, in more chronic forms, a concurrent neutrophilic inflammation might be found.
- The final diagnosis is made by confirming the high triglyceride (TG) content in the fluid, and the same criteria reported for chylothorax can be applied. The vast majority of chylous effusions have triglyceride concentrations >100 mg/dl (1.1 mmol/l).

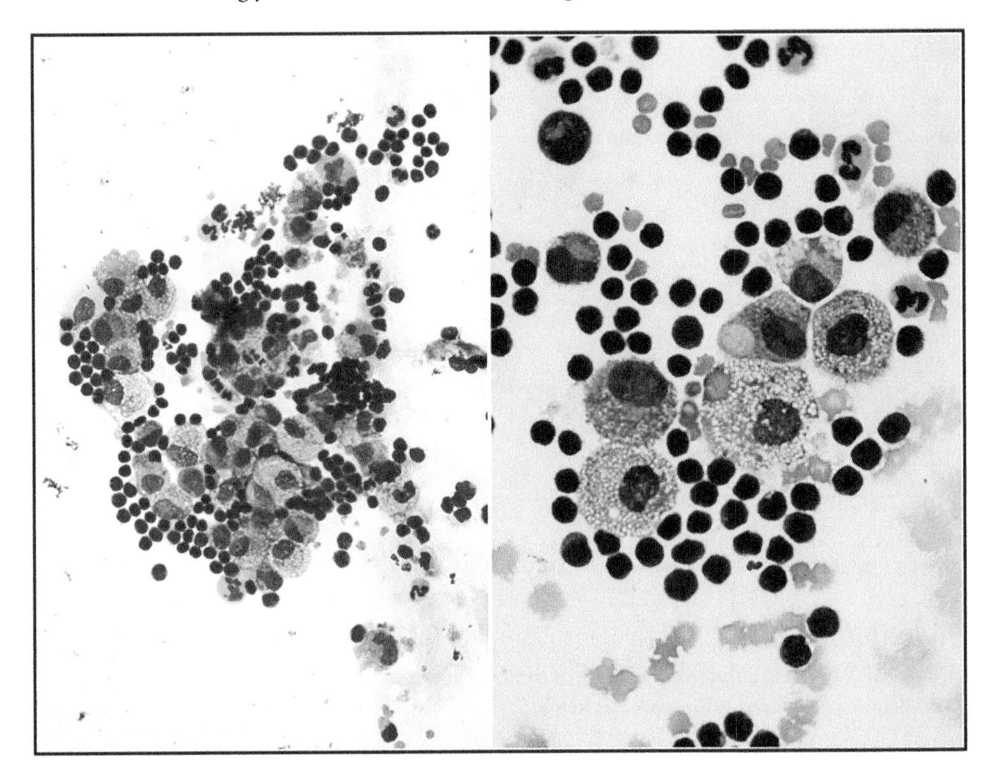

Fig. 3.40. Cat. Abdominal effusion. Chyloabdomen. Predominance of small lymphocytes with lower numbers of macrophages containing small, clear, punctate vacuoles. Wright-Giemsa.

Keratin-induced sterile peritonitis

Rare type of peritonitis secondary to the rupture of an epidermal or dermal cyst present in the abdominal cavity.

Clinical features

- Epidermoid and dermoid cysts arising within the intestinal wall have been described in dogs and cats.
- Epidermoid and dermoid cysts are rare congenital lesions derived from pluripotent cells:
    - Epidermoid cysts are lined by stratified squamous epithelium and the cavity contains a mixture of cholesterol, keratinocytes and degenerating keratinaceous amorphous material.
    - Dermoid cysts contain in their lining adnexal structures such as hair follicles, sebaceous glands and sweat glands.

- The keratinaceous content of these cysts is a strong irritant and causes inflammation (peritonitis) when released into the abdominal cavity.
- Clinical signs are variable and usually relate to the presence of fluid in the abdominal cavity and to the inflammation caused by the release of keratin into the peritoneal cavity.

Cytological features

- Cellularity and protein concentration are usually high, in the range of an exudate.
- The background can be pale basophilic and variably haemodiluted.
- Following the rupture of the cyst, numerous squamous epithelial cells can be seen in the cytological preparations of the effusion. They are usually large, angular to polygonal and have an abundant pale basophilic cytoplasm. When present, the nuclei are central, small and can be pyknotic. Cholesterol crystals may also be observed.
- Inflammatory cells are mostly neutrophils that tend to be non-degenerate. Macrophages may be seen in low numbers.

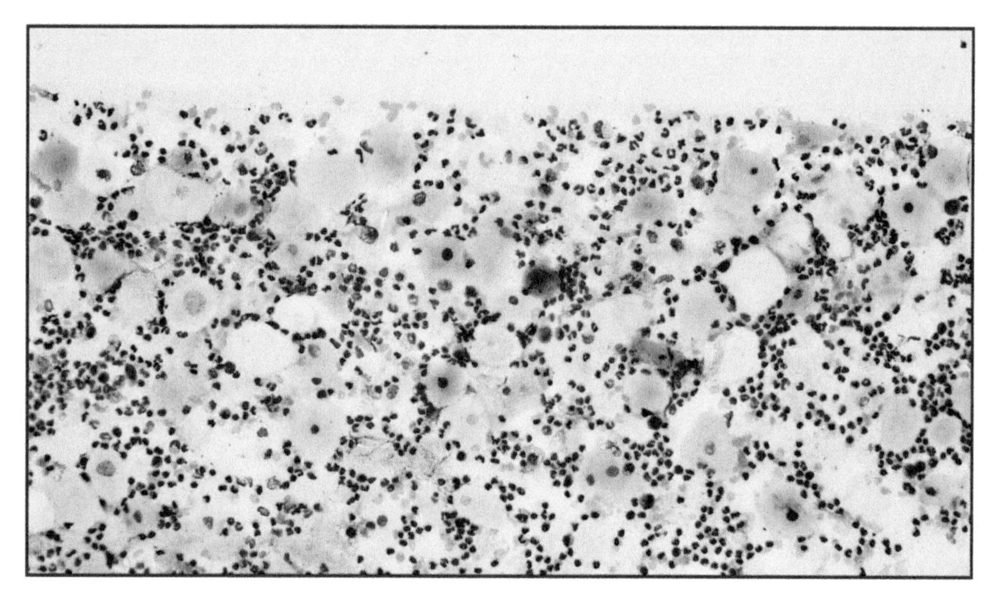

Fig. 3.41. Dog. Abdominal effusion. Keratin-induced peritonitis secondary to the rupture of an intestinal epidermoid cyst. Numerous squamous epithelial cells are seen in between the neutrophils. Wright-Giemsa.

Peritonitis secondary to reproductive tract tears

Inflammation of the female or male intraabdominal genital tract may occasionally be associated with peritonitis.

Causes

- Female:
  - Ruptured pyometra: uncommon cause of septic peritonitis. It usually occurs prior or during surgery due to increased friability of the uterus.
  - Seminoperitoneum: usually secondary to traumatic breeding causing a tear in the uterine wall.

- Male:
  - Rupture of prostatic abscesses: this is quite common and could be life threatening.
  - Seminoperitoneum: complication of vasectomy.

Cytological features

- Macroscopic appearance of the fluid: variably coloured and haemodiluted and usually turbid.
- Cellularity and TP are usually high in the range of an exudate.
- Ruptured pyometra and prostatic abscesses: most of the cells are neutrophils. They can display a variable degree of degeneration and may contain phagocytosed bacteria (cocci or rods). Macrophages are usually present in lower numbers and may display leucophagia, erythrophagia or contain amorphous phagosomes.
- Seminoperitoneum: Neurophils often predominate, with lower numbers of macrophages. The neutrophils may be mildly degenerate and macrophages are frequently vacuolated. Haemorrhage might occur and signs of red blood cell degradation can be present (e.g. erythrophagia and macrophages containing haemosiderin and/or haematoidin crystals). Free in the background or within the inflammatory cells, spermatozoa might be seen. They have small basophilic heads, and the tails are often detached.

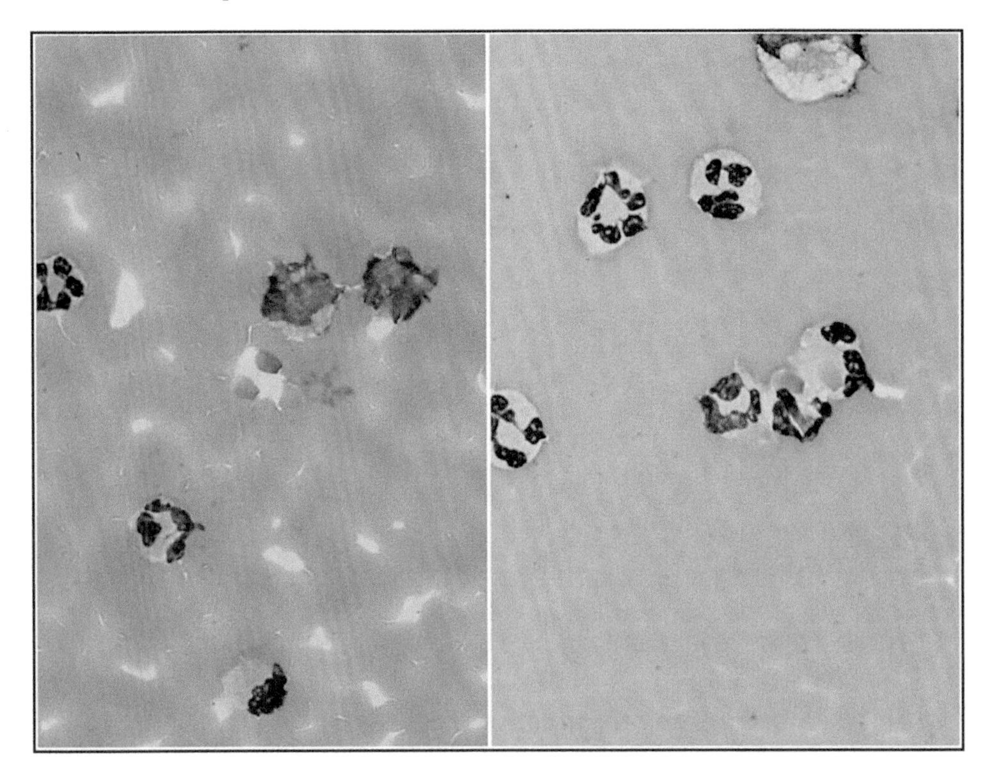

Fig. 3.42. Dog. Abdominal effusion. seminoperitoneum. Head of spermatozoa are seen in the background or within the inflammatory cells. Wright-Giemsa. (*Courtesy of Alice Pastorello.*)

Further reading

DiDomenico, A.E., Stowe, D.M. and Lynch, A.M. (2020) What is your diagnosis? Abdominal fluid from a dog. *Veterinary Clinical Pathology* 49(1), 164–166.

3.7.5 Peritoneal neoplastic effusions (effusions from cell exfoliation)

Exfoliation of neoplastic cells and/or reactive mesothelial cells into the abdominal cavity can lead to the accumulation of variably cellular effusions.

- The term 'neoplastic effusion' should only be used to describe effusions when a neoplastic cell population has been identified on cytology.
- Neoplastic effusions can present either as transudates or exudates. There are no specific numerical parameters for neoplastic effusions.
- Neoplastic cells often do not exfoliate in the abdominal fluid. For this reason, absence of tumour cells does not exclude an underlying neoplasia. False-negative results are relatively high, with a reported sensitivity of fluid cytology for neoplasia of 64% in dogs and 61% in cats.
- In dogs, neoplastic abdominal effusions are most commonly associated with carcinomas, followed by round-cell tumours. Sarcomatous effusions are rare.
- In cats, neoplastic effusions by epithelial and round cell tumours have similar frequency.

Pathophysiology

The accumulation of fluid in the body cavities secondary to neoplasia may be due to:

- Increased hydrostatic pressure: the tumour may cause venous compression leading to a transudative effusion.
- Compression of the lymphatics: this usually leads to the accumulation of chyle.
- Increased vascular permeability: secondary to the effects of cytokines and vasoactive amines released by the tumour.
- Inflammation associated with the tumour: this usually leads to the formation of an exudate.

Epithelial Tumours

- Primary epithelial tumours of the abdominal cavity include GI, biliary, hepatocellular, pancreatic, adrenal and urogenital carcinomas.
- Metastatic epithelial tumours: examples include mammary carcinoma, anal sac adenocarcinoma and pulmonary carcinoma.

Cytological features

- Cellularity and protein concentration: variable.
- Background: clear to pale basophilic and variably haemodiluted.
- The cell morphology of different epithelial tumours that exfoliate in the ascitic fluid is very similar one to another and the identification of their lineage is often difficult.
- Neoplastic epithelial cells usually exfoliate in cohesive clusters. The form of the clusters varies depending on the tissue of origin: they can form rafts, papilloid arrangements, sheets, balls, etc.
- Cells morphology may vary from cuboidal to polygonal or columnar.
- The cytoplasm is variable in amount, basophilic, and may contain single or multiple, variably sized clear vacuoles. Urothelial cells from urinary tract carcinomas may contain typical large pink vacuoles of secretory material named Malamed-Wolinska bodies.
- Nuclei are usually round and have variable chromatin patterns.

- Criteria of malignancy are also variable. In some carcinomas, such as the ovarian papillary carcinoma, cells can be relatively uniform in size and shape. In others, cell pleomorphism, anisokaryosis and anisocytosis can be more pronounced.
- To follow, only the cytological description of the more common epithelial tumours that may be found in ascitic fluid is provided.

Ovarian carcinoma

Ovarian carcinoma can exfoliate and disseminate in the peritoneal cavity as carcinomatosis and produce ascites.

Cytological features

- Cellularity: often moderate to high.
- Background: haemodiluted.
- The neoplastic cells are often arranged in papillary patterns, although some individualized cells may be present. The papillary clusters can be round, oval or branching. The intercellular spaces are often not visible.
- Cells have round to oval, paracentral nuclei, fine chromatin and generally poorly visible small nucleoli. The cytoplasm is moderate in amount and pale basophilic.
- Anisocytosis and anisokaryosis are usually mild, but in some cases, they might be more prominent.

Differential diagnoses

- Papillary mesothelial hyperplasia
- Mesothelioma
- Metastases from other papillary carcinomas

Ovarian teratomas

Tumours arising from the ovarian germ cells. They are composed of abnormal tissue derived from at least two, and often all three, germinal layers.

Clinical features

- Benign or malignant forms are possible. Benign teratomas are more common.
- Uncommon in domestic animals, but most frequently described in the bitch.

Cytological features

- In literature, a cytology case of a malignant teratoma with associated ascites and pleural effusion is described in a 1-year-old bitch.
- Cellularity and protein concentration: high in the range of an exudate.
- Neoplastic cells were in cohesive clusters. Rarely, acinoid formations were found.
- Cells appeared pleomorphic, round or oval with abundant and variably vacuolated cytoplasm.
- Nuclei were round and had finely stippled chromatin. They contained large, often multiple, irregularly shaped nucleoli.
- Occasional squamous epithelial cells appearing keratinized were also observed.

- Multinucleated cells and mitotic figures were common. Anisocytosis and anisokaryosis were marked. Bacteria were not detected.
- Numerous non-degenerate neutrophils were also present.

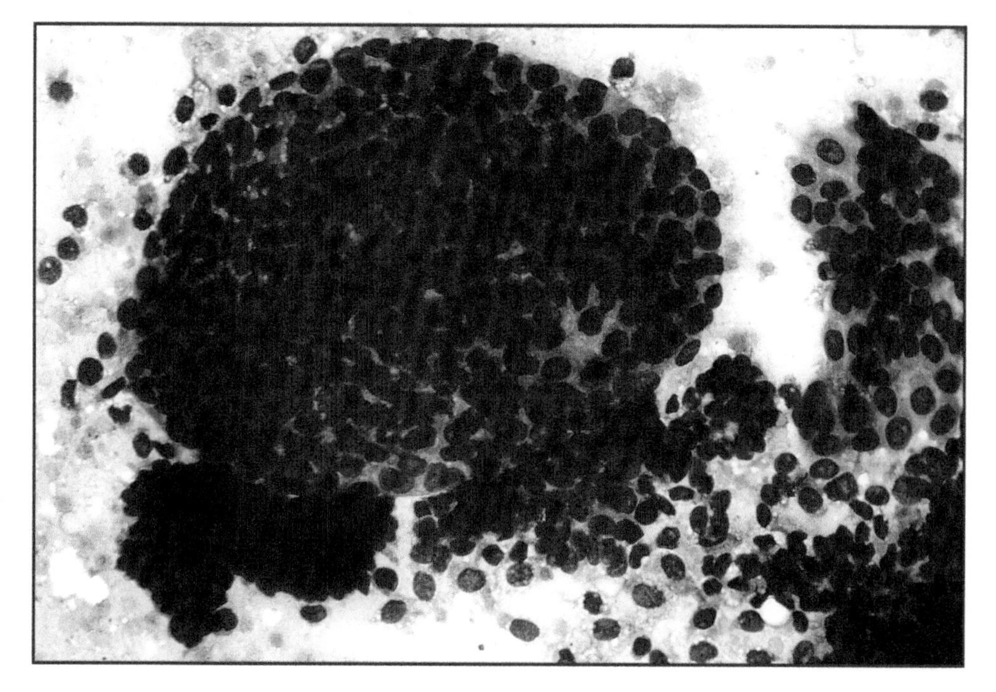

Fig. 3.43. Dog. Abdominal effusion. Ovarian carcinoma. The neoplastic cells are arranged in cohesive clusters. They are cuboidal and display minimal features of atypia. Wright-Giemsa. (*Courtesy of Walter Bertazzolo and Ugo Bonfanti.*)

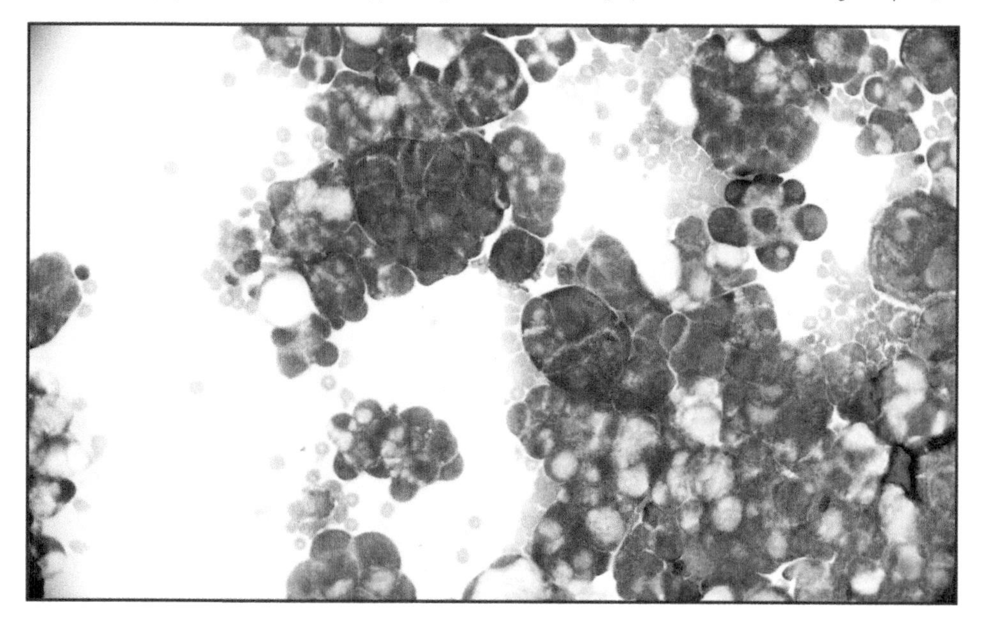

Fig. 3.44. Dog. Abdominal effusion. Metastatic mammary carcinoma. The neoplastic cells are arranged in cohesive clusters or balls and display marked features of atypia. Wright-Giemsa.

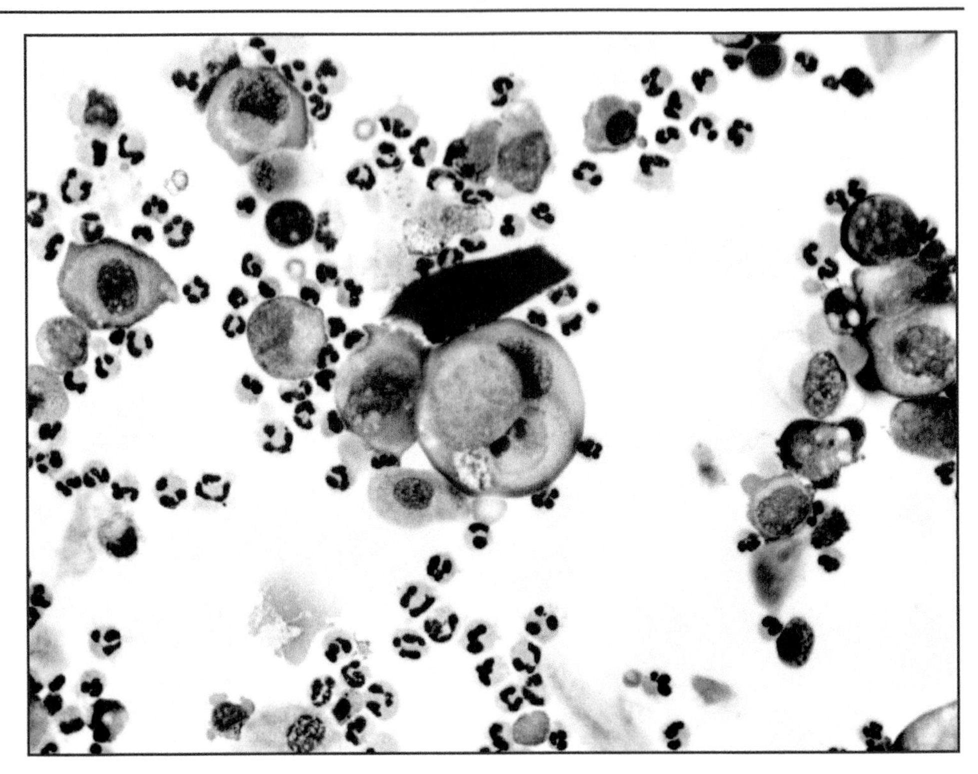

Fig. 3.45. Dog. Abdominal effusion. Urothelial carcinoma. Pleomorphic neoplastic epithelial cells are seen including one containing Melamed-Wolinska bodies. Wright-Giemsa.

Further reading

Bertazzolo, W., Bonfanti, U., Mazzotti, S. and Gelain, M.E. (2021) Cytologic features and diagnostic accuracy of analysis of effusions for detection of ovarian carcinoma in dogs. *Veterinary Clinical Pathology* 41(1), 127–132.

Elena Gorman, M., Bildfell, R. and Séguin, B. (2010) What is your diagnosis? Peritoneal fluid from a 1-year-old female German Shepherd dog. Malignant teratoma. *Veterinary Clinical Pathology* 39(3), 393–394.

Round Cell tumours

Lymphoma

Clinical features

- Lymphoma in the abdominal cavity may be part of a multicentric form or could arise primarily in a visceral organ, e.g. alimentary lymphoma and hepatosplenic lymphoma.

Cytological features

- Cells exfoliate individually in the ascitic fluid. In a rare case report in a dog, the neoplastic cells were also found forming variably sized clusters with distinct cell borders. This was demonstrated to be caused by an up-regulation of the adhesion molecule ICAM-1.
- Neoplastic lymphoid cells that exfoliate in the effusion are generally medium to large and monomorphic.
- The cytoplasm is scant to moderate and basophilic. In cats, this could contain small clear, punctate vacuoles. Depending on the subtype, fine azurophilic granules might be found in the cytoplasm.
- Nuclei are medium-large, round, eccentric and have finely stippled chromatin. One to multiple, small and round, variably prominent nucleoli might be seen. Mitoses can be found.
- Variable numbers or mixed leucocytes may be present. In same cases of GI lymphoma, rupture of the abdominal wall may occur causing a secondary septic neutrophilic peritonitis.

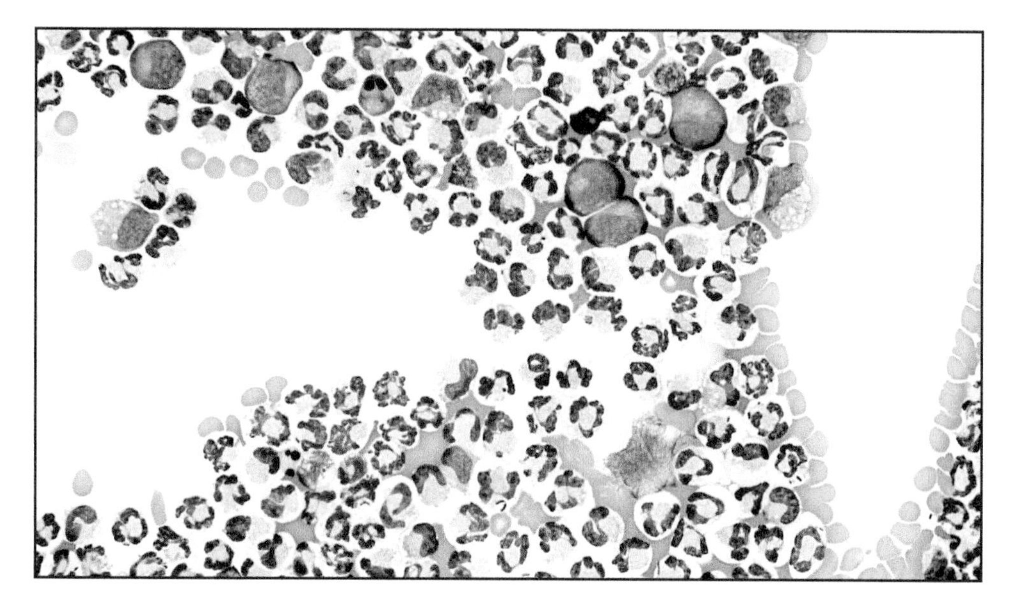

Fig. 3.46. Dog. Abdominal effusion. Lymphoma. Occasional large lymphoid cells admixed with neutrophils. Some of the neutrophils contain phagocytosed bacteria. Wright-Giemsa.

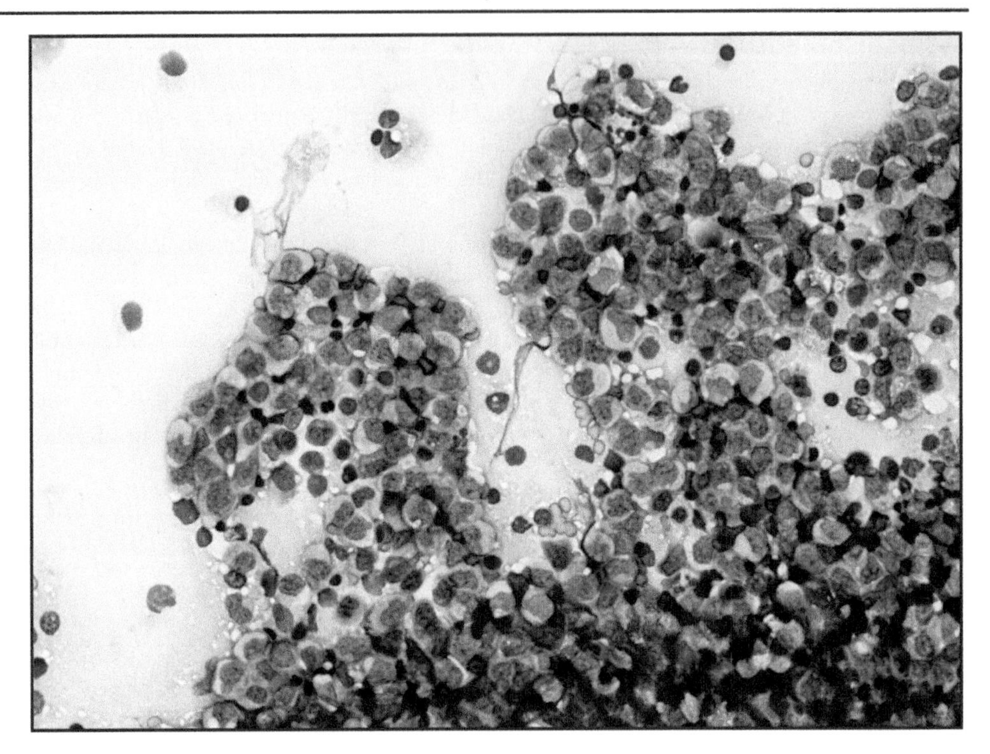

Fig. 3.47. Cat. Abdominal effusion. Lymphoma. Numerous monomorphic large lymphoid cells are seen. Wright-Giemsa.

Mast cell tumour

Clinical features

- Intracavitary abdominal mast cell tumours could be primary (visceral) or metastatic from a primary cutaneous mass.
- Visceral mast cell tumour is more common in cats than dogs.
- In cats, visceral mast cell tumours most commonly arise in the spleen or less frequently in the GI tract.
- In dogs, visceral mast cell tumour typically originates in the GI tract.

Cytological features

- Cellularity and protein concentration: variable.
- Background: variably haemodiluted. It may contain free purple granules.
- The neoplastic mast cells are similar to those observed in other locations. Anisokaryosis and anisocytosis may be variable, and multi-nucleated cells may be present or absent. The degree of granulation is also variable.
- The cytoplasm is usually moderate in amount and contains variable numbers of purple granules.
- Nuclei are round to oval, most commonly eccentric or paracentral.
- Variable numbers of eosinophils may also be present.

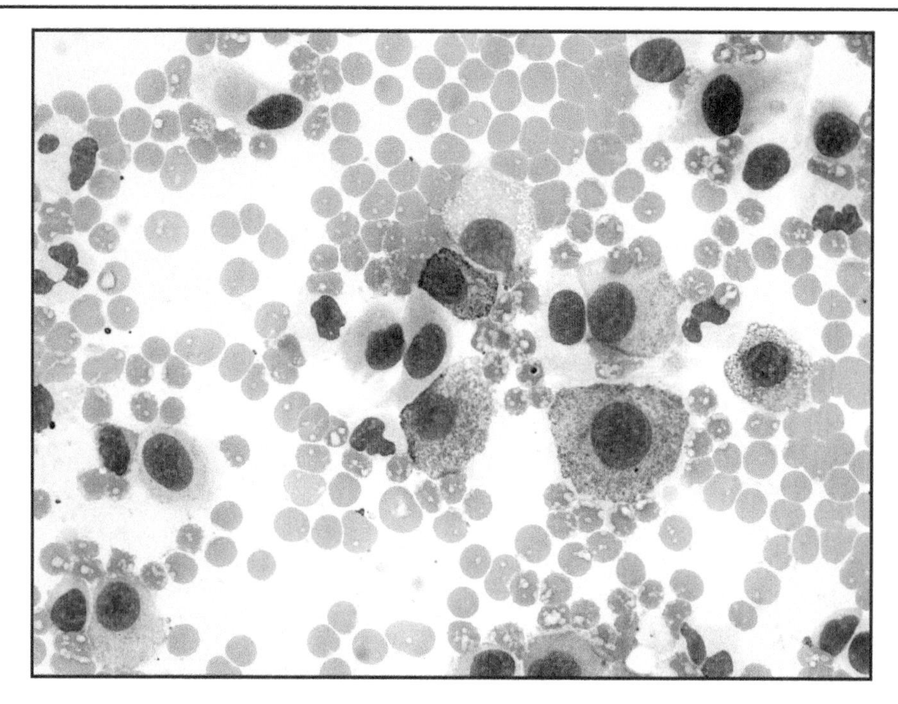

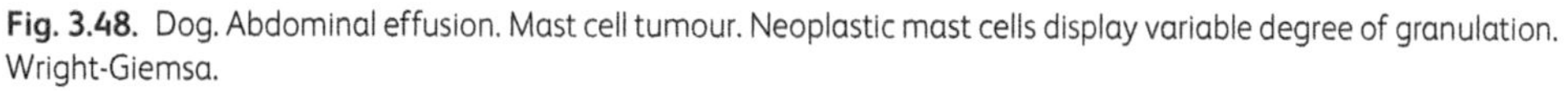

Fig. 3.48. Dog. Abdominal effusion. Mast cell tumour. Neoplastic mast cells display variable degree of granulation. Wright-Giemsa.

Mesenchymal Tumours

- Mesenchymal tumours in the abdominal cavity can be primary or metastatic.
- They may sometimes cause ascites, but the neoplastic cells rarely exfoliate in the fluid.
- Sarcomas in the abdominal cavity can be primary or metastatic.
- Primary abdominal visceral sarcomas: e.g. soft-tissue sarcoma, haemangiosarcoma, histiocytic sarcoma.
- The most common abdominal visceral soft-tissue sarcoma in dogs include the following: stromal sarcoma (spleen), leiomyosarcoma (spleen, small intestine, pylorus, cecum, bladder and ureter), fibrosarcoma (spleen, small intestine, kidney), myxosarcoma (spleen), peripheral nerve sheath tumour (spleen).
- Neoplastic cells can exfoliate in the effusion during organ rupture (e.g. haemangiosarcoma) or from peritoneal foci of sarcomatosis.
- Cytologically, the identification of the tissue of origin can be very challenging, although the clinical history and imaging findings may help.

Cytological features

- Cellularity and protein concentration: variable.
- Background: variably haemodiluted from mild iatrogenic blood contamination to haemoabdomen (e.g. splenic rupture associated with haemangiosarcoma).
- Different types of sarcoma may appear morphologically similar and the identification of their lineage is often difficult.
- Neoplastic mesenchymal cells can exfoliate individually or sometimes in small loose aggregates. They may be associated with a small amount of pink extracellular matrix.

- Cells can vary from spindle shaped to plump oval. They are often mononucleated but binucleated and multinucleated forms may be present.
- The cytoplasm is basophilic, may form tails that project away from the nucleus and occasionally can contain small clear vacuoles. Some types of sarcomas, such as haemangiosarcomas and histiocytic sarcomas, can display erythrophagia.
- Nuclei are often large, oval, round or irregularly shaped. The chromatin has a variable pattern, from finely to coarsely stippled. One to multiple, variably sized and shaped nucleoli can be visible.
- Prominent anisocytosis and anisokaryosis and variable N:C ratio are common.

Mesothelioma

Mesothelioma is an aggressive neoplasm that arises from the mesothelial cells that line the serosal surface of the body cavities.

Clinical features

- Rare neoplasm more frequently seen in dogs than cats.
- It can present as diffuse or localized thickening of the mesothelium, plaques or discrete nodules.
- Dogs: effusions can be monocavitary, bicavitary or tricavitary. In a recent study that included 34 dogs, 16 patients had a monocavitary effusion (mostly pleural), 12 dogs had a bicavitary effusion (mostly pleural and pericardial) and 5 dogs had a tricavitary effusion.
- Cats: peritoneal mesotheliomas are less frequent than thoracic forms.
- Mesotheliomas are subclassified as:
  - Epithelioid.
  - Sarcomatous (fibrous).
  - Biphasic (or mixed).

Cytological features

- Cellularity and protein concentration: variable. Effusions can be transudates, exudates or haemorrhagic effusions.
- Background: variably haemodiluted.
- Cells can be individualized or in cohesive clusters, often forming variably sized balls. Cell crowding and nuclear moulding may be noticed.
- Cells are most frequently round to slightly polygonal. Occasionally, the neoplastic cells could be spindle shaped, probably reflecting the sarcomatous/fibrous variant.
- Nuclei are generally large, round to oval and often central to paracentral. They can be hyperchromatic, and the chromatin is finely to coarsely stippled. One to multiple, small to large, round or irregular prominent nucleoli may be present.
- The cytoplasm is variable in amount. In some of the cells, it is scant, in others, it is abundant and may contain one to multiple, small to large vacuoles. Fringed margins may be observed.
- Anisokaryosis and anisocytosis are usually prominent, and multi-nucleated cells are common.

Differential diagnoses

- Carcinomatosis
- Reactive mesothelial hyperplasia/dysplasia
- Sarcomatosis (for sarcomatous/fibrous variant)

Pearls and Pitfalls

- The differentiation between mesothelioma, carcinoma and reactive/dysplastic mesothelial cells can be very difficult on cytology and small biopsies. In some cases, further testing (e.g. IHC, electron microscopy) might be required for a definitive diagnosis (refer to chapter 9).

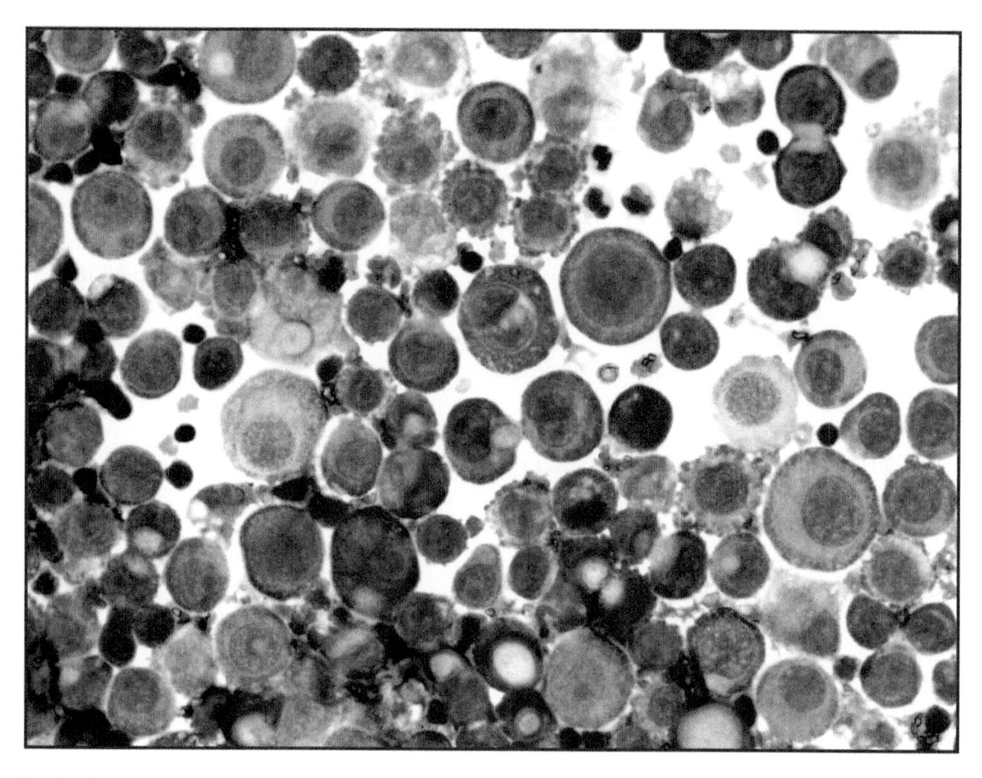

Fig. 3.49. Dog. Abdominal effusion. Mesothelioma. Neoplastic mesothelial cells exfoliate individually. They are round and display marked anisocytosis, anisokaryosis and have prominent nucleoli. Occasional membrane blebbing is observed. Wright-Giemsa.

3.7.6 Microbiology testing of peritoneal fluids

Processing and recommendations of abdominal fluids for culture are similar to pleural fluids.

3.8 Pericardial Effusions

Pericardial effusion (PE) usually forms when there is an imbalance between the production and reabsorption of the physiologic pericardial fluid. When diagnosed, the first step is to evaluate its haemodynamic impact.

Although cytology is not very sensitive for disease aetiology, analysis is usually rewarding in case of bacterial infections and exfoliated malignant effusions. In one study in dogs, fluid analysis identified the cause of the PE in only 12.8% of cases.

Clinical features

- If the fluid builds up slowly, the pericardium can stretch and adapt. This allows the accumulation of a larger amount of fluid before the diastolic function of the heart is compromised.
- Fast accumulation of fluid leads to cardiac tamponade. The heart is compressed and the atrial and ventricular fillings are impaired causing the venous blood to pool into the splanchnic and systemic circulations.
- Clinical signs associated with acute presentation include weakness or collapse, hypotension, cardiogenic shock, dyspnoea or even death.
- Signs associated with chronic cardiac tamponade include collapse, exercise intolerance, anorexia, vomiting, tachypnoea, weakness and lethargy.
- PE can be associated with concurrent pleural effusion and ascites.

3.8.1 Pathophysiology

- Increase of the microvascular pressure caused by hypervolemic states e.g.:
  - Congestive heart failure (CHF).
  - Renal failure.
- Decreased colloid osmotic pressure secondary to hypoalbuminaemia e.g.:
  - Protein losing nephropathy (PLN).
  - Protein losing enteropathy (PLE).
  - Malnutrition.
  - Liver failure.
- Increased permeability of the capillary vessels e.g.:
  - Inflammation.
  - Infection.
- Cell exfoliation:
  - Neoplasia.
- Haemorrhage:
  - Idiopathic.
  - Haemorrhagic neoplasia.
  - Trauma.
  - Coagulopathy.
- Chyle.

Based on the characteristic of the fluid, TNCC and TP, PEs can be classified in transudates (protein-poor and protein-rich), exudates, haemorrhagic and chylous fluids. The effusion could be infectious or non-infectious.

Causes

- Dogs:
  - Neoplasia: haemangiosarcoma (most frequently), mesothelioma, chemodectoma, ectopic thyroid carcinoma.
  - Idiopathic pericarditis.
  - Coagulopathy.
  - Rupture of left atrium in patients with severe mitral valve regurgitation.
- Cats:
  - Cardiac heart failure: more frequently due to hypertrophic cardiomyopathy, followed by unclassified and restrictive cardiomyopathy.
  - Neoplasia.
  - Idiopathic.
  - FIP.
  - Uraemia/fluid overload.
  - Pericardioperitoneal hernia.

Further reading

Cagle, L.A., Epstein, S.E., Owens, S.D., Mellema, M.S., Hopper, K. *et al.* (2014) Diagnostic yield of cytologic analysis of pericardial effusion in dogs. *Journal of Veterinary Internal Medicine* 28(1), 66–71.

3.8.2 Pericardial transudates

As in other cavities, the accumulation of a poorly cellular fluid in the pericardial space is defined as transudation. The transudate could be protein-poor or protein-rich, based on the underlying cause.

Clinical features

- The severity of the clinical signs depends on the rate at which the fluid accumulates in the pericardial sac. Acute forms are associated with signs of cardiac tamponade; chronic forms tend to be more compensated (see Section 3.8).
- It can be associated with concurrent pleural effusion and ascites.

Causes

- Hypoproteinemia: this can cause the accumulation of a protein-poor transudate. Most commonly associated with:
  - Protein-losing nephropathy (PLN).
  - Protein-losing enteropathy (PLE).
  - Hepatic failure.
- CHF: this can lead to the accumulation of a protein-rich transudate. It is often seen with hypertrophic cardiomyopathy.
- FIP (cats).
- Uraemia.
- Peritoneopericardial hernia.
- Non-exfoliating neoplasia.

Cytological features

- Macroscopic appearance of the fluid: colourless/yellow/pink and clear.
- Background: clear with low numbers of erythrocytes.
- Cellularity: low.
- Protein concentration: usually high in FIP and effusion caused by cardiovascular disease and low when secondary to hypoalbuminaemia.
- Nucleated cells usually consist of a mixture of segmented neutrophils, monocytoid cells -/ macrophages and small lymphocytes. Neutrophils are generally non-degenerate although *in vitro* swelling may occur.
- Infectious agents are not found.

3.8.3 Pericardial exudates

Pericardial exudates in dogs and cats are rare and represent approximately 5% of all pericardial effusions. They are caused by inflammation. The cytokines and vasoactive amines released during the inflammatory process cause increased permeability of the vessels, allowing protein-rich fluids and cells to enter and accumulate in the pericardial sac.

Clinical features

- As for pericardial transudates, the severity of the clinical signs depends on the rate at which the fluid accumulates. Acute forms are associated with signs of cardiac tamponade; chronic forms tend to be more compensated.
- It can be associated with concurrent pleural effusion and ascites.
- Uncommon in dogs and rare in cats.

Neutrophilic exudate

Most commonly, neutrophilic pericardial effusions are associated with an underlying infectious aetiology. Rarely, sterile forms have been described, whose cause was not identified.

Causes

- Haematogenous bacterial and fungal colonization (more common).
- Migrating foreign bodies.

Cytological features

- Macroscopic appearance of the fluid: it can be variably coloured, blood stained and often turbid.
- Cytological findings are similar to exudates described in other locations.
- Cellularity and TP: high.
- Background: variably haemodiluted.
- The majority of the cells are often neutrophils. In septic causes, neutrophils appear variably degenerate and may contain bacteria. Infectious agents can also be found free in the background.
- In more chronic forms, other inflammatory cells such as macrophages, lymphocytes and plasma cells might also be present.
- Examples of infectious agents isolated from PE include:
  - Bacteria: *Bacteroides* spp., *Actinomyces* spp., *Streptococcus canis* and *Pasteurella* spp.
  - Fungi/yeast: *Coccidioides* spp. (dog).

Eosinophilic exudate

- Uncommon type of PE. It was described in an 11-year-old cat with concurrent low-airway eosinophilic inflammation.
- The underlying cause was not determined.

Cytological features

- The fluid had a high cellularity and protein concentration and was classified as an exudate.
- It contained a vast predominance of eosinophils (approximately 79%), low numbers of non-degenerate neutrophils, macrophages and a few small lymphocytes. Infectious agents were not found.

Further reading

Prado Checa, I., Woods, G.A., Oikonomidis, I.L., Paris, J., Culshaw, G.J. *et al.* (2021) Eosinophilic pericardial effusion in a cat with complex systemic disease and associated peripheral eosinophilia. *Journal of Veterinary Cardiology* 35, 55–62.

3.8.4 Pericardial effusions from ruptured or leaky vessels or organs

Haemorrhagic effusion

Accumulation of haemorrhagic fluid in the pericardial sac, most commonly associated with idiopathic pericarditis and neoplasia.

Causes

- Idiopathic haemorrhagic PE: it occurs without an apparent cause. Most commonly observed in large-breed dogs.
- Haemorrhagic neoplasia: e.g. haemangiosarcoma.
- Erosion of blood vessels: e.g. neoplasia.
- Trauma.
- Rupture of the atrial wall.
- Coagulopathy: e.g. rodenticide toxicity, haemophilia and *Angiostrongylus vasorum.*
- Iatrogenic.

Idiopathic pericarditis (haemorrhagic)

Accumulation of haemorrhagic fluid into the pericardial sac.

Clinical features

- Fluid accumulation is usually slow, and patients usually have clinical signs related to chronic cardiac tamponade (see Section 3.8).
- Pericardial effusion can be associated with concurrent pleural effusion and ascites.
- More common in dogs than cats.
- Idiopathic pericarditis is the most common cause of PE in dogs after haemangiosarcoma.
- The cause is unknown but is thought to be associated with pericardial inflammation secondary to viral or immune-mediated disease. The inflammation seems to target the pericardial blood vessels, causing their damage and secondary haemorrhage.
- Over-represented canine breeds: large canine breeds are over-represented. In one study, Golden Retriever, German Shepherd, Great Dane, Great Pyrenean and Saint Bernard dogs were found to be predisposed.

Cytological features

- Macroscopically, the fluid has the appearance of frank blood.
- Background: heavily haemodiluted.
- Beside the blood-derived leucocytes, variable numbers of macrophages and reactive/hyperplastic mesothelial cells are seen. In acute forms, these cells may not be found or may be present in low numbers. In established effusions, they are more numerous.
- Macrophages usually have abundant and vacuolated cytoplasm. They often show signs of red blood cell degradation. In the early phases, erythrophagia predominates. In long-standing effusions, macrophages more typically contain haemosiderin granules or haematoidin crystals. The latter are orange and refractile. Their most typical form is rhomboid, but needle-like forms may be found.
- Mesothelial cells can be very numerous. They exfoliate singly or in clusters. They can be mononucleated or sometimes binucleated. Nuclei are round to oval and variably positioned within the cell. One to multiple nucleoli may occasionally be seen. The cytoplasm is moderate in amount, moderately or occasionally deeply basophilic and may contain vacuoles. Fringed outlines are not uncommon. Mesothelial cells may contain haemosiderin granules or haematoidin crystals. Anisokaryosis and anisocytosis and N:C ratio are variable.

Pearls and Pitfalls

- The diagnosis of idiopathic pericarditis is attempted by combining the clinical signs, imaging results (negative echocardiography for cardiac neoplasia) and haemorrhagic effusion. On cytology, the absence of exfoliated neoplastic cells in a haemorrhagic effusion does not rule out cardiac neoplasia.
- In one study, it has been shown that measurement of serum cardiac troponin I (cTnI) can help in distinguishing between haemangiosarcoma and idiopathic PE. In that study, dogs with HSA had significantly higher concentrations of cTnI (2.77 ng/dL; range: 0.09–47.18 ng/dL) than did dogs with idiopathic pericardial effusion (0.05 ng/dL; range: 0.03–0.09 ng/dL).

Differential diagnosis

- Mesothelioma.

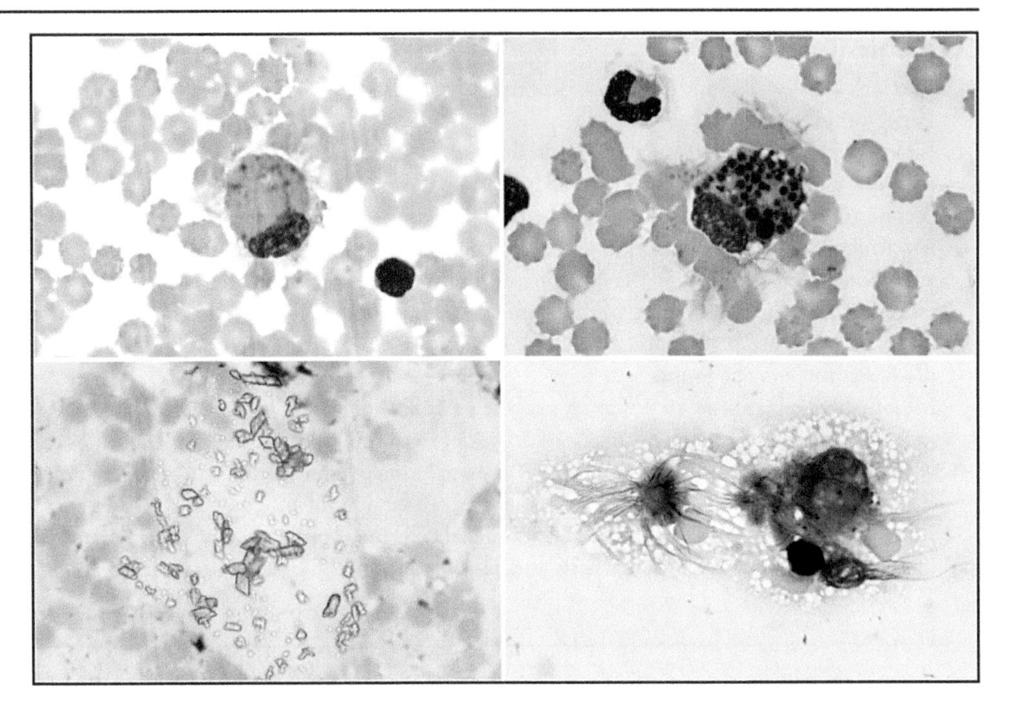

Fig. 3.50. Pericardial haemorrhagic effusion. Erythrophagia (top left); macrophage containing haemosiderin granules (top right); golden rhomboid shaped haematoidin crystals (bottom left); golden strand-like haematoidin crystals (bottom right). Wright-Giemsa.

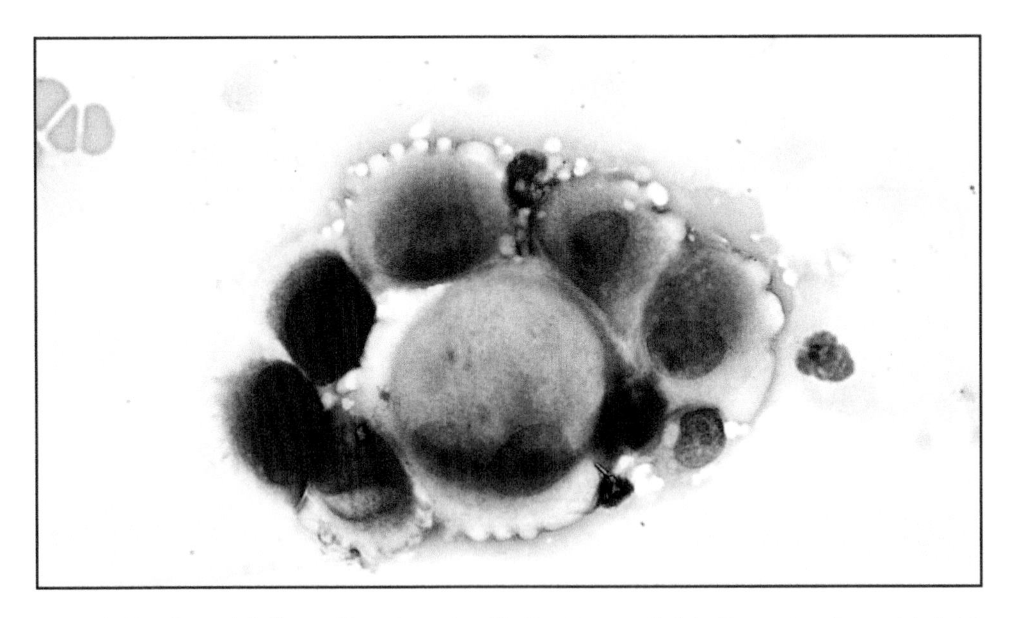

Fig. 3.51. Dog. Pericardial effusion. Idiopathic pericarditis. Reactive mesothelial cells, occasionally associated with haematoidin crystals. Wright-Giemsa.

Chylous effusion

- Leakage of lipid-rich lymph into the pericardial sac.
- Rare condition described in several canine cases in veterinary literature.
- Often believed idiopathic.
- Cytological features and diagnostic criteria are similar to those described in chylothorax and chyloabdomen.

3.8.5 Neoplastic pericardial effusions (effusions from cell exfoliation)

- Tumours of the heart and pericardium are rare with a reported incidence in dogs between 0.12% and 4.33%. They occur most frequently in adult/old dogs, with the exception of lymphoma, which may also affect younger patients.
- They can be benign or malignant, primary or metastatic, with haemangiosarcoma being the most common cardiac tumour in dogs, followed by aortic body tumours (chemodectoma and paraganglioma), lymphoma and ectopic thyroid carcinoma. Other tumours that have been rarely described in this location include cardiac myxoma/myxosarcoma, pericardial mesothelioma, mast cell tumour, rhabdomyoma/rhabdomyosarcoma, osteosarcoma, chondrosarcoma, fibroma/sarcoma, leiomyoma/sarcoma, melanoma, blastoma, granular cell tumour and lipoma.
- In cats, cardiac tumours are much less common than in dogs and tend to be malignant. Two retrospective studies on feline cardiac tumours found lymphoma to be the most common neoplasia in this district.
- In dogs, clinical signs associated to cardiac tumours can vary from mild to severe and can sometimes be life threatening. They are independent of the tumour type and are generally caused by altered cardiovascular function secondary to the mass effect and/or local haemorrhage/effusion into the pericardial space.
- Over-represented canine breeds: German Shepherd dogs, Golden Retrievers, Boxers, Bulldogs, Boston Terriers, Scottish Terriers, English Setters, Afghan Hounds, Flat-Coated Retriever, Irish Water Spaniels, French Bulldogs and Salukis.

Only the tumours that are most common and may occasionally exfoliate in the pericardial fluid are described in the section below.

Pearls and Pitfalls

Based on a large retrospective study on 259 dogs with PE, it has been shown that echocardiographic evidence of a mass did not result in a significant increase in the diagnostic utility of cytology of the pericardial fluid.

Haemagiosarcoma

Clinical features

- Most frequent primary tumour of the heart in the canine species. In the cat, it is uncommon.
- Most commonly arising from the right atrium and forming a mass. It can present as a solitary tumour or occur concurrently with a splenic mass.
- Age: 7–15 years old (dog).
- Clinical signs are commonly due to cardiac tamponade secondary to PE.

- Diagnosis is only rarely achieved via cytology of the primary mass due to the high frequency of non-representative/haemodiluted samples and potential risk (arrhythmia, haemorrhage). According to one study that evaluated the diagnostic utility of pericardial fluid analysis, false negative results were very frequent (74%) in particular when the HCT of the effusion was > 10%.
- A study has shown that dogs with cardiac haemangiosarcoma have higher plasma cTnI than dogs with idiopathic effusions. A plasma cTnI concentration >0.25 ng/ml had a sensitivity of 81% and specificity of 100% for cardiac haemangiosarcoma.
- Over-represented breeds: Golden Retrievers and German Shepherd Dogs.

Cytological features

- Pericardial effusion is frequently haemorrhagic and neoplastic cells often do not exfoliate in the fluid.
- Background: large amount of blood.
- Nucleated cells include mixed blood-derived leucocytes, macrophages and mesothelial cells. In more chronic effusions, macrophages and sometimes mesothelial cells may contain haemosiderin granules and/or haematoidin crystals.
- When the neoplastic cells are present in the cytology preparations, their morphology would mirrors that of haemangiosarcomas arising in other locations.
- Cells are variably spindle shaped and can exfoliate singly or in small aggregates. They have large, round-to-oval nuclei, coarse chromatin and variably prominent nucleoli. The cytoplasm is basophilic and can contain small clear vacuoles. Erythrophagocytosis may occur. Cells margins are often poorly defined. Anisokaryosis and anisocytosis are often prominent, and mitoses might be seen.

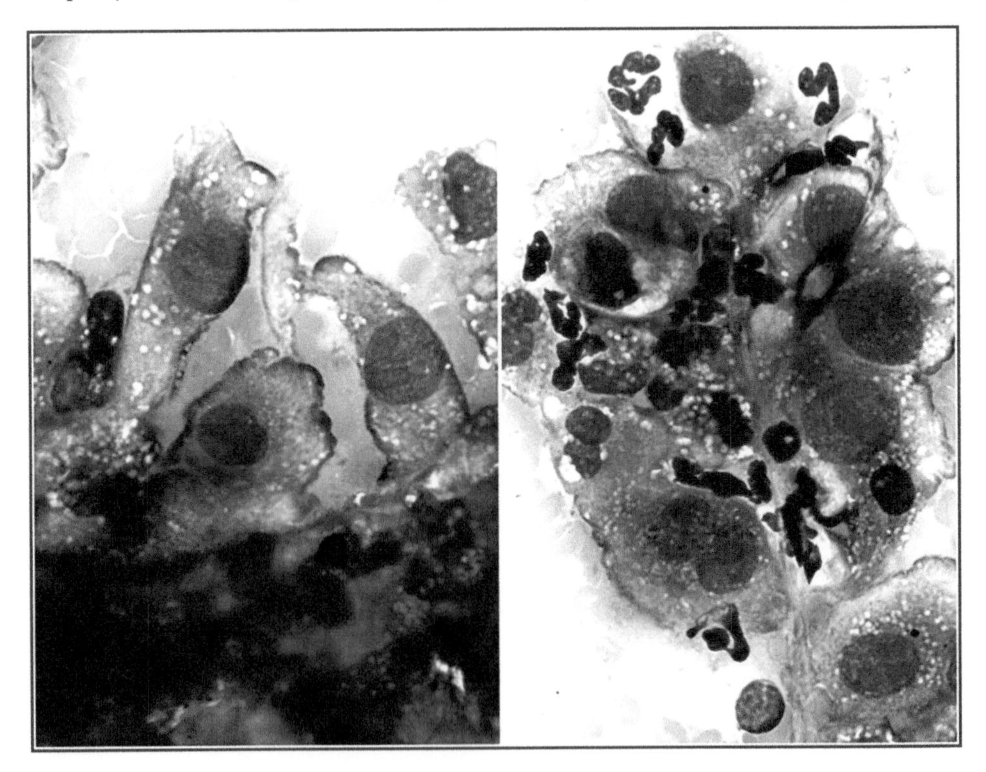

Fig. 3.52. Dog. Pericardial effusion. Cardiac haemangiosarcoma. Neoplastic cells are plump-spindle shaped and display marked atypia. They are admixed with a few inflammatory cells. Wright-Giemsa. (*Courtesy of Giuseppe Menga.*)

Lymphoma

Clinical features

- Most common cardiac tumour in the cat, infrequently reported in dogs.
- Age: 2–10 years. Median age: 5 years (cat).
- According to a retrospective study on seven feline pericardial lymphoma, 6/7 patients were FeLV positive.
- It may cause discrete masses or may form more diffuse lesions.
- It can be associated with PE, in which case the clinical signs are most typically caused by cardiac tamponade.

Cytological features

- Background: variably haemodiluted.
- Neoplastic lymphoid cells can exfoliate in the effusion and a diagnosis can be reached on cytology.
- Lymphoid cells are mostly intermediate to large in size.
- Nuclei are mainly medium-large and eccentric with stippled chromatin. Round nucleoli may be visible.
- The cytoplasm is usually scant to moderate, variably basophilic, with distinct borders and may contain clear intracytoplasmic vacuoles or fine azurophilic granules (LGL lymphoma).
- Mitotic figures may be seen.

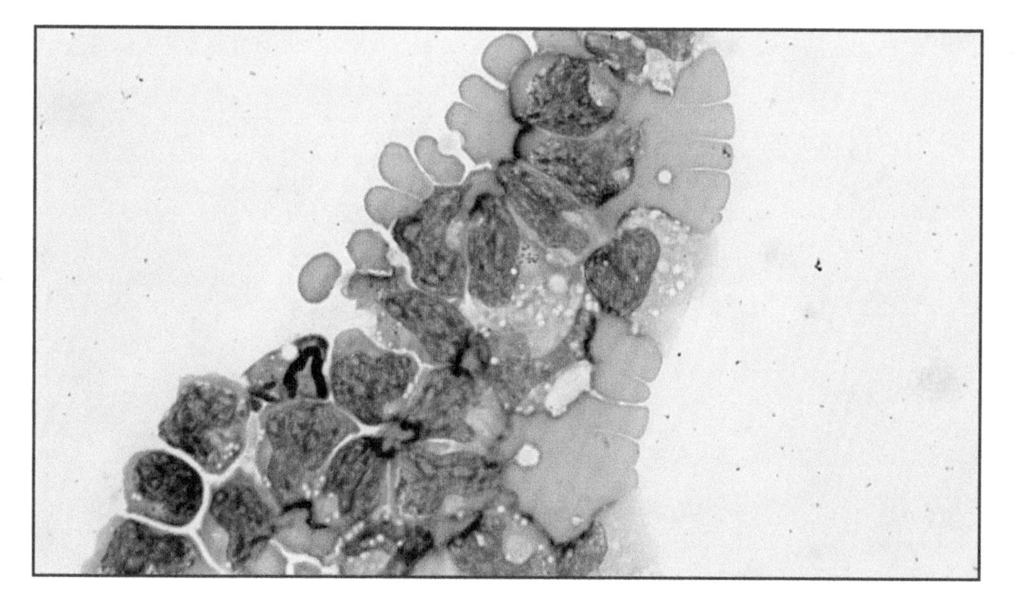

Fig. 3.53. Dog. Pericardial effusion. Large granular lymphocyte lymphoma. Neoplastic cells are large, monomorphic and contain fine azurophilic granules. Wright-Giemsa.

Further reading

Amati, M., Venco, L., Roccabiaca, P., Santagostino, S.F. and Bertazzolo, W. (2014) Pericardial lymphoma in 7 cats. *Journal of Feline Medicine and Surgery* 16(6), 507–512.

Chun, R., Kellihan, H.B., Henik, R.A. and Stepien, R.L. (2010) Comparison of plasma cardiac troponin I concentrations among dogs with cardiac hemangiosarcoma, noncardiac hemangiosarcoma, other neoplasms, and pericardial effusion of nonhemangiosarcoma origin. *Journal of American Veterinary Medical Association* 237(7), 806–811.

Jall, D.J., Shofer, F., Meier, C.K. and Sleeper, M.M. (2007) Pericardial effusion in cats: a retrospective study of clinical findings and outcome in 146 cats. *Journal of Veterinary Internal Medicine* 21(5), 1002–1007.

Treggiari, E., Pedro, B., Dukes-McEwan, J., Gelzer, A.R. and Blackwood, L. (2017) A descriptive review of cardiac tumours in dogs and cats. *Veterinary Comparative Oncology* 15(2), 273–288.

4 Synovial Fluid

4.1 Anatomy, Physiology and Composition

The articular or joint capsule is a fibrous structure richly supplied with blood vessels, nerves and lymphatics that encases the joint. It consists of two layers:

- Fibrous layer (outer) – consists of white fibrous tissue, known as the capsular ligament.
- Synovial layer (inner) or synovium – a highly vascularized layer of serous connective tissue.

The synovium (also called synovial membrane) is a specialized connective soft-tissue membrane with highly permeable fenestrated capillaries that lines the inner surface of the articular capsule and the cartilage, which covers the two bone ends. It contains three main cell types:

- Type A cells: histiocytic-macrophagic cells with phagocytic activity.
- Type B cells: secretory fibroblast-like synoviocytes producing most of the constituents of the synovial fluid responsible for its viscosity.
- Type C cells: transitional or stem cell-like cells with properties of both A and B cells.

The synovial fluid contained within the synovium is an ultrafiltrate of blood from synovial vessels supplemented by molecules produced by the B cells. It is a hypocellular fluid, mainly composed of hyaluronic acid, lubricin (water soluble glycoprotein), proteinases and collagenases.

The synovial fluid has three main functions:

- Lubrication of joint surfaces.
- Supplying nutrients and oxygen to articular chondrocytes.
- Removal of waste products and carbon dioxide.

4.2 Sampling Techniques

Indications

Arthrocentesis is commonly performed to investigate swollen joints. However, this diagnostic procedure is also performed in the presence of periodic shifting lameness, stiff or abnormal limb function associated with fever, joint deformity associated with lameness, pyrexia or leucocytosis of unknown origin, even if joint disease is not apparent. It is also indicated to monitor response to therapy for arthritis.

Materials

- Clippers, disinfectant and sterile gloves.
- Syringe: 2.5–5 ml depending on the size of the patient.

DOI: 10.1079/9781789247787.0004

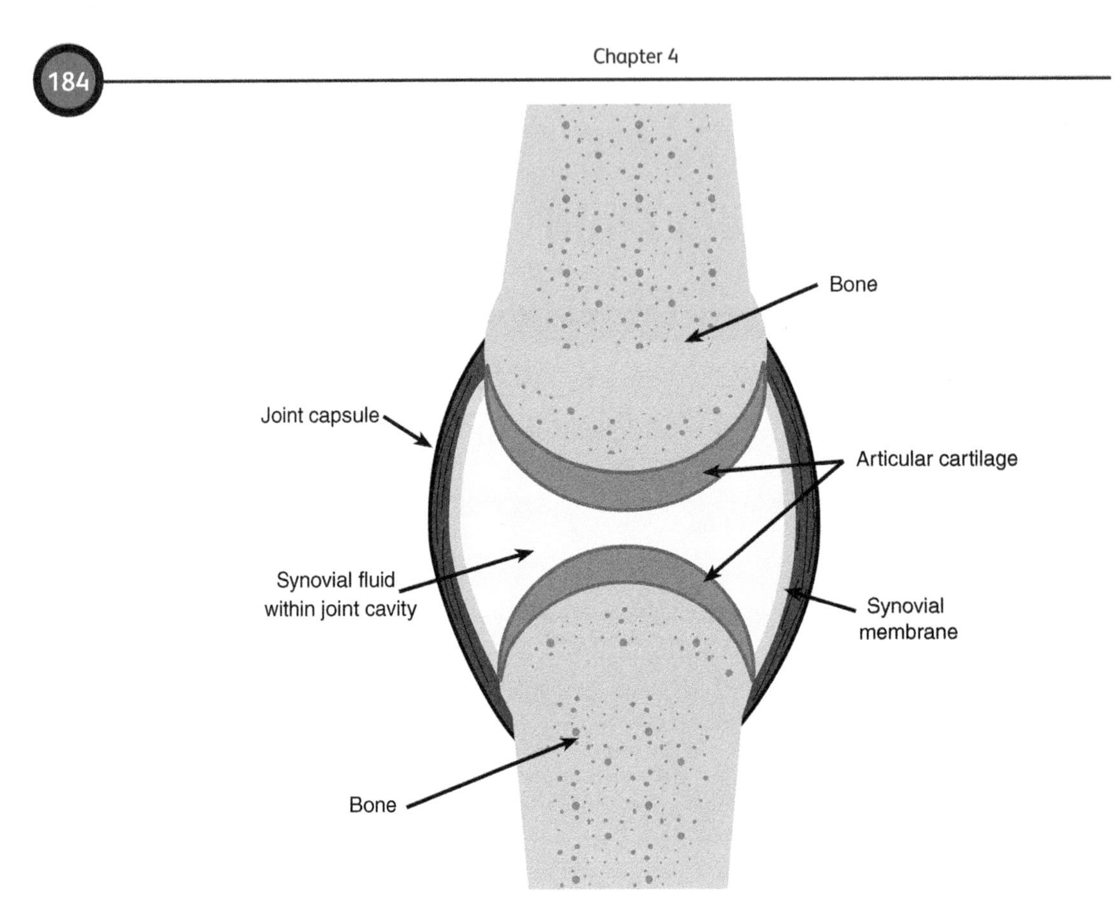

Fig. 4.1. Joint anatomy. (*Courtesy of Nic Ilchyshyn.*)

- Needle: the size of the needle depends on the size of the patient and deepness of the joint cavity. The following are most commonly used:
  - 21–22 G (most dogs) to 23–25 G (smaller joints or smaller dogs and cats).
  - 0.5–1.5 in (most joints) to 3 in (hip joint).
- Tubes:
  - EDTA tube for cytology and total cell count. This can also be used for PCR testing.
  - Plain tube for total protein measurement and microbiology.
  - Heparin tube: for mucin clot test.
- Glass slides:
- Enrichment media and/or blood culture bottles for microbiology.

Patient preparation

- Use of chemical restraint is common and aims to avoid excessive movement during the procedure. This is under clinician discretion and largely depends on the temperament of the animal and tolerance for discomfort.
- A lateral recumbency is usually adopted, and the joint to be sampled is positioned uppermost. Palpation of the joint during manual flexion and extension helps identifying the insertion point.
- The area of insertion of the needle should be clipped and aseptically cleaned.

Technique

Collection of synovial fluid varies to some degree depending on the joint sampled. General indications are listed below:

- Identify the appropriate insertion site.
- Attach the needle to the syringe and pass it gently through the joint until correct position is reached. Pay attention not to scratch the articular surface during the advancement of the needle.
- Aspirate the synovial fluid and then release the suction before needle and syringe are withdrawn from the joint, in order to minimize blood contamination. Selected joints (e.g. shoulder and stifle) have higher potential space for fluid accumulation than others (e.g. carpus and tarsus).

Complications (rare)

- Cartilage injury.
- Iatrogenic infections.
- Iatrogenic haemorrhage.

Contraindications

- Cellulitis/dermatitis overlying the joint of interest.
- Bacteriaemia.
- Severe coagulopathy.

Pearls and Pitfalls

- At least four joints should be sampled whenever there is the suspicion of immune-mediated polyarthritis, favouring tarsal and carpal joints, even in the absence of detectable swelling or pain.
- Diagnostic imaging should be performed before arthrocentesis to avoid potential confounding factors (e.g. iatrogenic haematomas and haemoarthrosis).
- In case only a limited amount of synovial fluid is collected, cytological examination (direct smear) should be prioritized over other tests.

4.3 Sample Handling, Analysis and Slide Preparation

4.3.1 Sample handling

- Once the synovial fluid has been collected, this should be analysed as soon as possible. However, this type of sample is relatively stable when stored at 4°C, at least for the first 24 h.
- The sample should be collected, divided and aliquoted in the following tubes:
  - EDTA tube: used mainly for cytology preparations. The anticoagulant avoids clotting formation and preserves cell morphology. It is also used for cell count and PCR testing when required.
  - Plain sterile tube: used for measurement of total protein. It is also used for culture and sensitivity testing.

- Heparin tube: preferred sample for mucin clot test.
- Enrichment media and blood culture bottles: used for bacterial culture as they increase the likelihood of retrieving organisms.

4.3.2 Sample analysis

Routine synovial fluid examination includes:

- Macroscopic evaluation.
- Total cell count.
- Total protein concentration.
- Mucin clot test.
- Cytological evaluation.
- Other tests.

Macroscopic evaluation

The fluid is first grossly evaluated for volume, colour, turbidity and viscosity. In normal instances, synovial fluid should be present in very small amounts and be clear to straw colour and reasonably viscous.

- Volume:
  - It depends on multiple factors including the size of the animal, the joint from which it is collected, and the distension of the joint capsule.
  - It varies from a few drops in cats and small dogs to higher volumes in larger patients, especially in case of articular diseases characterized by joint effusions.
  - The joint capsule should not be drained.
- Colour and turbidity:
  - When pink or red, it indicates the presence of erythrocytes or free haemoglobin. This may be due to genuine haemorrhage or blood contamination during the sampling. In case of iatrogenic haemorrhage, sudden appearance and uneven distribution of blood in the synovial fluid during aspiration is usually noted.
  - A golden-yellow colour (xanthochromia) is usually associated with prior haemorrhage.
  - A white or opaque/turbid colour usually suggests increased cellularity. This may also be accompanied by the presence of suspended flecks of material.
- Viscosity:
  - It correlates with the concentration and quality of mucinous proteins within the fluid. It can be assessed subjectively by pulling a small amount of fluid from a tube with a wooden stick or by stretching small amounts of fluid between two fingers. If it forms a long string before breaking, it is considered normal. It is usually reported as normal, decreased or markedly decreased. A viscometer can also be used.
  - Reduced viscosity is often associated with inflammation (enzymatic hyaluronic acid degradation), increased leakage of serum or joints lavage and decreased production of hyaluronic acid and lubricin by injured synovial cells. EDTA may reduce sample viscosity.
  - Sample viscosity may also be subjectively assessed when examining the cytological preparations. This will be discussed later in the chapter.

Total cell count

- It is performed on the EDTA sample after gently mixing the fluid.
- It can be performed using a manual counting chamber or an automated haematology analyser. There may be some discrepancy between the two methods, but this is not significant enough to affect clinical interpretation.

- Nucleated cell count may be significantly affected by fluid viscosity and consequent cell clumping; therefore, incubation for 5–30 min with hyaluronidase (a few drops of a 150 IU/ml solution) might be required for the most viscous samples. The obtained cell count should be corrected for the dilution factor due to the addition of hyaluronidase. Automated methods have a higher limit of detection for erythrocyte count (usually 10,000 cells/μl) than manual methods but obtaining an accurate erythrocyte count is clinically not very relevant.
- Cell count may also be estimated when examining the cytological preparations. A manual differential cell count on a minimum of 100 cells may also be performed when required.
- Normal canine joints fluids are expected to have <3000 nucleated cells/μl, but cellularity is often lower, in particular in cats (<1000 nucleated cells/μl). This corresponds to one or two cells per high-power field (40X) when examined on the microscope, although it depends on the thickness of the smear.

Total protein concentration

- It can be assessed with a refractometer, but sample viscosity may be a problem; therefore, quantitative biochemical assay may be preferred and it is also a more accurate method.
- Normal protein values are generally <25–30 g/l but can be occasionally higher.
- Inflammation is a common cause for elevation of total protein. This may also be spuriously high when measurement is performed from EDTA tube, especially if a short sample is submitted.

Mucin clot test

- This test, not routinely performed in most diagnostic laboratories, aims to assess the hyaluronic acid quantity and quality.
- It is performed on test tubes or glass slides by adding and gently mixing one or two drops of undiluted synovial fluid (preferably from heparin tube) to four to eight drops of 2% acetic acid, and then assess clot formation. Reduced clot formation (friable clot or no clot formation) can occur with any type of inflammation due to decreased quality/amounts of hyaluronic acid as a consequence of the proteases released by the neutrophils.

Cytological evaluation

- Direct slides are prepared preferably from the EDTA sample.
- Smears should be spread as thinly as possible and dried rapidly.
- Slides are stained by any type of Romanowsky stain.
- Concentrated preparation may also be considered, in particular when the cell count is very low or when infectious agents are suspected.
- Cytological evaluation aims to assess the following:
  - Total cell count (estimate).
  - Differential cell count.
  - Morphology of the cellular elements.
  - Presence of infectious agents.

4.4 Normal Cytology of the Synovial Fluid

The cytological features of normal synovial fluid samples are summarized below:

- Cellularity: the body of the direct smear usually contains up to two cells per field at high magnification (40×).
- Background: usually amphophilic, granular or forming crescents to reflect the high-protein content. Erythrocytes and nucleated cells may be arranged in rows (windrowing arrangement).

- Erythrocytes: absent or present as the result of iatrogenic haemorrhage at the time of sampling. In iatrogenic haemorrhage, platelets may also be observed.
- Nucleated cells:
  - Based on a manual differential count of at least 100 nucleated cells, the following cell types may be recorded:
    - Dogs:
      - Large mononuclear cells predominate (60-97%).
      - Of these, <10% may be vacuolated.
      - Lymphocytes: present in variable percentages.
      - Neutrophils: <5-10% (in non haemodiluted samples).
      - Eosinophils: absent.
      - Rare spindloid/synovial lining cells.
    - Cats:
      - Large mononuclear cells predominate (61-100%) and are mainly large and non vacuolated.
      - Neutrophils: <5%.
      - Rare spindle/synovial lining cells.

Pearls and Pitfalls

With delayed processing or with pre-treatment of fluid with hyaluronidase, the vacuolated large mononuclear cells may increase in percentage (up to 14–18%).

- Incidental sampling of underlying bone structures may result in the presence of occasional osteoblasts.

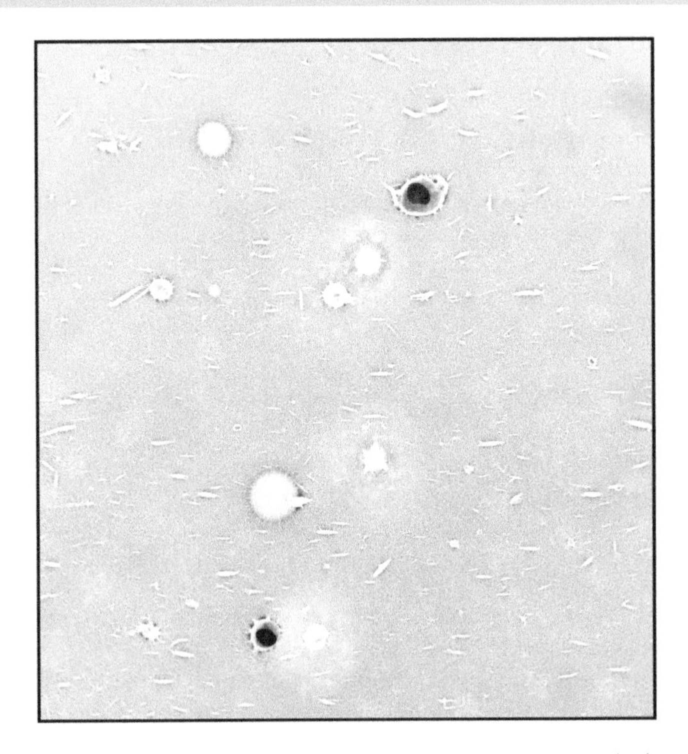

Fig. 4.2. Dog. Synovial fluid. Rare large mononuclear cells on granular proteinaceous background, considered unremarkable findings. Wright-Giemsa.

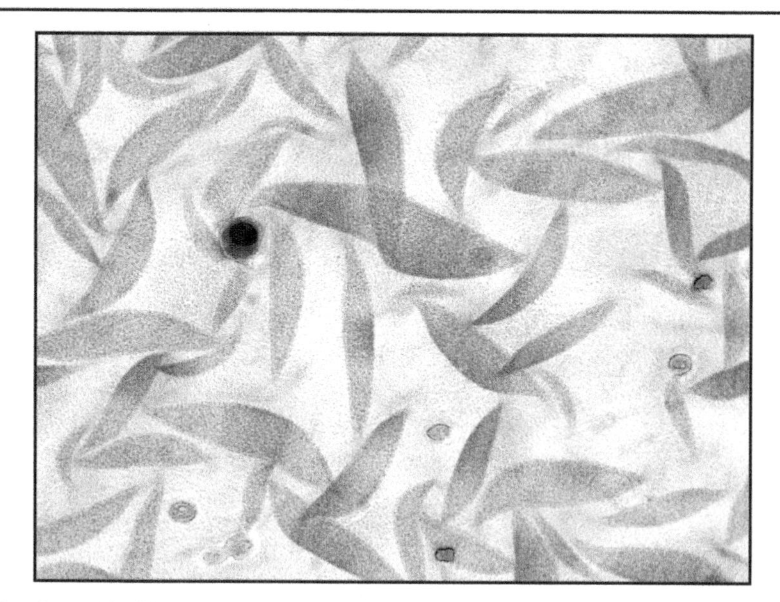

Fig. 4.3. Dog. Synovial fluid. Proteinaceous material in the background forming characteristic crescents. Wright-Giemsa.

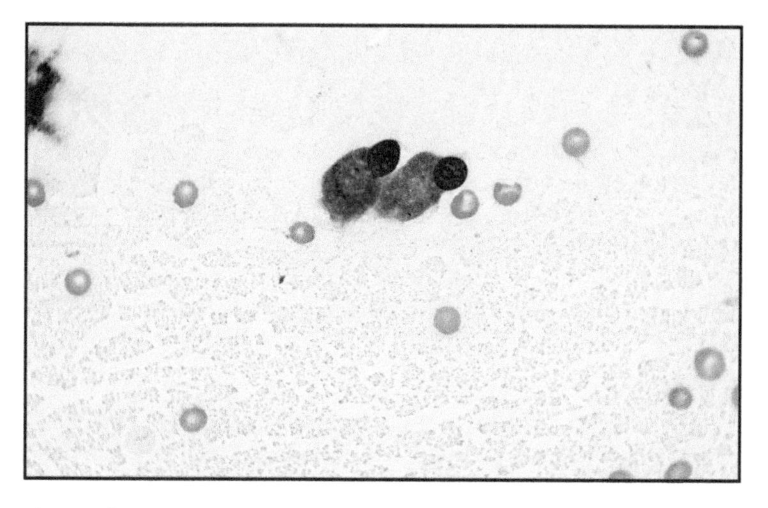

Fig. 4.4. Dog. Synovial fluid. Osteoblasts as result of accidental sampling from near bone structures. Wright-Giemsa. Note their typical deeply basophilic cytoplasm and their very eccentrically located round nuclei.

Further reading

Pacchiana, P.D., Gilley, R.S., Wallace, L.J., Hayden, D.W., Feeney, D.A. *et al.* (2004) Absolute and relative cell counts for synovial fluid from clinically normal shoulder and stifle joints in cats. *Journal of American Veterinary Medical Association* 225, 1866–1870.

4.5 Degenerative Joint Disease

Pathologic process characterized by degeneration of the articular cartilage, with secondary changes in associated joint structures.

Clinical features

- Very common form of arthritis in dogs of any age and breed; likely underdiagnosed in cats due to the lack in clinical signs.
- Chronic condition characterized by loss of joint cartilage, thickening of the joint capsule and new bone formation around it.
- Well-established causes in dogs (see full list in the table below) and mainly related to primary and specific problems with selected joints. In cats, the primary cause often cannot be found.
- Clinical signs vary depending on the severity of the disease and the joints involved. They most commonly include reluctance to exercise, decrease in overall activity, stiffness, lameness, inability to jump, changes in gait and pain on manipulation with possible behavioural changes (aggression, discomfort). In cats, clinical signs are often less obvious.
- In dogs and cats, the appendicular joints most commonly affected are hips, stifles and elbows.
- Diagnosis of DJD is usually made by a combination of history, physical examination and various imaging modalities.
- Progressive disease and treatment options can only aim to slow down the process.
- Over-represented canine breeds:
  - Rottweiler, Golden Retriever and Labrador Retriever, due to increased risk of cruciate ligament rupture.
  - Larger breeds such as Mastiff, Boxer, Italian Corso, German Shepherd Dog, Golden, Labrador Retriever and Bernese Mountain dog, due to higher risk of hip and elbow dysplasia.
  - Smaller breeds such as Pomeranian, Chihuahua, Yorkshire Terrier and French Bulldog, due to higher odds of developing patellar luxation.

Causes

- Primary DJD: largely idiopathic, but age and obesity can play a role. It appears to be more common in cats; however, it is also possible that unrecognized factors may be responsible for this pathology in this species.
- Secondary DJD: triggered by an underlying pathology or injury. It represents the most common form in dogs. Primary causes include:
  - Osteochondritis dissecans.
  - Elbow dysplasia.
  - Hip dysplasia.
  - Avascular necrosis of the femoral head.
  - Chronic patellar luxation.
  - Joint instability (e.g. caused by ligament damage).
  - Chronic bicipital tenosynovitis.
  - Trauma.
  - Nutritional disorders.

- Genetic disorders (e.g. osteochondrodysplasia and mucopolysaccharidoses).
- Underlying neoplasms.
- Inflammatory arthropathies.

Cytological features

- Fluid is clear; viscosity and total protein are within the reference range to slightly decreased. Cellularity is usually normal or variably increased (1000–10,000 cells/µl).
- Background: clear-to-pale amphophilic-basophilic and finely granular (proteinaceous).
- Red blood cells may be present as a result of iatrogenic haemorrhage or concurrent genuine haemorrhage.
- Mild increase in mononuclear cells, likely a mixture of macrophages, synovial lining cells and lymphocytes. A significant percentage of large mononuclear cells (>10%) is often moderately to heavily vacuolated. In some cases, the cellularity may not be increased, but a high proportion of vacuolated mononuclear cells is found.
- Neutrophils are generally within reference limit (<5–10%) but, in some cases, they may be mildly increased in percentage (e.g. ruptured cranial cruciate ligament).
- Small lymphocytes may also increase.
- Osteoclasts and chondrocytes may be found, indicating erosion of cartilage and exposure of underlying subchondral bone.

Differential diagnoses

- Rheumatoid arthritis
- Septic arthritis treated chronically or with suboptimal doses of antibiotics
- Waxing and waning immune-mediated polyarthritis (usually accompanied by increased numbers of neutrophils)
- Calicivirus infection (cat – one case reported in literature)

Pearls and Pitfalls

The terms osteoarthrosis and osteoarthritis are often used interchangeably to refer to DJD. Scientific literature in English language is dominated by the use of the term '*osteoarthritis*' for the most common pathological condition, namely DJD. Strictly taken, this application is incorrect because the suffix '-itis' implies the presence of inflammation and this should not be a primary feature of DJD. *Osteoarthrosis*, on the other hand, should be considered a more appropriate term, as it indicates a degenerative process. However, recent studies have shown that inflammation of the synovium plays an important role in DJD pathogenesis, refuting the concept expressed above. The acronym OA often used to refer to DJD seems to be a *salvage* solution of the existing terminological disturbance.

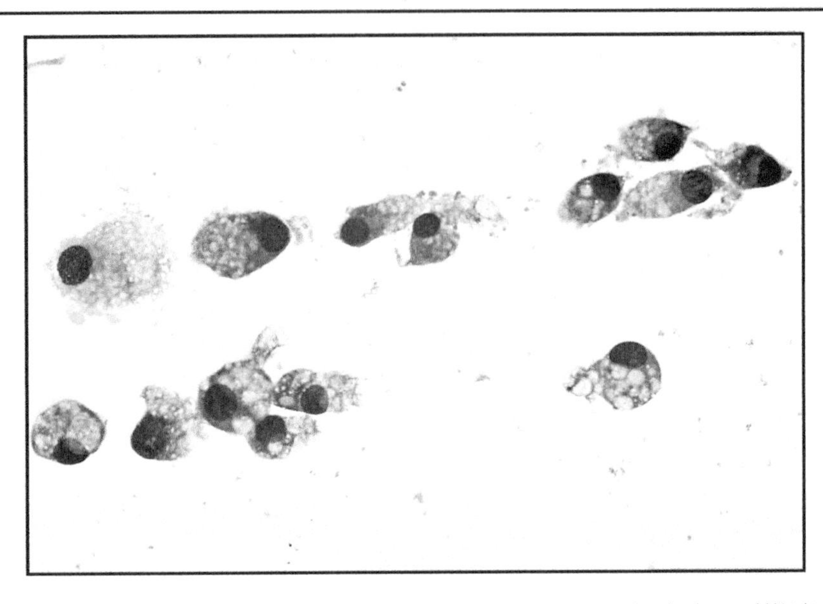

Fig. 4.5. Dog. Synovial fluid. DJD. Vacuolated large mononuclear cells lining in rows, on a clear background. Wright-Giemsa.

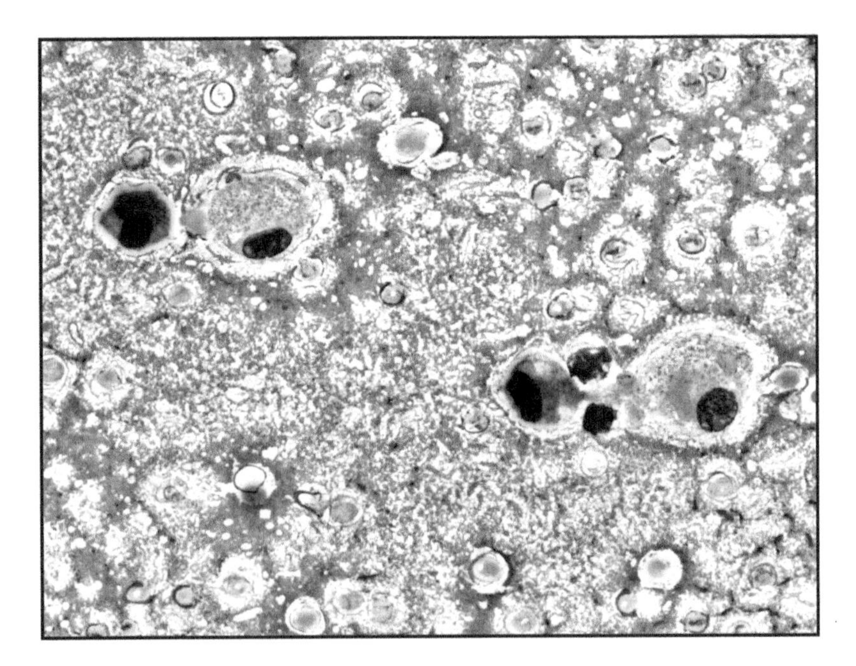

Fig. 4.6. Dog. Synovial fluid. DJD. Vacuolated large mononuclear cells on a granular proteinaceous background with occasional red blood cells. Wright-Giemsa.

Further reading

Anderson, K.L., Zulch, H., O'Neill, D.G., Meeson, R.L. and Collins, L.M. (2020) Risk factors for canine osteoarthritis and its predisposing arthropathies: a systematic review. *Frontiers Veterinary Science* 7, 1–16.
Berembaum, F. (2013) Osteoarthritis as an inflammatory disease (osteoarthritis is not osteoarthrosis!). *Osteoarthritis Cartilage* 21(1), 16–21.
Lascelles, B.D.X. (2010) Feline degenerative joint disease. *Veterinary Surgery* 39, 2–13.

4.6 Inflammatory Joint Disease

Also known as arthritis, it is an inflammatory process that involves the joint structures. It can be due to infectious or non-infectious causes, which differ for clinical presentation, treatment and prognosis. There is some degree of overlapping in the cytological presentation of these conditions. The final diagnosis relies on the combination of the clinical picture and results of diagnostic investigations. In dogs, unlike in cats, primary immune-mediated disorders are much more common than infectious causes.

Causes:

- Infectious:
  - Bacteria (more common).
  - Viruses.
  - Rickettsia.
  - Fungi/yeasts.
  - Protozoa.
  - Parasites.
- Non-infectious:
  - Non-erosive immune-mediated arthritis (more common).
  - Erosive arthritis.

4.6.1 Infectious causes

4.6.1.1 Bacterial arthritis

Clinical features

- Most common form of infectious arthritis in both dogs and cats.
- Often follows an infecting penetrating wound or joint surgery, the latter being particularly common in dogs. Haematogenous spread is also possible but less frequent.
- In dogs, reported predisposing risk factors for septic arthritis include pre-existing osteoarthritis, stifle surgery, comorbidities (e.g. urinary tract infection, diabetes mellitus, dermatopathy and bacterial endocarditis) and prosthetic joints. These may affect the success of the therapy and may increase the risk of recurrences.
- Usually monoarticular with acute onset. In case of haematogenous spread, multiple joints might be affected. The latter is a rare event and is seen mostly in neonates or immunocompromised patients. If an inflammatory polyarthritis is diagnosed, an immune-mediated component of the arthritis is most likely, which may also be associated with underlying infectious causes.
- Most typical clinical signs include heat, swelling and pain in the affected joints and reluctancy to walk. Animals may also be systemically ill, febrile, anorexic and depressed. Polyarticular arthritis due to haematogenous spread is more commonly seen in immunocompromised patients and in selected conditions including bacterial endocarditis and urinary tract infections.
- More commonly affected joints:
  - Dog: stifle and elbow.
  - Cat: carpus, hock and interphalangeal joints.
- Male, large and giant breed adult dogs are most commonly affected; however, this condition can be seen in animals of any age, sex and breed.
- Early diagnosis and treatment are crucial, as irreversible damage to the articular cartilage can occur. Therapeutic management of septic arthritis is usually successful, involving various approaches including antibiotic therapy, arthrocentesis, joint lavage and synovectomy.

Cytological features

- Fluid is often cloudy/turbid. Total protein is usually elevated, and viscosity of the fluid may be reduced. Cellularity is often markedly increased (>50,000 cells/μl).
- Background: clear to variably pink and finely granular (proteinaceous). The pink colour may be less homogenous and intense with clear spaces, as a result of the reduced viscosity.
- Red blood cells may be present as a result of iatrogenic haemorrhage or genuine concurrent haemorrhage.
- Most nucleated cells are neutrophils. Occasionally but not always, neutrophils show signs of degeneration including swollen and pale nuclei with loss of typical nuclear lobulation, and loss of definition of cytoplasmic borders (karyolysis).
- Bacteria (rods and/or cocci) may be seen. When found intracellularly, a septic arthritis is confirmed.

Selected bacteria are recognized as the most common causes of septic arthritis. These include:

- Dog: *Staphylococcus* spp. (most frequently *S. pseudointermedius* and *S. aureus*, but with coagulase-negative *Staphylococci* also recovered), *Streptococcus* spp. (most frequently *Streptococcus canis* but also *S. equi* subsp. *zooepidemicus*), *Pasteurella* spp., *Pseudomonas aeruginosa*, *Bacillus* spp., *Erysipelothrix rhusiopathie*, *Enteroccoccus faecalis*, *Borrelia burgdorferi*, *Bartonella* spp., *Corynebacterium* spp., *Salmonella* spp.
- Cat: *Pasteurella* spp., L-form bacteria, *Escherichia coli*, *Streptococcus* spp., *Bacteroides* spp., *Bartonella* spp. and *Mycoplasma* spp.

Staphylococcus spp. and *Streptococcus* spp.

Most common Gram-positive organisms recovered from septic arthritis in dogs. Both organisms can be part of normal commensal flora and become significant as part of systemic infections in young or immunocompromised patients, associated with penetrating wounds or extension of localized infection. A case series of kittens affected by *Streptococcus canis*, with severe systemic infection including polyarthritis, has been reported.

Pasteurella spp. and *Escherichia coli*

Gram-negative rod-shaped bacteria, common cause of cat bite wounds penetrating single joints, in particular the carpus, hock and interphalangeal joints. Cats often show systemic clinical signs.

Mycoplasma spp. (*M. gateae, M. felis*)

Bacteria generally with low pathogenic potential. They may be associated with erosive and non-erosive polyarthritis and tenosynovitis in cats and possibly in dogs, in particular in debilitated or immunosuppressed animals, as a result from haematogenous spread. These bacteria are not usually visible on cytological preparations. As these organisms may be challenging to recover on routine culture, specific culture with specialized media or alternative diagnostic methods (e.g. PCR) may be required for identification. In cats with suspected immune-mediated polyarthritis, specific diagnosis or empirical treatment should be considered ahead of immunosuppression.

L-forms of bacteria

Cell wall deficient bacteria similar to *Mycoplasma* spp. They are often the result of direct inoculation through bite wounds. They can cause fever, cellulitis and subcutaneous abscesses. Damage to articular cartilage and subchondral bone may occur. Cytology of synovial fluid shows mixed inflammation. Definitive diagnosis may require electron microscope evaluation. In cats, this type of infection should be considered when arthritis is associated with cellulitis, subcutaneous abscesses and draining tracts, but is culture-negative.

Borrelia burgdorferi (Lyme disease)

In dogs, the acute form usually manifests as polyarthritis. Fever may be present at this stage but not always. The lameness may affect the joint closer to the point of infection or cause shifting lameness. Despite the transient clinical signs of arthritis, inflammation of the tissues may persist. Coinfections with other arthropod-borne diseases should be considered. Organisms are almost never, if ever, detected by standard cytology.

Pearls and Pitfalls

- Bacterial organisms are rarely visualized on cytological preparations of septic arthritis cases. Therefore, their absence on cytology does not exclude sepsis. Culture also has low sensitivity when compared with clinical criteria. Collection of synovial fluid prior to starting antimicrobial therapy, use of blood culture vials or enrichment media and inclusion of anaerobic culture may increase the likelihood of identifying a bacterial organism. Some studies argue that culturing a biopsy of the synovium may yield growth when synovial fluid culture is negative. However, there is insufficient evidence to justify this more invasive procedure as routine practice.
- Antibiotic therapy prior to synovial fluid culture is associated with a higher incidence of false-negative results.
- All cats with inflammatory joint disease should be tested for feline immunodeficiency virus (FIV) and feline leukaemia virus (FeLV), since immunosuppression may be an important predisposing factor for infectious arthritis. FeLV has also been implicated in the development of periosteal proliferative polyarthritis. Immunocompromising conditions may also be considered in dogs with evidence of septic polyarthritis.
- Stain precipitate and granular proteinaceous background should be discriminated from bacteria, which usually are more regular in shape and size.
- Selected infectious agents may be impossible to detect with standard culture and may require special growing condition (e.g. *Mycoplasma* spp.). Molecular diagnostics (PCR) and serology are other possible considerations.

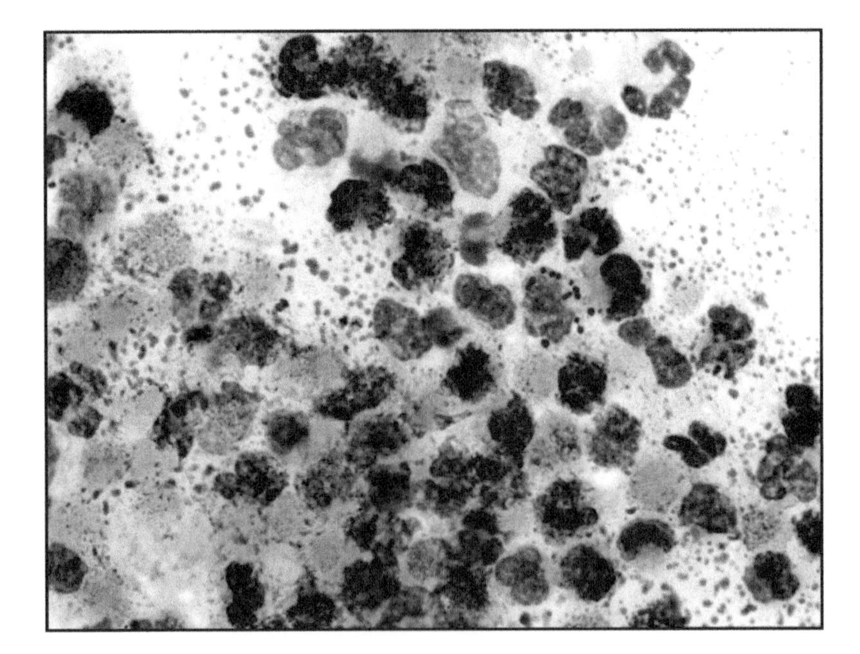

Fig. 4.7. Dog. Septic arthritis. Numerous neutrophils with marked signs of degeneration, occasionally containing intracellular bacteria (cocci). Wright-Giemsa.

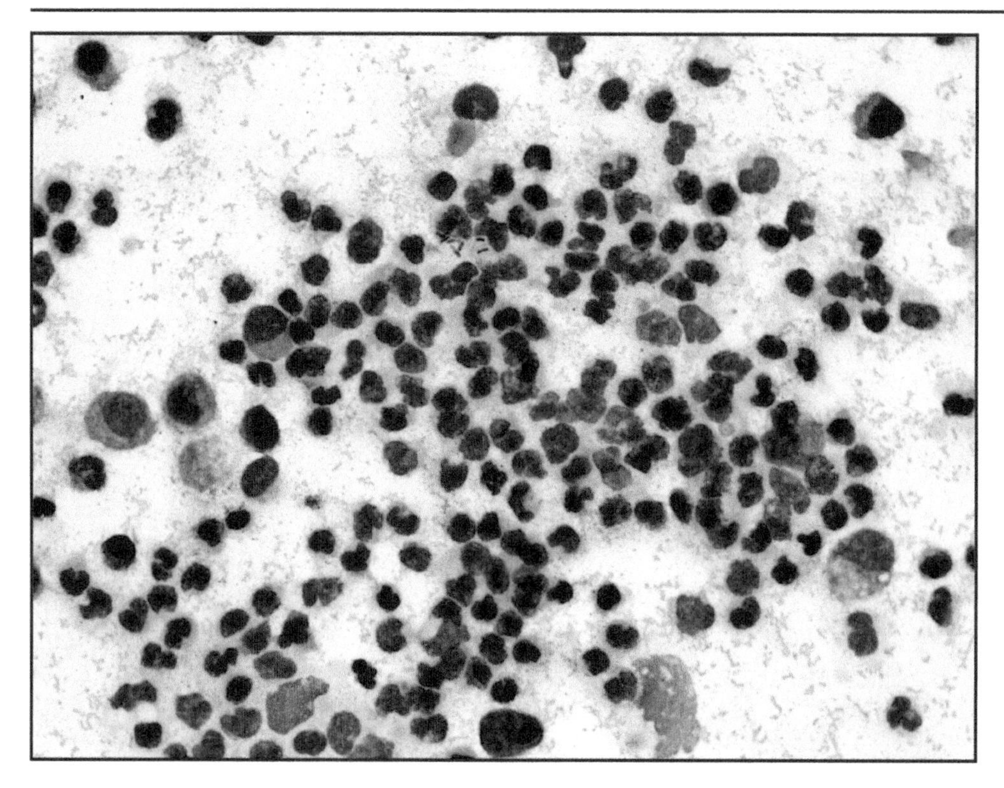

Fig. 4.8. Dog. Septic arthritis. Numerous neutrophils with signs of degeneration, occasionally containing intracellular bacteria (rods). Wright-Giemsa.

4.6.1.2 Rickettsia infections

Clinical features

- Infections caused by *Anaplasma* spp. and *Ehrlichia* spp. (*E. canis*, *E. chaffensis*, *E. ewingii*) have been reported in both dogs and cats. *Rickettsia rickettsii* (Rocky Mountain spotted fever) has been reported in dogs.
- Clinical signs may vary depending on the causative infectious agent and include fever, inappetence, lameness, thrombocytopenia and/or neurological signs.

Cytological features

- Cellularity is variably increased and total protein is usually elevated.
- Background: clear to pale basophilic, finely granular (proteinaceous) and variably haemodiluted.
- Cells are predominantly neutrophils. They generally do not show signs of degeneration.
- Intracellular morulae may be seen in a small percentage of canine cases, mostly in the leucocytes and very rarely in synovial cells. Morulae are round, lightly basophilic inclusions within the cytoplasm of neutrophils (*E. ewingii*, *A. phagocytophilum*) or mononuclear cells (*E. canis*).

Pearls and Pitfalls

- Cross-reactivity between organisms can occur on serology testing; therefore PCR testing is preferred.

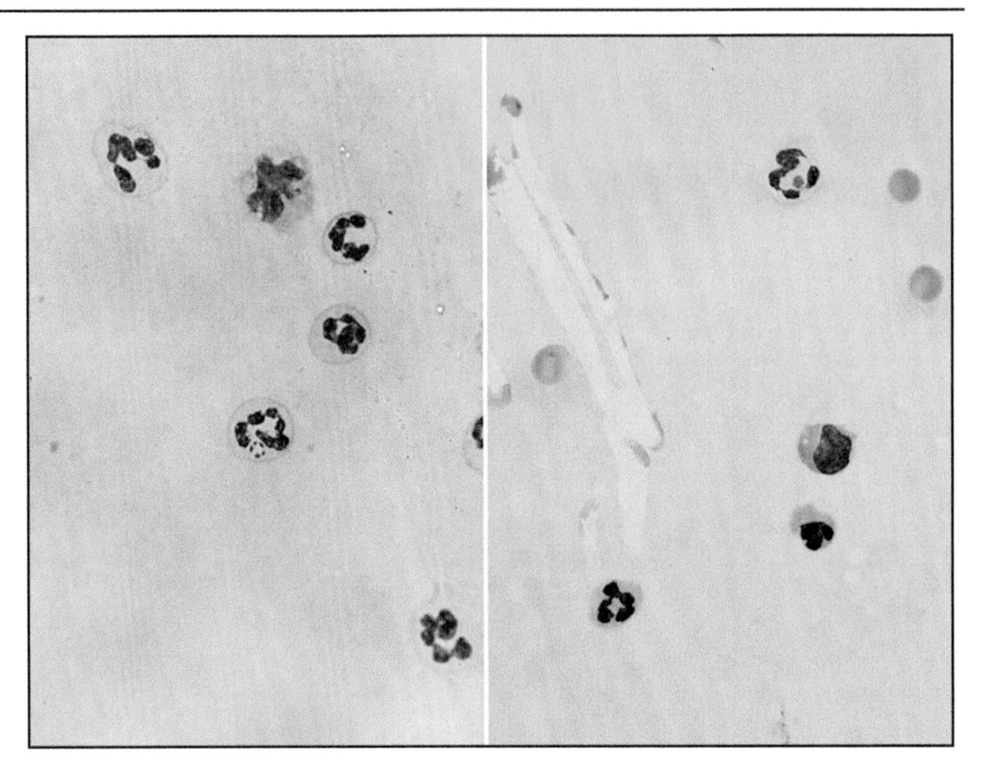

Fig. 4.9. Dog. Synovial fluid. (Left) ***Anaplasma phagocytophilum*** infection. Morula seen in a neutrophil. Wright-Giemsa. (*Courtesy of Ulrika Falkenö.*) (Right) ***Ehrlichia ewingii*** infection. Morula found in a neutrophil. Wright-Giemsa. (*Courtesy of Jim Meinkoth.*)

4.6.1.3 Viral infections

- Canine distemper virus (CDV) infection and vaccination have been proposed as possible triggers of immune-mediated polyarthritis.
- In cats, virus-induced polyarthritis has been mostly frequently described in association with feline calicivirus infection (FCV) or vaccination, but also with FeLV, feline syncytial forming virus (FeFV) and feline coronavirus (FCoV).
- FCV-induced arthritis is more common in young cats and has mostly been associated with field strains, but cases are also reported post first vaccination (unclear if due to field strains or altered strains from the modified live vaccine). The polyarthritis is self-limiting and may be associated or not with signs of systemic infection, including fever and other typical signs of calicivirus infection. Cellularity is increased with a predominance of mononuclear cells. Neutrophils may also be increased. Leucophagocytosis may be observed.

4.6.1.4 Fungal and yeasts infections

This may occur in dogs and cats as localized or more frequently as part of systemic infection. Possible organisms include *Blastomyces* spp., *Coccidioides immitis*, *Cryptococcus* spp., *Histoplasma capsulatum*, *Candida* spp. and *Aspergillus* spp. Neutrophilic inflammation is the most common cytological abnormality.

- Diagnosis of fungal arthritis can be straightforward when the organisms are detected on cytology, but their number may be low and not always be present in the sample.

- Testing for fungal disease in endemic areas should be considered when there is clinical suspicion due to presence of other consistent clinical signs of systemic infection, particularly ahead of immunosuppression.
- Use of serological techniques (e.g. antigen testing) or molecular techniques such as PCR can be considered in such cases.

4.6.1.5 Protozoal infections

Mono- or polyarthritis have been reported in dogs affected by canine visceral Leishmaniasis. These include erosive and non-erosive forms. Synovial fluid samples show increased numbers of nucleated cells, including neutrophils and mononuclear cells, sometimes containing *Leishmania* spp. amastigotes. Protozoal organisms are rarely found, and testing for suspected protozoal disease should be considered in endemic areas or in patients with relevant travel history.

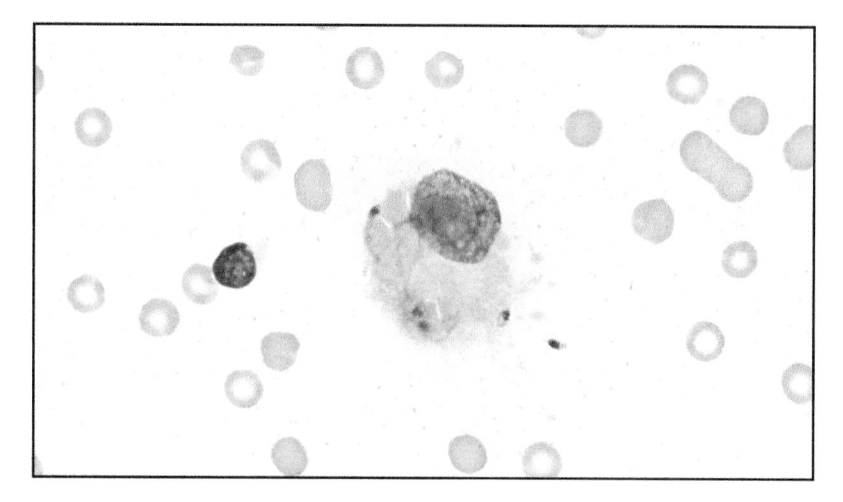

Fig. 4.10. Dog. *Leishmania* spp. infection from a synovial fluid. Large mononuclear cell containing *Leishmania* amastigotes. Wright-Giemsa. (*Courtesy of Alice Pastorello.*)

4.6.1.6 Parasite infestations

Microfilariae have been rarely observed in synovial fluid of dogs accompanied by mild, mononuclear to mixed inflammation.

Further reading

Lemetayer, J. and Taylor, S. (2014) Inflammatory joint disease in cats. Diagnostic approach and treatment. *Journal of Feline Medicine and Surgery* 16, 547–562.

Phillips, T.F. and Bleyaert, H.F. (2022) Retrospective evaluation of 103 cases of septic arthritis in dogs. *Veterinary Records* 190(5): e938.

4.6.2 Non-infectious causes

Clinical features

- Depending on the presence/absence of erosive lesions at the level of the articular cartilage, sterile arthritis can be classified in:
  - Erosive.
  - Non-erosive (more common).
- Commonly observed in dogs but rare in cats.
- Largely immune mediated, they are mainly caused by a type III hypersensitivity reaction with deposition of antigen-antibody complexes in the synovial blood vessels walls, eliciting a secondary inflammatory response. Emerging evidence confirms concurrent cell mediated or genetic mechanisms.
- Usually affecting multiple joints and with acute onset. The joints most commonly affected vary.
- Swelling, heat, pain in the affected joints and reluctancy to walk are common. Animals may also be systemically ill, febrile, anorexic and depressed. Neck or back pain may be present when associated with meningoencephalitis. Lymphadenopathy may also occur.
- Selected breed and age predispositions are described and vary depending on the specific condition. However, non-infectious arthritis can be seen in animals of any age, sex and breed.
- The prognosis is usually good, with favourable response to immunosuppressive therapy.

Causes

- Non-erosive polyarthritis:
  - Immune-mediated polyarthritis (IMPA) (types 1–4).
  - Drug-associated polyarthritis.
  - Vaccine-associated polyarthritis.
  - Polyarthritis-meningitis syndrome.
  - Polyarthritis-polymyositis syndrome.
  - Polyarthritis associated with systemic lupus erythematosus (SLE).
  - Lymphoplasmacytic gonitis.
  - Juvenile-onset polyarthritis of Akitas.
  - Synovitis-amyloidosis of Shar Peis.
- Erosive polyarthritis:
  - Canine rheumatoid arthritis.
  - Greyhound polyarthritis.
  - Felty's syndrome.
  - Feline progressive polyarthritis.

Cytological features

- Cellularity is often markedly increased (often >100,000 cells/µl). Total protein is usually elevated, and viscosity of the fluid may be reduced.
- Background: clear to pale basophilic to amphophilic and finely granular (proteinaceous). The pink colour may be less homogenous and intense, with clear spaces, as result of the reduced viscosity.

- Red blood cells may be present as a result of iatrogenic haemorrhage or genuine concurrent haemorrhage.
- Large predominance of neutrophils (often >90%). They are usually segmented and do not show signs of degeneration.
- In polyarthritis associated with SLE, ragocytes and lupus erythematosus (LE) cells may be present:
  - Ragocytes: neutrophils that contain variable numbers of irregular, dark-purple intracytoplasmic structures that are considered being phagocytosed immune complexes or nuclear particles.
  - LE cells: phagocytic neutrophils or monocytoid mononuclear cells containing relatively large-pink homogenous cytoplasmic inclusions that distend the cytoplasm and compress the nuclei. These inclusions consist of degenerated nuclear material.
- In erosive forms, fragments of cartilage may be present and a higher proportion of small lymphocytes may be observed.

Pearls and Pitfalls

- Since polyarthritis may be subclinical and the animal may not show joint swelling or pain, four or more joints in particular distal, should be sampled and analysed in order to confirm/rule out this condition.
- Erosive arthritis is characterized by the presence of radiographic changes consistent with subchondral bone destruction. It is important to note that radiographic changes can take up to 6 months to appear. Therefore, dogs with apparently non-erosive forms of chronic polyarthritis should be periodically re-evaluated for erosive changes.
- The severity of inflammation observed on cytology is not associated with the clinical outcome.
- Cytological findings may be different among joints; they can be partially masked by concurrent immuno-suppressive treatment and can fluctuate during the disease.

Immune-mediated polyarthritis

- Immune-mediated process involving multiple joints and commonly observed in the canine species and very rare in cats.
- Age: young to middle-aged dogs.
- Canine breed predisposition: medium and large-breed dogs and Cocker Spaniels.
- It includes four types:
  - Type 1: idiopathic and diagnosed by exclusion of other possible causes or specific disease/breed association. It is common in dogs and accounts for approximately 50–65% of all idiopathic polyarthritis cases.
  - Type 2: triggered by a concurrent inflammatory process distant to the joint (e.g. urogenital tract, respiratory tract and skin). It has been linked to various vector-borne diseases. It accounts for approximately 13–25% of all cases of IMPA.
  - Type 3: associated with gastroenteritis or hepatopathy, including colitis, idiopathic inflammatory bowel disease, chronic-active hepatitis and cirrhosis. It has been theorized that disease of the gut leads to an increase in intestinal permeability to potential antigens, which then stimulate the production of immune complexes.
  - Type 4: associated with malignant neoplasms remote from the joint. Examples include mammary carcinoma, squamous cell carcinoma, heart base tumours, leiomyoma and

feline myeloproliferative diseases. Neoplasia may act as an antigenic stimulus against which antibodies are formed, leading to circulating immune complexes that deposit in the joint spaces.

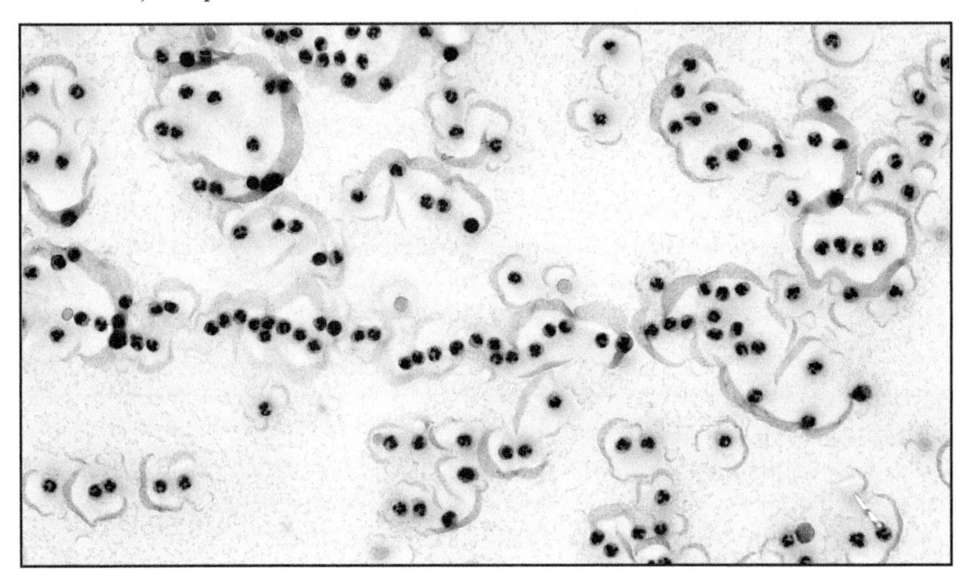

Fig. 4.11. Dog. Immune mediated polyarthritis. Note the prevalence of non-degenerate and segmented neutrophils on a proteinaceous granular background. Wright-Giemsa.

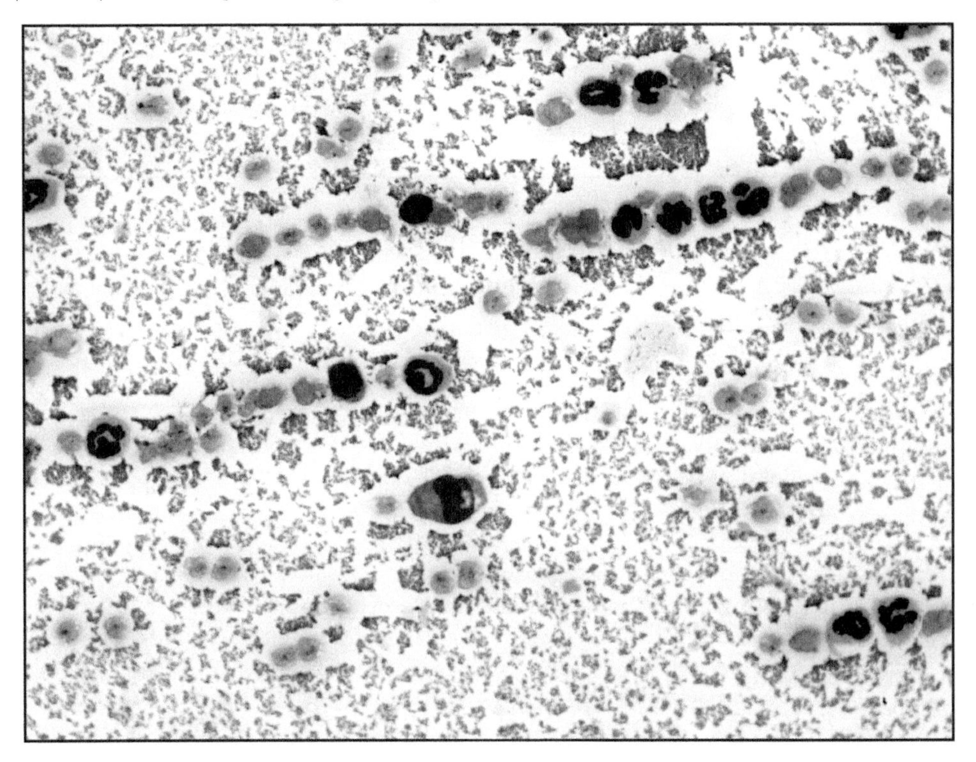

Fig. 4.12. Dog. Immune mediated polyarthritis. Neutrophils and red blood cells showing characteristic wind rowing arrangement. Wright-Giemsa.

Drug-associated polyarthritis

- Immune-mediated condition commonly linked to antibiotics, such as sulfonamides, cephalosporins, penicillin, erythromycin and lincomycin.
- This condition may be associated with fever, thrombocytopenia, neutropenia, hepatopathy, haemolysis and keratoconjunctivitis sicca.
- Clinical signs usually resolve within 2–7 days of discontinuing the drug.
- Over-represented canine breeds: Doberman Pinchers, Miniature Schnauzer and Samoyeds are prone to systemic hypersensitivity reactions to sulfonamides.

Vaccine-associated polyarthritis

- Condition associated with recent administration of polyvalent-modified live virus vaccine. It is usually transient and resolve in a few days.
- Over-represented canine/feline breeds: it has been described in a group of young Weimaraners and as transitory form in cats vaccinated against feline calicivirus. Akita dogs appear to be predisposed to this condition and suffer a longer disease course. This may be related to the heritable juvenile-onset polyarthritis of Akitas.

Polyarthritis-meningitis syndrome

- Immune-mediated condition characterized by non-erosive sterile polyarthritis associated with steroid responsive meningitis arteritis (SRMA).
- Clinical signs often include fever, cervical rigidity and stiff gait. Lameness and joint swelling are not always present.
- Diagnosis also requires cerebrospinal fluid (CSF) analysis, which shows neutrophilic pleocytosis, increased protein and high levels of IgA.
- Over-represented canine breeds: Bernese Mountain dog, Boxer, Corgi, German Shorthaired Pointer, Newfoundland and Weimaraner.

Polyarthritis-polymyositis syndrome

- Immune-mediated condition characterized by non-erosive sterile polyarthritis associated with focal or generalized inflammatory myopathy, leading to muscle atrophy and fibrosis.
- Diagnosis requires identification of myositis in two or more individual muscles via histopathology and sterile inflammation in the joints.
- Described in dogs, in particular Spaniels.

Systemic lupus erythematosus (SLE)

- Chronic autoimmune disease that may cause non-erosive polyarthritis in dogs, very rare in cats.
- It is a result of a combination of abnormal immune activity (type II, III and IV hypersensitivity reactions), loss of self-tolerance and multifactorial antigenic triggers.
- Clinical signs can be separated in two main categories (major and minor) based on their importance in contributing to the diagnosis of SLE.
- Major signs include polyarthritis, glomerulonephritis, haemolytic anaemia, leucopaenia, thrombocytopenia, characteristic skin lesions and polymyositis. Minor signs include fever, central nervous signs, oral ulcerations, lymphadenopathy, pericarditis and pleuritis.
- Over-represented canine breeds: mixed-breed young adult dogs as well as German shepherd, Shetland sheepdog, Beagle, Afghan hound, Irish setter, Old English sheepdog, Cocker Spaniel, Collie and Poodle.
- Diagnosis is commonly made when the patient shows three or more separate manifestations of autoimmunity and high-positive antinuclear antibody titre (ANA test).

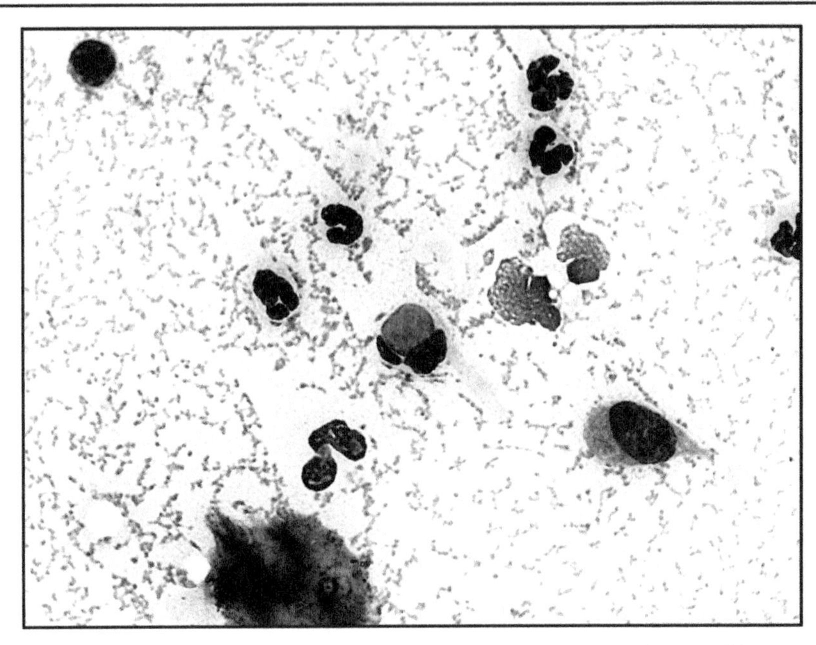

Fig. 4.13. Dog. Synovial fluid. SLE. LE cell in the centre of the picture. Wright-Giemsa. (*Courtesy of Giuseppe Menga.*)

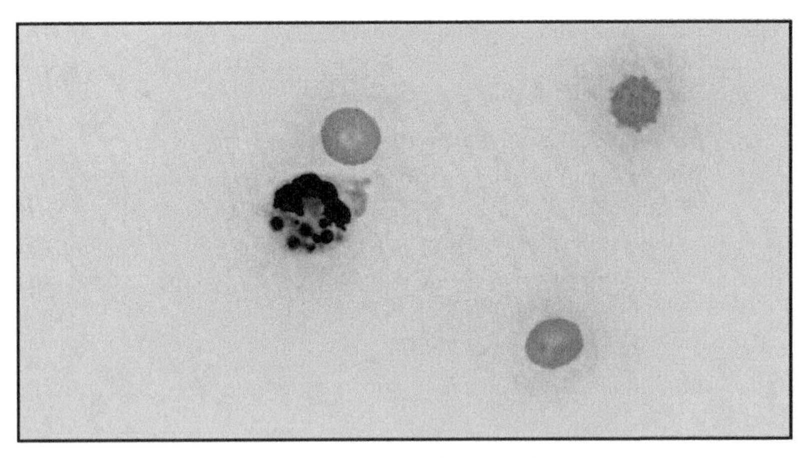

Fig. 4.14. Dog. Synovial fluid. SLE. Ragocyte in the centre of the picture. Wright-Giemsa.

Lymphoplasmacytic gonitis

- Rare inflammatory condition, likely immune mediated, affecting the knee joint.
- Linked to a small proportion of dogs that eventually develop or have been diagnosed with cruciate ligament rupture.

Juvenile-onset polyarthritis of Akitas

- Rare condition described in young Akitas and characterized by neutrophilic sterile arthritis, cyclical pain, generalized lymphadenopathy and non-regenerative anaemia.
- Concurrent meningitis may occur.

Synovitis-amyloidosis of Shar Peis

- Joint involvement of familial amyloidosis. This may precede or may be concurrent to glomerular disease.
- Tarsal joints are more often involved and the joint disease can be either monoarticular or pauciarticular.

Canine rheumatoid arthritis

- Main, but overall rare form of erosive polyarthritis in dogs.
- Tarsal, carpal and phalangeal joints are most commonly affected.
- Dogs are often seropositive for rheumatoid factor (RF) and may have a low positive or transient ANA titre.
- Age: middle-aged dogs.
- Over-represented canine breeds: mainly reported in small breeds.

Greyhound polyarthritis

- Rare form of erosive polyarthritis described in young Greyhounds.
- Extensive necrosis of deep articular cartilage zones with relative sparing of the more superficial surface cartilage is often observed.

Felty's syndrome

- Disease triad initially observed in humans and characterized by rheumatoid arthritis, neutropenia and splenomegaly. Rarely reported in dogs.

Feline progressive polyarthritis

- Two uncommon immune-mediated disorders causing joint damage and destruction are described in cats, most commonly male and individuals positive to feline syncytium forming virus (FeSFV):
  - Feline periosteal proliferative polyarthritis: observed in young adult male cats. It is characterized by fever, lethargy, lymphadenopathy, stiff gait, joint pain and swelling, particularly of the carpus and hock. Within a few months from the clinical onset, radiographic changes with periosteal proliferation occur and may be severe, including new bone formation. Synovial fluid analysis reveals neutrophilic inflammation.
  - Feline rheumatoid-like arthritis is a deforming arthritis resembling rheumatoid arthritis in humans and dogs. Mainly observed in middle-aged and older cats. Siamese cats may be over-represented. Cats do not show systemic signs, but lameness and joint deformity develop slowly over months. This disease is aggressive, destructive and irreversible. Synovial fluid reveals mixed inflammation. This condition is commonly associated with the presence of circulating RF.

Further reading

Johnson, K.C. and Mackin, A. (2012) Canine immune-mediated polyarthritis. *Journal of the American Animal Hospital Association* 48(1), 12–17.

Lemetayer, J. and Taylor, S. (2014) Inflammatory joint disease in cats. Diagnostic approach and treatment. *Journal of Feline Medicine and Surgery* 16, 547–562.

4.7 Haemarthrosis

Haemorrhagic event into the joint cavity secondary to ruptured blood vessel.

Clinical features

- Clinical signs vary depending on the severity of the process, its cause, and the joint involved.
- It could be primary (e.g. trauma and coagulopathy) or may be associated with degenerative and inflammatory arthropathies. When primary, it is usually more severe.

Causes

- Trauma.
- Coagulation defect: congenital (e.g. haemophilia) or acquired (e.g. rodenticide toxicosis).
- Underlying neoplasm.
- Degenerative arthropathies (usually mild).
- Arthritis (usually mild).

Cytological features

- Variable numbers of red blood cells are present, often arranged in rows (windrowing arrangement).
- Signs of erythrophagia, haemosiderophagia and/or presence of haematoidin crystals are common.
- Platelets are usually absent unless it is a per-acute event, or there is concurrent iatrogenic haemorrhage during the sampling.
- Leucocytes, in particular neutrophils, are usually present and are at least partially blood derived. With time, haemarthrosis will eventually elicit an inflammatory response.

Pearls and Pitfalls

- Genuine and iatrogenic haemorrhage can be differentiated at the time of sampling. In case of blood contamination, it should be noted sudden appearance and uneven distribution of blood in the synovial fluid during aspiration. In case of prior haemorrhage, the fluid will appear either homogenously haemodiluted and cloudy or will have golden-yellow colour (xanthochromia).
- Erythrophagocytosis may occur *in vitro* and may be the result of delayed fluid analysis; therefore, preparation of fresh direct smears (which can be sent to an external laboratory together with the fluid) is always encouraged, as it will allow identification of transit artefacts. Spurious erythrophagocytosis may also be secondary to sample centrifugation/cytocentrifugation.
- Risk of blood contamination may be reduced by using minimal negative pressure for retrieval of the fluid and gently releasing the negative pressure of the syringe before withdrawing the needle from the joint capsule.

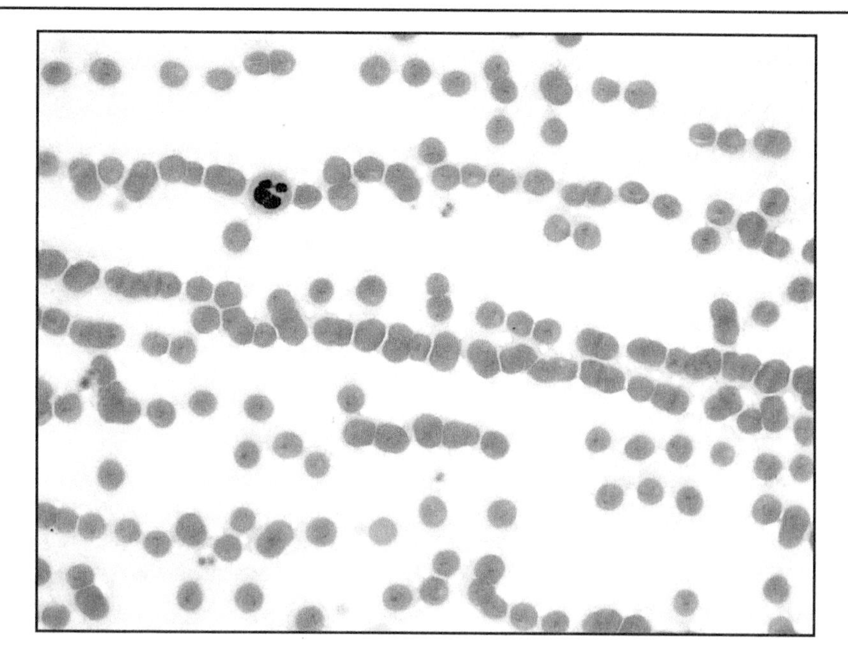

Fig. 4.15. Dog. Synovial fluid. Iatrogenic blood contamination. Numerous red blood cells arranged in lines, occasional platelets on a clear background. Wright-Giemsa.

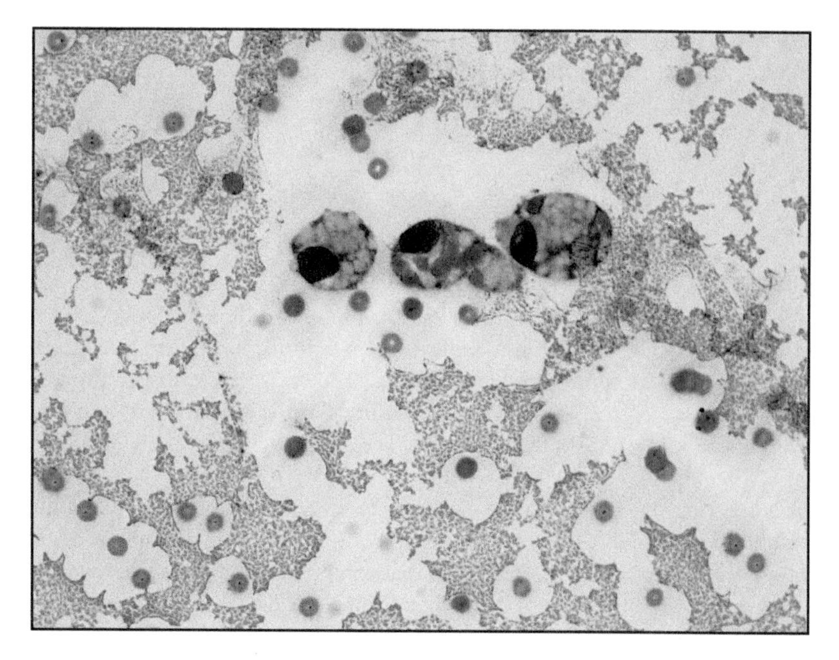

Fig. 4.16. Dog. Synovial fluid. Haemarthrosis. Foamy vacuolated macrophages displaying erythrophagia. Wright-Giemsa.

4.8 Exogenous/Endogenous Material Deposition

Accumulation of exogenous or endogenous material in joint space.

Clinical features

- Deposition of uric acid crystals in the synovium (also known articular gout) has been recently reported in four dogs and one cat. Causes are likely multifactorial and include diet (purine rich food) and hormonal state (ovariohysterectomized animals). Clinical signs include lameness, often intermitting or shifting. Warmth, swelling, pain response and disuse atrophy are also generally observed. Erosive changes may occur. Prognosis is variable, and recurrence after treatment is common.
- Accumulation of calcium pyrophosphate crystals (also known as pseudogout) in the articular cartilage has been reported in a few dogs. Its cause is unknown, and most cases are considered idiopathic.
- Injectable material (e.g. corticosteroids, hyaluronic acid, antibiotics, autologous serum, platelet-rich plasma and stem cells) used in the management of joint disease may accumulate in the joint space in dogs and cats.
- Metallosis is referred as fibrosis, local necrosis or loosening of a device secondary to metal-on-metal wear with subsequent release of metallic particles into the surrounding soft tissue. This has been described in a few dogs that underwent hip replacement.
- Synovial lipomatosis is a rare disorder of the synovium characterized by the extensive and diffuse synovial proliferation of fatty tissue. It has been reported in a few dogs, all Bullmastiff, that had partial cranial cruciate ligament rupture. It is associated with joint swelling and pain. It is hypothesized that these situations may induce an inflammatory articular stage where the released pro-inflammatory substances promote hyperplasia of the synoviocytes and adipocytes.

Cytological features

- Gout in dogs does not seem to be associated with increased total nucleated cells. However, a few neutrophils may be observed. In the only cat reported having gout, neutrophils were significantly increased in numbers. Urate crystals appear as needle-shaped brownish structures, which show negative birefringence, meaning that the refractive index of perpendicular waves is smaller than that of parallel ones. These crystals may be individualized or forming groups/bundles.
- Pseudogout is accompanied by mild elevation of mononuclear cells (in particular macrophages) and neutrophils. The mononuclear cells often contain multiple clear, square or rhomboid-shaped crystals of variable sizes that exhibit mild birefringence under polarized light and do not stain by von Kossa's method. These can also be seen in the background.
- Cytological appearance of intra-articular injectable material and its consequence on synovial fluid are poorly described. An increase in neutrophils has been reported in association with gentamicin sponge implantation in the canine stifle.

- Metallosis may result in the presence of dark colour synovial fluid with unremarkable/low total cell count (<1000/μl) and decreased viscosity. On microscopy, there is evidence of black and basophilic granular amorphous materials presumably metal foreign material and necrosis, not refractile under polarizing light.
- Synovial lipomatosis is characterized by the presence of adipocytes and/or lipid vacuoles associated with normal synoviocytes on a typical proteinaceous background. Extra-articular fatty tissue contamination may appear similar and therefore diagnosis cannot be based on cytology only.

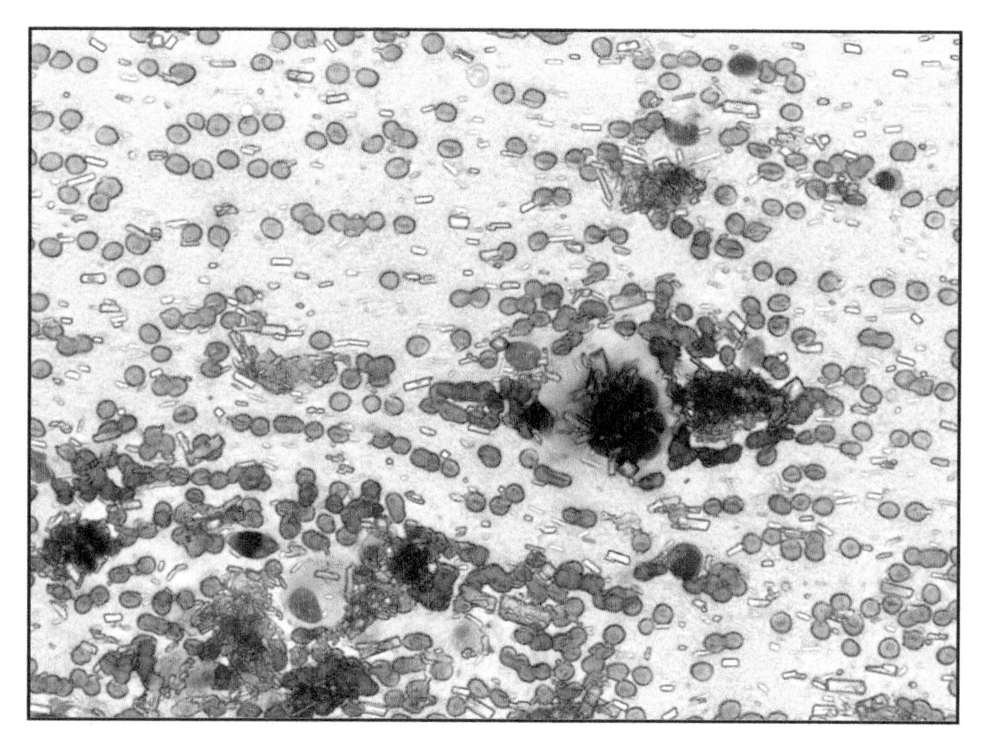

Fig. 4.17. Dog. Synovial fluid. Pseudogout. Numerous square-shaped crystals associated with small numbers of large mononuclear cells on a lightly basophilic and haemodiluted background. Wright-Giemsa.

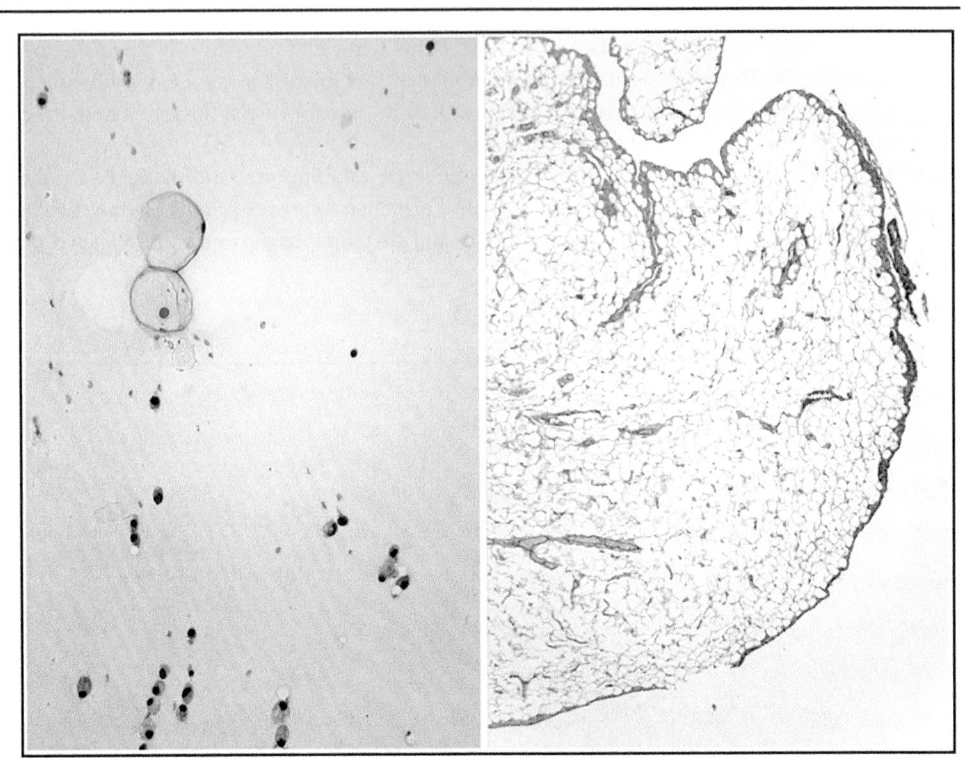

Fig. 4.18. Dog. Synovial lipomatosis. (Left) Mature adipocytes admixed with vacuolated synoviocytes/macrophages. Wright-Giemsa. (Right) Adipocytes are lined by a thin layer of fibrovascular tissue and synoviocytes. Haematoxylin and Eosin. (*Photos courtesy of Beatriz Agulla, Josep Pastor and Roser Velarde.*)

Further reading

Forsyth, S.F., Thompson, K.G. and Donald, J.J. (2007) Possible pseudogout in two dogs. *Journal of Small Animal Practice* 48, 174–176.

Hayes, G., Gibson, T. and Moens, N.M. (2016) Intra-articular implantation of gentamicin impregnated collagen sponge causes joint inflammation and impaired renal function in dogs. *Veterinary and Comparative Orthopaedics and Traumatology* 29(2), 159–163.

Kim, H.-S., Hwang, H.J., Kim, H.-J. and Do, S.-H. (2022) Case report: articular gout in four dogs and one cat. *Frontiers in Veterinary Science* 9, 752774.

Sandoval, K., Miller, B., Carvajal, J., Mendoza, P., Roberts, J.F. *et al.* (2021) What is your diagnosis? Coxofemoral synovial fluid in a dog. *Veterinary Clinical Pathology* 50(3), 459–461.

4.9 Synovial Cysts

Fluid-filled herniations of the synovial membrane.

Clinical features

- Synovial cysts usually communicate with the adjacent joint but may also arise from tendon sheaths and bursae.
- Cats: most commonly observed in geriatric patients and with pre-existing and usually bilateral DJD. The most commonly affected joint is the elbow, but cysts may extend distally and proximally to the carpus and shoulder, respectively. They have also been rarely reported in other locations including the digits.
- Dogs: rare and mainly reported in the vertebrae arising from the articular facet joints and compressing the spinal cord. Reported also in the carpus and elbow.
- Presumed to be the result of increased intra-articular pressure causing herniation of the synovium.
- Typically but not always in communication with the joint space.
- In cats, clinical signs include slowly progressive unilateral enlargement of the joint, with or without lameness. The swelling can be multilobulated, cystic, fluctuant or firm.
- These lesions may slowly increase in size, but otherwise have a good prognosis. Recurrence after surgical excision may occur. Regression over time has also been reported.
- In cats, the type B synoviocytes present within the cysts may undergo neoplastic transformation into myxoma.

Cytological features

- Macroscopic appearance: clear, colourless or slightly blood tinged and viscous. The viscosity is usually comparable to a normal synovial fluid or slightly decreased.
- Cellularity: within the normal limit for a synovial fluid or slightly increased.
- Background: clear to pale amphophilic-basophilic and finely granular (proteinaceous).
- Low numbers of mononuclear cells, likely a mixture of macrophages and synovial lining cells and lymphocytes are present. They can either appear quiescent or have abundant and foamy cytoplasm, especially when associated with underlying DJD.

Differential diagnosis

Ganglion cyst

Pearls and Pitfalls

- A ganglion cyst is a fluid-filled structure not lined by synovial cells. They also contain a viscous fluid. They seem to occur due to escape of synovial fluid from the joint/tendon sheath without herniation of the synovial membrane or due to mucinous degeneration of periarticular connective tissue.
- Other poorly cellular cystic lesions that may be encountered around joints include:
  - Hygroma: fluid-filled lesion that develops as a result of repeated trauma or pressure over a bony prominence.
  - Seroma: collection of clear fluid found in areas of prior trauma, such as surgical sites.

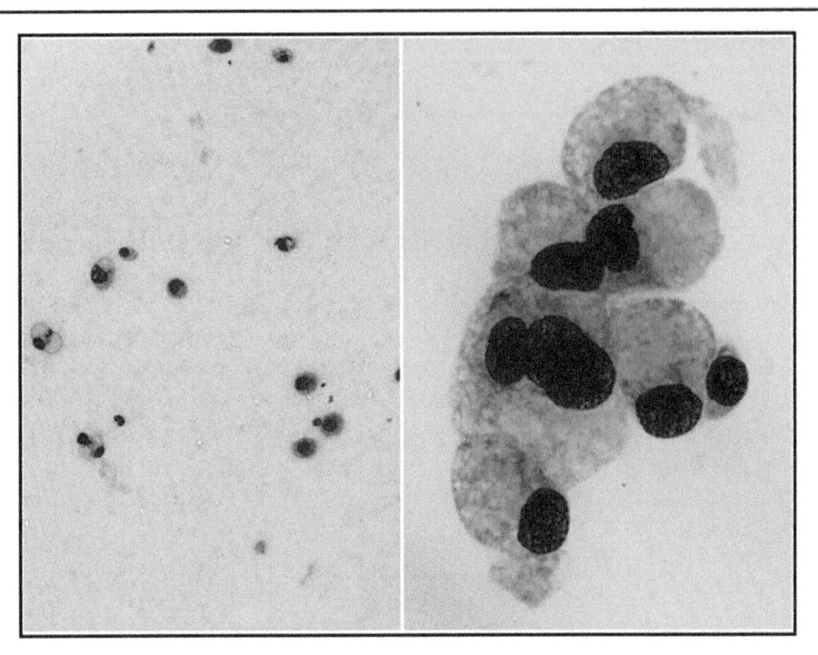

Fig. 4.19. Cat. Synovial cyst at the level of the elbow. Vacuolated large mononuclear cells on a granular proteinaceous background. Wright-Giemsa.

Further reading

Craig, E.L., Krimer, P.M. and O'Tool, A.D. (2020) Synovial cysts and myxomas in 16 cats. *Veterinary Pathology* 57(4), 554–558.
Dickinson, P.J., Sturges, B.K., Berry, W.L., Vernau, K.M., Koblik, P.D. *et al.* (2001) Extradural spinal synovial cysts in nine dogs. *Journal of Small Animal Practice* 42(10), 502–509.
Hittmair, K.M., Maedl, I., Reifinger, M. and Mayrhofer, E. (2010) Synovial cyst of the fifth digit in a cat. *Journal of Feline Medicine and Surgery* 12(2), 175–178.

4.10 Neoplasms

Tumours involving the joints could be primary or metastatic and are more frequently malignant. With exception for lymphomas and carcinomas, neoplastic cells are usually not present in the synovial fluid and diagnosis is generally achieved by fine-needle aspiration (or solid biopsy) of the mass.

General clinical features

- Histiocytic sarcoma and soft-tissue sarcomas are the most common neoplasms affecting the joints in dogs and cats.
- Lymphoma and metastatic carcinomas (e.g. urothelial carcinoma, bronchoalveolar carcinoma and mammary carcinoma) have also been reported.
- Primary joint tumours present as solitary lesions in weight-bearing joints in middle-aged to older animal.
- Clinical signs vary. Lameness is frequent. Their onset is often gradual and may mimic DJD. Depending on the type of tumour, systemic signs may also be present.
- Both benign and malignant lesions may be associated with bone lysis around the joint. Advanced imaging will help to establish the extent of the tumour.

Cytological features

- Synovial fluid changes are poorly described; however, neoplastic cells rarely exfoliate in the synovial fluids. Signs of degenerative or inflammatory arthropathies may be observed. The specific cytological features described below refer to direct aspiration of the mass (FNA).

Histiocytic sarcoma

Clinical features

- Malignant neoplasia arising from interstitial dendritic cells (DCs). It can arise within the joints (intra-articular) and/or adjacent to the joints (periarticular) of the appendicular skeleton.
- Most common tumour affecting the joints in dogs. It often presents as a particular mass at the level of the stifle and elbow (with or without surgical repair). It is also rarely reported in the joints of cats, in particular at the level of the tarsi.
- The prognosis is poor compared with other joint tumours. However, the outcome is more favourable compared with histiocytic sarcomas (HS) in other districts if localized. Early detection and treatment of articular HS is potentially curative. Invasion of bone, metastases to lymph nodes, lungs, liver and spleen are reported and are associated with poor prognosis.
- Over-represented canine breeds: Rottweiler, Golden Retriever, Labrador Retriever and Flat-coated Retriever. Bernese Mountain dog seems to be less affected in this district.

Cytological features

- Cellularity is variable often high.
- Background: clear to lightly basophilic and variably haemodiluted.
- Neoplastic histiocytic cells are pleomorphic and can be bi- or multinucleated. They are usually round to oval, slightly elongated and occasionally with small cytoplasmic tails. They mainly exfoliate individually.
- Nuclei are round to oval, often large, with coarse, granular or clumped chromatin. They are eccentric to paracentral. Multiple prominent and irregularly shaped nucleoli are frequently seen.
- The cytoplasm is lightly, occasionally moderately basophilic and moderate in amount. It may contain clear intracytoplasmic vacuoles or include small phagosomes.
- Neoplastic cells can display erythrophagocytosis.
- Cytological features of atypia are often prominent. Anisocytosis and anisokaryosis are variable to marked, and the N:C ratio is variable. Binucleation and/or multinucleation and frequent mitotic figures are often seen. In some cases, the pleomorphism is less prominent and anisokaryosis and anisocytosis are modest.
- Concurrent increase in leucocytes, in particular lymphocytes and neutrophils may be present.

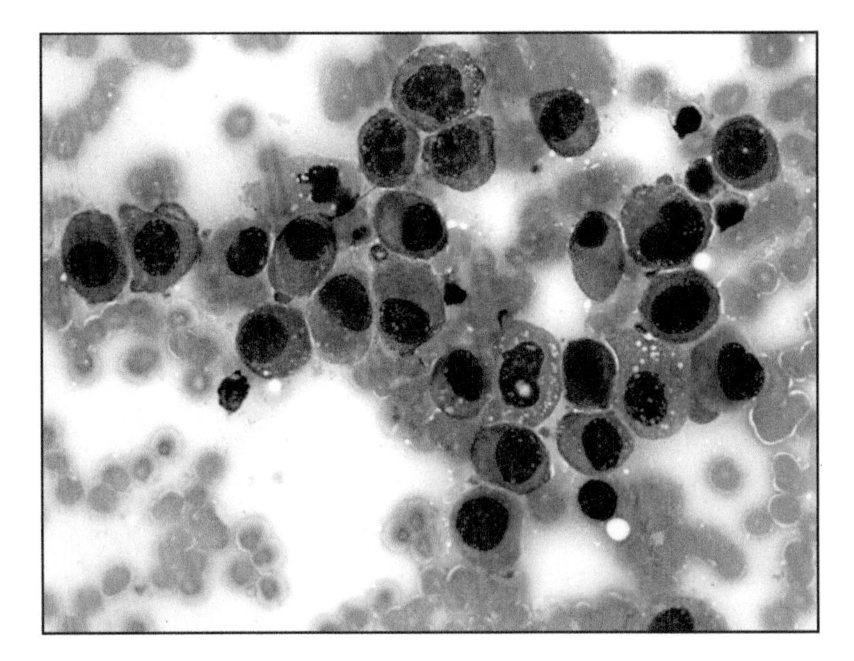

Fig. 4.20. Dog. Articular joint. Histiocytic sarcoma. Neoplastic cells appear roundish, slightly vacuolated, and display marked cytological features of atypia (anisokaryosis, binucleation, atypical mitoses). Wright-Giemsa.

Synovial sarcoma

Clinical features

- Malignant mesenchymal neoplasm infrequently diagnosed at the level of the joints in both dogs and cats and likely arising from synovial type B cells.
- It presents as an infiltrative mass within the joint. The stifle is the most reported site.
- Clinical behaviour has been reported to be highly variable. This might be due to the fact that many different sarcomas have been misdiagnosed as synovial sarcoma. Metastatic rate may be similar to those of other canine soft-tissue sarcomas.

Cytological features

- Background: clear to lightly basophilic and variably haemodiluted.
- Neoplastic cells appear round to oval. They are often arranged in apparently cohesive clusters and sometimes associated with extracellular pink amorphous material. Perivascular arrangement may occur.
- Nuclei are round to oval, often large, with coarse, granular or clumped chromatin. They are variably located within the cells. Multiple prominent and irregularly shaped nucleoli are frequently seen.
- The cytoplasm is lightly, occasionally moderately basophilic, and moderate in amount. It may contain sporadic clear intracytoplasmic vacuoles or fine-pink granules. Small cytoplasmic projections may be observed.
- Cytological features of atypia may vary and include anisocytosis, anisokaryosis and mitotic figures.

Pears and Pitfalls

- HS and other sarcomas affecting the joint share several morphological features and cannot be accurately distinguished on cytology or histopathology. The generic term 'joint associated sarcoma' may therefore be more appropriate in cytology until immunohistochemical studies are performed. Neoplastic cells in HS express both vimentin and CD18. Neoplastic cells in synovial sarcoma express vimentin and a small percentage may express cytokeratin. Variable expression of smooth muscle actin is also reported.
- In human medicine, the gold standard for the diagnosis of synovial sarcoma is the demonstration of a gene translocation specific for this tumour type. It has also been proven that the cell of origin of this neoplasm is not a synoviocyte, but a pluripotent mesenchymal stem cell that occurs throughout the body; therefore, the term 'synovial sarcoma' is preferred over 'synovial cell sarcoma'. In veterinary medicine, the exact origin of these cells has not been proven and specific gene translocation has not been found yet; therefore, the term 'cytokeratin-positive joint associated sarcoma' may be preferred.

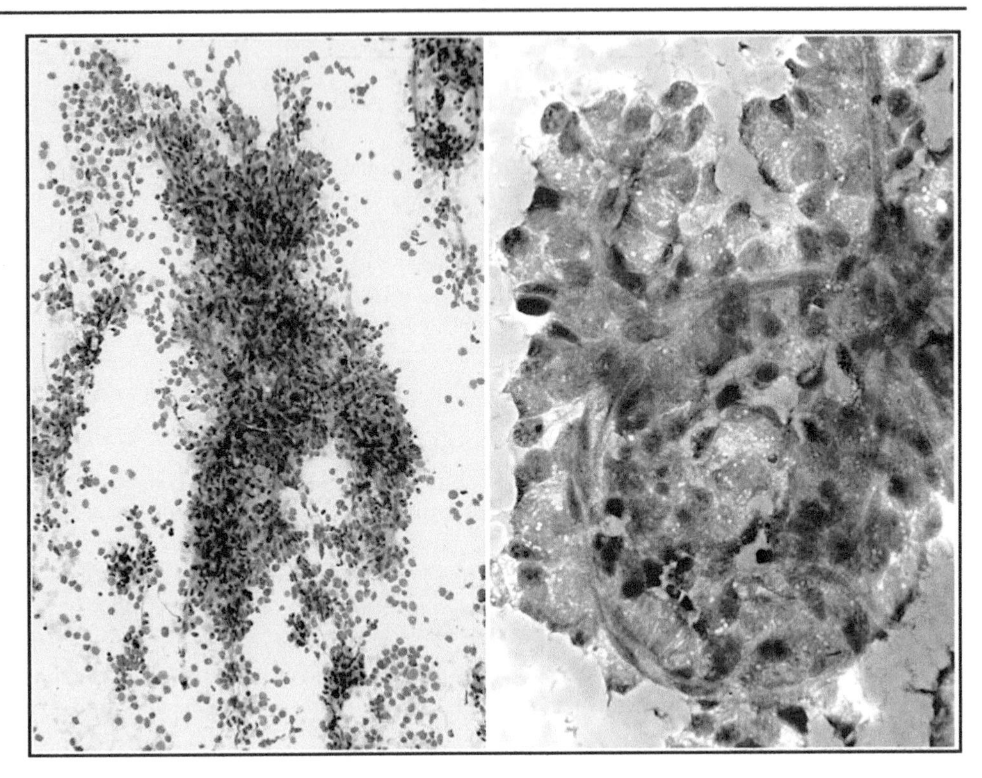

Fig. 4.21. Dog. Joint. Synovial sarcoma. Variably cohesive cohesive clusters of neoplastic cells with perivascular arrangement. Wright-Giemsa.

Other mesenchymal tumours

- Benign tumours include synovial haemangioma, periarticular fibroma and synovial myxoma.
- Malignant forms include malignant fibrous histiocytoma, chondrosarcoma, osteosarcoma, fibrosarcoma, haemangiosarcoma, perivascular wall tumour, peripheral nerve sheath tumour, liposarcoma, myxosarcoma and undifferentiated sarcoma.
- Cytological features are similar to what observed on the skin/subcutis.
- In some cases, the identification of the tumour lineage may require immunohistochemical studies.

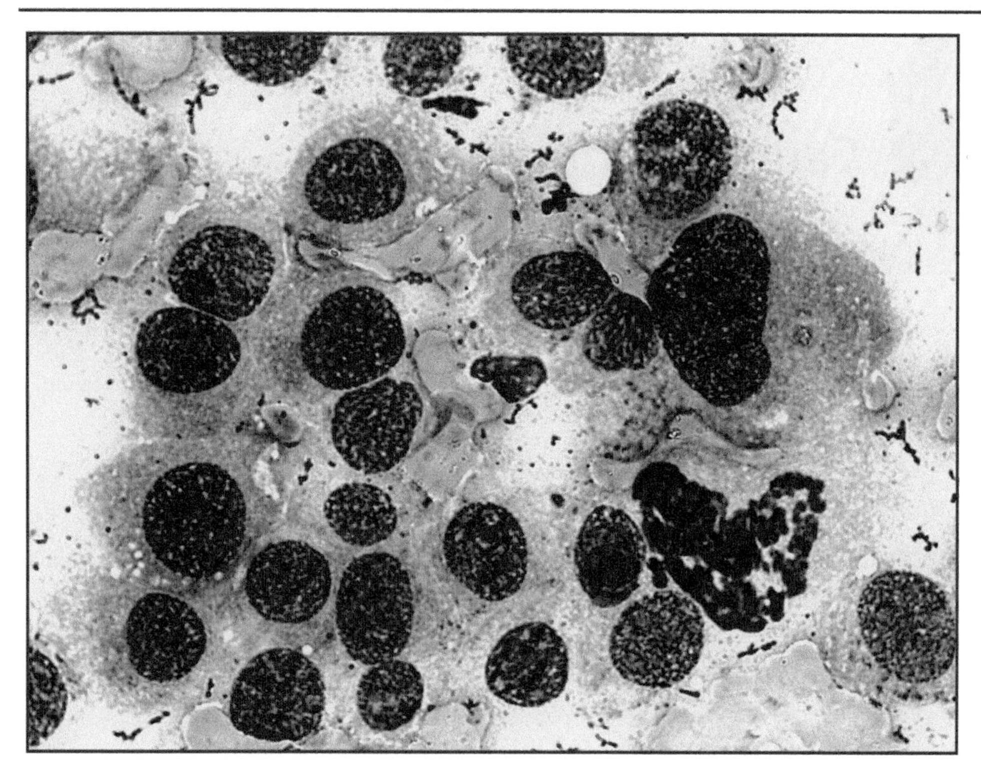

Fig. 4.22. Dog. Joint. Osteosarcoma. Neoplastic cells are round, with basophilic cytoplasm, rarely containing pink granules. Nuclei are large in size, round, paracentral to eccentric, with clumped chromatin and prominent nucleoli. Wright-Giemsa. (*Courtesy of Giuseppe Menga.*)

Lymphoma

Extremely rare in both dogs and cat, as only one case in each species has been described in literature and clinical information are therefore very limited.

Further reading

Burr, H.D., Keating, J.K. and Clifford, C.A. (2014) Cutaneous lymphoma of the tarsus in cats: 23 cases (2000–2012). *Journal of American Veterinary Medical Association* 244(12), 1429–1434.

Lahmers, S.M., Mealey, K.J., Martinez, S.A., Haldorson, G.J., Sellon, R.K. *et al.* (2002) Synovial T-cell lymphoma of the stifle in a dog. *Journal of American Veterinary Medical Association* 38, 165–168.

Monti, P., Barnes, D., Adrian, A.D. and Rasotto, R. (2018) Synovial cell sarcoma in a dog: a misnomer – cytologic and histologic findings and review of the literature. *Veterinary Clinical Pathology* 47, 181–185.

Moore, P.F. (2014) A review of histiocytic diseases of dogs and cats. *Veterinary Pathology* 51(1), 167–184.

5 Cerebrospinal Fluid

The cerebrospinal fluid (CSF) (liquor) is a hypocellular, clear and colourless fluid, mainly produced by the choroid plexus. It flows through the ventricular system down to the subarachnoid space, where it is reabsorbed.

5.1 Anatomy and Physiology

The CNS is isolated from the body and the systemic circulation, but it interfaces with systemic fluids at the level of:

- Blood-brain barrier (BBB).
- Blood-CSF barrier.
- CSF-brain barrier.

The CSF is produced by specialized epithelial cells that line the choroid plexus present in the ventricles. The choroid plexus represents areas of highly vascularized invaginations of the pia mater (innermost meningeal layer) into the ventricles. The cells producing the CSF are modified cuboidal ciliated ependymal cells. The CSF is then reabsorbed in the subarachnoid space into the venous system.

The CSF is present in:

- Ventricular system of the brain. This is made of four compartments:
  - Two lateral ventricles within the cerebral hemispheres.
  - Third ventricle in the midbrain.
  - Fourth ventricle that extends into the central canal of the upper cervical spinal cord.
- Subarachnoid space. This has CSF-built dilations called subarachnoid cisterns. One of these is the cisterna magna (posterior cerebellar-medullary cistern).
- Central canal of the spinal cord.

Once produced, it flows rostro-caudally from the lateral ventricles to the third ventricle, then to the fourth ventricle and finally caudally to the central canal of the spinal cord. From the fourth ventricle, the CSF can enter the subarachnoid space.

The CSF has multiple functions:

- Protection and support for the brain.
- Buoyancy: prevents the compression of vessels and cranial nerves by the brain against the internal surface of the bones of the skull.
- Regulation of intracranial pressure.
- Transport medium for chemical signals, nutrients, hormone-releasing factors (e.g. TRH), waste products, etc.

DOI: 10.1079/9781789247787.0005

Composition

The CSF derives from plasma filtration and membrane secretion. It contains almost no cellular elements and should not contain erythrocytes. Main constituents are:

- Proteins: usually present in very low concentration, but increase caudally. Albumin represents approximately 50–70% of all proteins. Other proteins include gamma-globulins.
- Glucose: 60–80% of blood glucose concentration. It derives from the plasma and is carried into the brain by facilitated transport or diffusion.
- Water and electrolytes: sodium (most abundant ion), potassium, chloride, calcium and magnesium.
- Neurotransmitters: these are produced by the neurons. They include GABA and glutamate.
- Enzymes: these can derive from the peripheral blood, neural tissue or neural tumours cells present in the CSF (e.g. CK and lactate dehydrogenase [LDH]).

Further reading

Di Terlizzi, R. and Platt, S. (2006) The function, composition and analysis of cerebrospinal fluid in companion animals: part I – function and composition. *Veterinary Journal* 172(3), 422–431.

5.2 Sampling Techniques

Indications

CSF analysis has an important role in the work-up of patients with neurological disease. It is sampled when inflammation, degenerative disease, trauma, haemorrhage or neoplasia are suspected.

It can be collected from:

- Cerebellar-medullary cistern (cisterna magna) (CMC).
- Caudal lumbar subarachnoid space.

Given the one-way direction of its flow (rostro-caudal), sampling caudally to the suspected lesion has proven to be more diagnostically useful.

Materials

- Clippers, disinfectant, and sterile gloves.
- Spinal needles:
  - Large dogs: 20-22 G (40-90 mm).
  - Small dogs and cats: small hypodermic needles (22G or 25G).
- Tubes:
  - Sterile plain tube for protein and enzymes measurements, serology and microbiology.
  - EDTA tube for cytology, total cell count and PCR.

Patient preparation

- General anaesthesia is required. A reinforced endotracheal tube may be used to avoid tracheal collapse during the maximum neck flexion (cerebellar-medullary cistern collection).
- The area must be clipped and cleaned aseptically.
- The patient is positioned in lateral recumbency:
  - Cerebellar-medullary cistern collection: the skull and cervical vertebrae are placed at the edge of the table and the skull is fully flexed, creating a 90° angle with the cervical spine. The nose should be elevated off the table so that the long axis of the muzzle is parallel to the table.
  - Lumbar collection: the pelvic limbs are fully flexed. The sternum should be elevated so that it is at the same level as the patient's vertebral column.
- No more than 1 ml of CSF per 5 kg bodyweight in dogs and cats should be collected.

Technique

- Cerebellar-medullary cistern collection:
  - Entry site: at the insertion of the imaginary lines drawn from the occipital protuberance to the dorsal arch of C2 horizontally and along the rostral aspect of the left and right wings of the atlas.
  - The needle (with the stylet in place) is kept parallel to the body of the mandible and advanced in slowly through the skin. As it advances, more resistance can be felt but not always, especially in small dogs and cats. Loss of resistance can be felt when the dura has been penetrated.
  - Once the dura is entered, the stylet is removed and the fluid is allowed to drip into the collecting tubes.

- To avoid cord damage, the stylet can be removed multiple times during the advancement to check for fluid accumulation in the hub of the needle.
- A minimum of 0.5 ml is required for protein measurement, cell count and cytology although larger volumes are preferred.

- Lumbar collection:
  - Entry site: L5–L6 in dogs and L6–L7 in cats.
  - The needle is inserted just caudally to the selected space and should be kept perpendicular to the dorsal laminae of the vertebrae. It is usually advanced until it enters in contact with the bone of the ventral aspect of the spinal canal. The stylet is then removed, and the fluid is allowed to drip into the collecting tubes. If no fluid appears in the hub of the needle, rotate very slightly the needle and/or withdraw it.
  - Lumbar collection is usually more difficult that sampling from the cerebellar-medullary cistern and iatrogenic blood contamination is more frequent.
  - The tail and pelvic limb muscles often twitch visibly when the subarachnoid space is entered.
  - The rate of fluid flow is usually slower than from the CMC, and the fluid quantity retrieved smaller.

Complications

- Subarachnoid haemorrhage.
- Cerebrum or cerebellum herniation: this usually occurs when the intracranial pressure is increased and may result in brainstem injury.
- Spinal cord injury.
- Haematomyelia.
- Meningitis.

Contraindications

- Increased intracranial pressure (ICP).
- Underlying coagulopathy.
- Intoxication.
- Atlanto-axial subluxation.
- Chiari-like malformation.
- Cervical trauma.

Pearls and Pitfalls

Diagnostic imaging of the brain and cervical spinal cord should be carried out before CSF sampling, in order to localize the lesion and plan the sampling site. It is also required to establish if the underlying pathology could increase the intracranial pressure, predisposing to brain herniation post sampling. If increased intracranial pressure is suspected, CSF should not be collected.

Further reading

Di Terlizzi, R. and Platt, S.R. (2009) The function, composition and analysis of cerebrospinal fluid in companion animals: part II – analysis. *Veterinary Journal* 180(1), 15–32.

Elias, A. and Brown, C. (2008) Cerebellomedullary cerebrospinal fluid collection in the dog. *Laboratory Animal (NY)* 37(10), 457–458.

5.3 Sample Handling, Analysis and Slide Preparation

5.3.1 Sample handling

- Once the CSF sample has been collected, this should be processed as soon as possible (ideally within 30 min), as cell count can decrease over time due to *in vitro* lysis, and cell morphology can deteriorate.
- Different studies have investigated the stability of CSF samples and had concluded that a delay up to 4–8 h (and possibly as long as 12 h) is unlikely to cause significant changes that would lead to alter the final diagnosis, especially when the protein concentration is >0.5 g/l (>50 mg/dl).
- The differential cell count is more likely to be affected by delayed analysis than the total nucleated cell count.
- If analysis is delayed, it has been suggested to separate the sample in two aliquots:
    - One unaltered aliquot: for protein concentration and total cell count.
    - One aliquot added to 10% volume of autologous serum: for differential cell count.
- If these are sent to an external laboratory, tubes should be clearly labelled specifying any addition to the CSF sample.
- The sample can be placed in:
    - EDTA tube: used for cell count and cytology. This prevents clotting of the sample in case of haemodilution. It can also be used used for ancillary tests (e.g. PCRs and PARR). EDTA sample is not suitable for protein measurement, as the additives present in this tube might interfere with the analysis causing false elevation of the protein concentration.
    - Plain tube: used for protein concentration and microbiology (when required).

Pears and Pitfalls

The use of formalin as a fixative is not advisable, as this alters cell morphology.

5.3.2 Sample analysis

Routine CSF analysis usually includes:

- Macroscopic evaluation.
- Quantitative measurements:
    - Protein measurement.
    - Total cell count.
- Cytological examination of concentrated stained slides.

Macroscopic evaluation

CSF should be a clear and colourless fluid.

- Colour: any change from the normal colourless appearance indicates an abnormality:
    - Pink/red discolouration: this usually reflects haemodilution. In these cases, the sample is centrifuged and:
        - If the supernatant is clear and the red blood cells form a small pellet at the bottom of the tube, the haemorrhage is likely to be iatrogenic or very acute (within hours).

    - If the supernatant is yellow or yellow-orange (xanthochromia), genuine previous haemorrhage is likely.
- Turbidity: increased turbidity is always regarded as abnormal. It is usually associated with increased cellularity (usually >500 cells/μl).

Quantitative measurements

Protein concentration:

- The majority of the CSF proteins come from plasma and consist of albumin (80–90%). Globulins are present in lower quantities.
- The choroid plexus can produce small quantities of proteins including transthyretin, transferrin and retinol-binding protein.
- Cisternal protein concentration is usually slightly lower than lumbar CSF protein concentration.
- Methods:
  - Clinical refractometer: due to the low protein concentration, this is inaccurate and is not used.
  - Urine dipstick: this could be used if a preliminary result is needed. However, it appears that only results ≥2+ truly reflect an increased protein concentration. Results lower than this may be false-positive. False-negative results are also possible.
  - Microprotein methodologies are used for quantitative measurement, as conventional protein methods are insensitive due to the low CSF protein concentration. Methods include:
    - Turbidimetric method.
    - Trichloroacetic acid method.
    - Dye-binding spectrophotometric methods: e.g. Pyrogallol red, Comassie Brillant Blue, etc. These are considered to be the most accurate.

Cell count:

- Manual counting is the most common method used in veterinary medicine. This requires the use of a Neubauer Improved or Fuchs-Rosenthal counting chamber.
- Automated cell count is less commonly used. Some haematology analysers are provided of separate assays for CSF analysis. Although these have proven to have high correlation with the manual counting, the correlation with the manual differential cell count is only moderate.
- Moreover, the high cost of specific quality control materials for CSF analysis usually does not justify the use of an automated method.

Cytology examination

Cytology is used for:

- Differential cell count.
- Morphological examination of the cellular elements.
- Search for infectious agents.

5.3.3 Slide preparation

- Due to the usually low cellularity, sample concentration is required:
  - Cytospin centrifugation: this is the most commonly used technique, especially in large laboratories. This method usually guarantees a good cell preservation. However, some studies have described an imprecise cellular yield and differential cell count on preparations obtained by cytocentrifugation.

- Sedimentation technique: this method has been described and can be adopted in case of necessity. Although cell morphology is less preserved than in slides obtained by cytocentrifugation, differential cell count appears more accurate.

Staining:

- Conventional Romanowsky stains are preferred for CSF analysis.

Pearls and Pitfalls

- Xanthochromia of the supernatant has also been associated with significantly increased protein concentration, hyperbilirubinaemia, CNS neoplasia and inflammation.
- CSF analysis has low specificity for the identification of the underlying disease. The possible cytological abnormalities are relatively limited if compared to the varieties of neurological disease that exist. Moreover, selected disorders causing neurological signs (e.g. congenital malformations, toxicities and nutritional disorders) are unlikely to cause CSF abnormalities.

5.4 Normal CSF Composition

A normal CSF sample should be clear and colourless and should contain a low amount of protein and low numbers of cells.

Cells numbers and types

- The reference interval for total nucleated cell count (TNCC) in CSF samples may vary depending on each laboratory. In literature, the most commonly reported RIs are as follows:
  - Dogs: 0–5 cells/μl.
  - Cats: 0–8 cells/μl.
- Normal nucleated cells in the CSF include:
  - Mononuclear cells: these represent the predominant cell type in CSF from dogs and cats. They consist of:
    - Small lymphocytes.
    - Monocytoid cells.
  - Non-degenerate neutrophils (<10% in dogs; <8% in cats).
  - Surface epithelial cells (ependymal cells), choroid plexus cells and meningeal lining cells may also occasionally be found (incidental finding).
- In dogs, the mononuclear cells are predominantly small lymphocytes, with fewer monocytoid cells.
- In cats, most mononuclear cells are monocytoid cells (69–100%) with a lower proportion of small lymphocytes.

Protein concentration

- Cisternal samples: usually <0.25–0.30 g/l.
- Lumbar samples: usually <0.45 g/l.

5.5 Cells Types and Non-cellular Material

Red blood cells

- Erythrocytes are not normally present in CSF samples.
- If present in normal CSFs, they usually reflect mild iatrogenic haemorrhage during sampling.
- True haemorrhage is also possible, but less common and usually accompanied by signs of red blood cell degradation (haemosiderin/siderophages) and xanthochromatic supernatant.

Lymphocytes

- Small lymphocytes are the predominant cell type in canine CSF and are similar to those found in the peripheral blood. They have small, round and dense nuclei and a small, pale cytoplasmic rim. Nucleoli are indistinct.
- Reactive lymphocytes may also be found in reactive or inflammatory CNS diseases. They are usually mixed in morphology and size. They are intermediate to large in size and have medium-large nuclei, finely stippled chromatin, occasionally small nucleoli and a small to moderate amount of moderately to deeply basophilic cytoplasm.

Monocytoid cells/macrophages

- Second most common cell type in canine CSF and most frequent mononuclear cells in feline CSF.
- They are similar to those found in the peripheral blood. They are larger than other leucocytes, have round-to-oval, occasionally reniform nuclei and a moderate amount of pale basophilic cytoplasm.
- Some of the cells can have a large amount of foamy/vacuolated cytoplasm and may occasionally contain amorphous phagosomes or display erythrophagia or leucophagia. Occasionally, they may contain fragments of myelin. They may sometimes be found in small groups.

Neutrophils

- Usually absent or present in very low numbers. According to some sources, they can account for up to 20% of the TNCC in absence of pleocytosis.
- Morphologically similar to those found in the peripheral blood.
- Increased numbers of neutrophils reflect an underlying inflammatory process, primary or secondary.
- They are most frequently non-degenerate. In bacterial infections, they can display a variable degree of degeneration (karyolysis).

Eosinophils

- Usually not found in CSF. When present, they indicate an underlying CNS pathology.
- Increased numbers may be seen in idiopathic eosinophilic inflammation, granulomatous meningoencephalitis (GME), fungal infection, parasite migration, etc.
- Eosinophils have a lobulated nucleus usually slightly larger and less segmented than the nuclei of neutrophils. They contain distinctive eosinophilic granules, which are rod shaped in cats and round in dogs.
- In some sources, eosinophilic pleocytosis is defined as a pleocytosis with >20% eosinophils.

Plasma cells

- Can be found in reactive or inflammatory CNS pathologies.
- They have small, round and eccentric nuclei with clumped chromatin and indistinct nucleoli. The cytoplasm is moderate in amount, moderately basophilic and often has a perinuclear paler area (Golgi zone).

Surface epithelial cells

- The ependymal cells that line the ventricles or the choroid plexus and the subarachnoid cells can occasionally exfoliate in low numbers in the CSF. These cells are all collectively referred to as *surface epithelial cells*.
- They can exfoliate singly or in small clusters.
- Their presence does not have any clinical significance.
- Cells are mononucleated and have a moderate N:C ratio. They have round-to-oval, eccentric nuclei with granular chromatin and indistinct nucleoli. The cytoplasm is moderate in amount, pale amphophilic and often has fine pink granulations.

Neoplastic cells

- The cell morphology depends on the lineage of the tumour.

Haematopoietic cells

Low numbers of mixed haematopoietic cells can be found if the needle is accidentally placed in the bone marrow present in the vertebral body.

Non-cellular material

Myelin

- This can be seen in the CSF with a variety of underlying CNS pathologies and its finding is non-specific, although it seems to be more common in samples from patients with intervertebral disc disease.
- Ribbon-like to granular, pale-pink amorphous material.
- It can occasionally be found within the macrophages.

Cartilage/chondrocytes

- If the needle is inserted too cranially, the CSF can be contaminated with chondrocytes and cartilage from the intervertebral disc.
- Cartilage appears as a pink to purple, variably fibrillar or diffuse amorphous material.
- Chondrocytes are plump-oval cells with round-to-oval, eccentric nuclei, granular chromatin and a moderate amount of pale basophilic cytoplasm, occasionally containing pink granules.

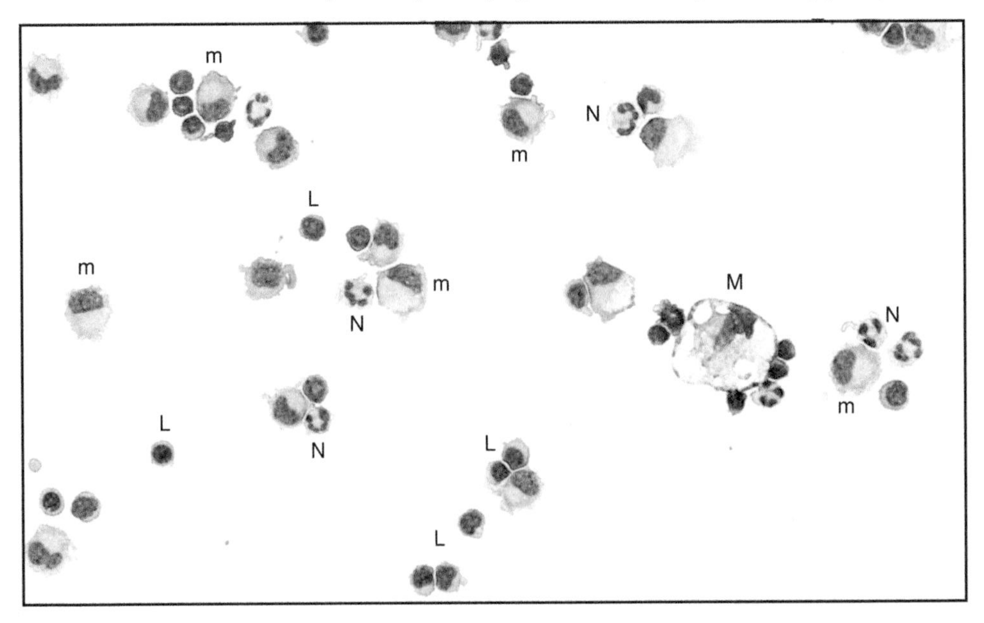

Fig. 5.1. Dog, CSF. (M) macrophage, (m) monocytoid cells, (L) small lymphocytes, (N) neutrophils. Wright-Giemsa.

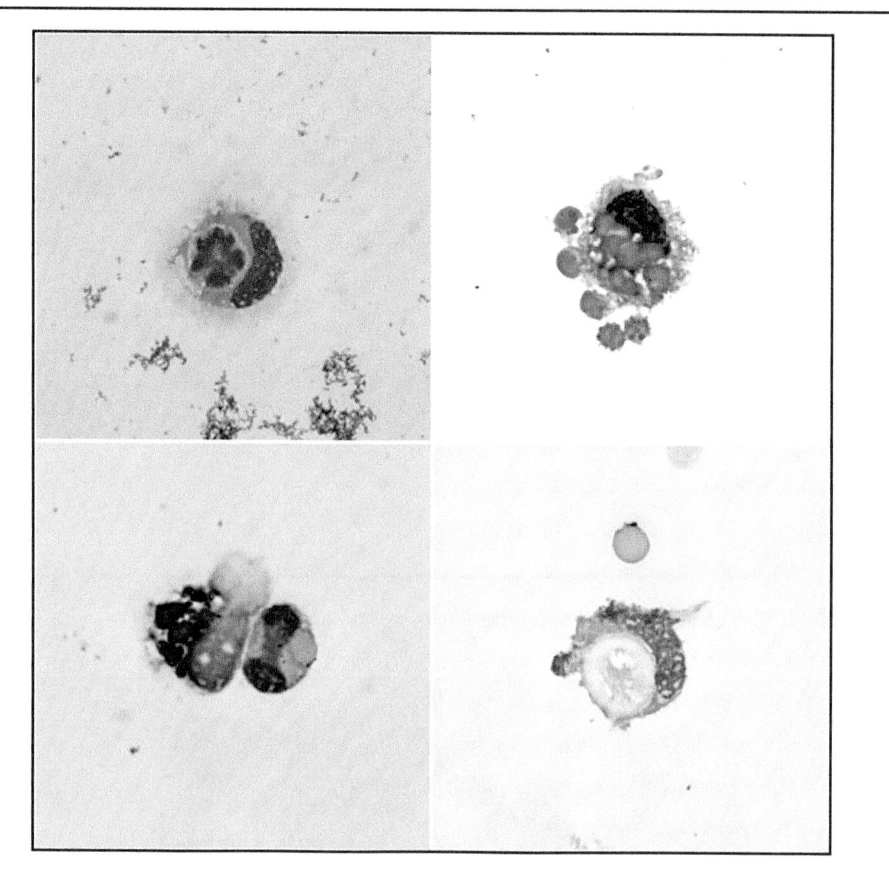

Fig. 5.2. Dog. CSF. Monocytoid cells displaying leucophagia (top left); erythrophagocytosis (top right); macrophage containing haemosiderin granules and a phagocytosed red blood cell (bottom left), macrophage containing myelin (bottom right). Wright-Giemsa.

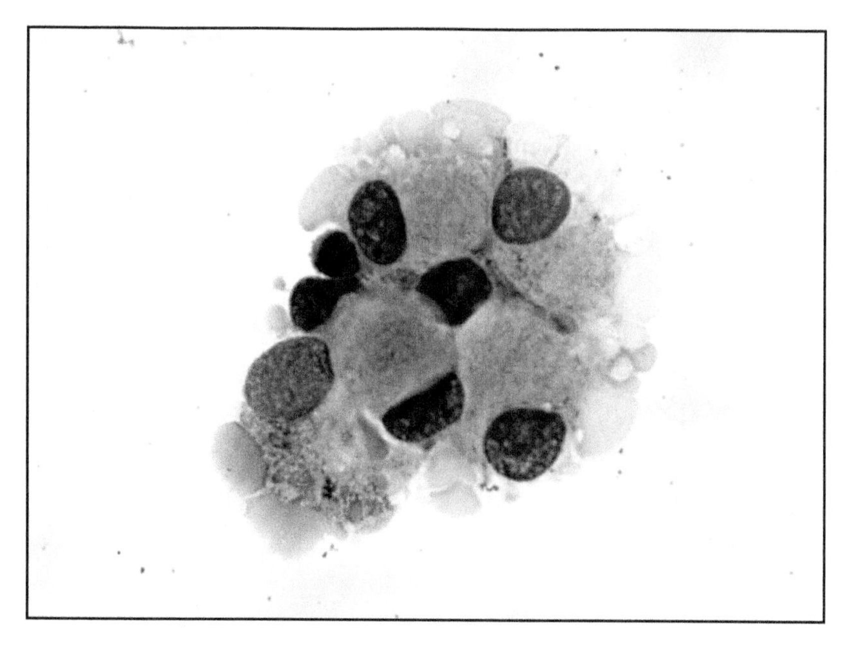

Fig. 5.3. Dog. CSF. Surface epithelial cells. Wright-Giemsa.

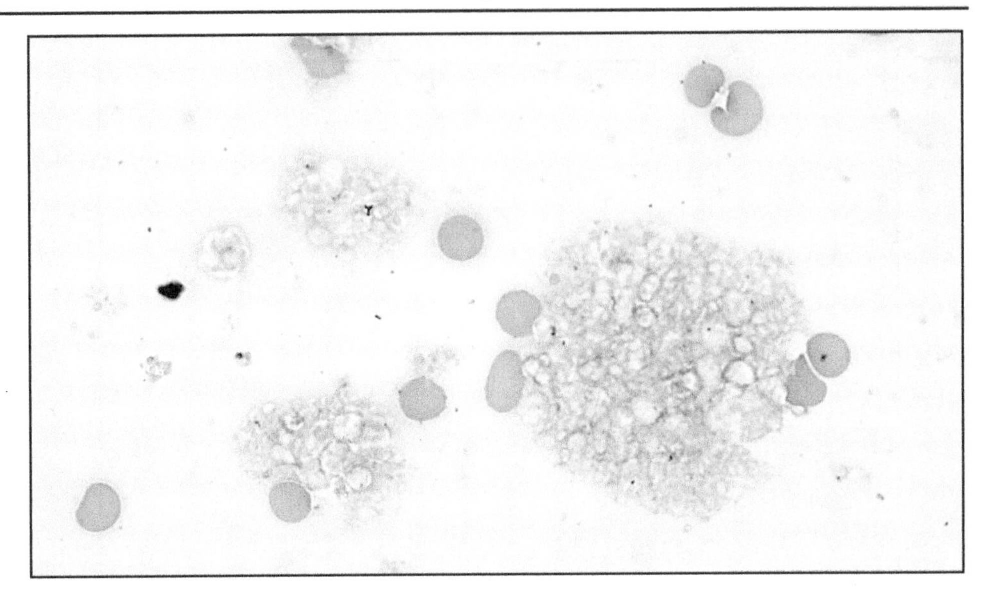

Fig. 5.4. Dog. CSF. Extracellular myelin. Wright-Giemsa.

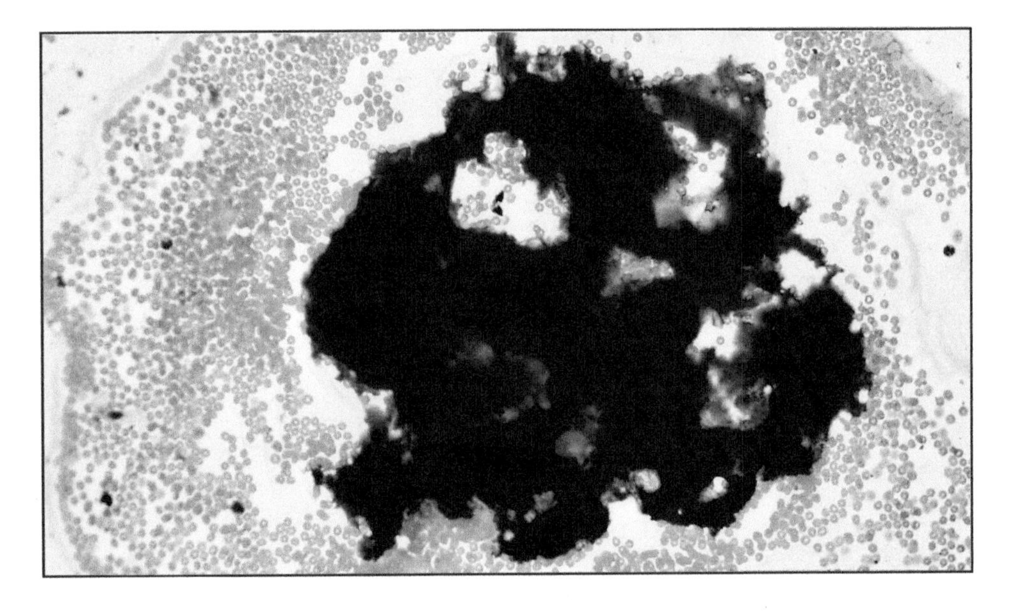

Fig. 5.5. Dog. CSF. Cartilage. Wright-Giemsa.

5.6 Introduction to CSF Abnormalities

A wide variety of conditions can affect the central nervous system, resulting in changes in the cerebrospinal fluid composition. Similarly, not all reactive, inflammatory or neoplastic pathologies in the CNS are accompanied by alteration of the CSF.

The main abnormalities that can occur in the CSF include:

- Increased protein concentration (with or without pleocytosis).
- Increased cellularity (pleocytosis).
- Abnormal leucocyte differential cell count (without pleocytosis).
- Presence of atypical/neoplastic cells.
- Presence of infectious agents.

Increased protein concentration

- The elevation of CSF protein can be associated with a variety of underlying pathologies and usually relates to an increased permeability of the BBB or increased synthesis of proteins or immunoglobulins in the CNS. Main causes include:
    - Inflammation.
    - Reactive CNS changes.
    - Neoplasia.
- An increased protein concentration not associated with a concurrent pleocytosis is termed *albuminocytologic dissociation* (ACD). This is a non-specific alteration that can also be caused by increased permeability of the BBB, increased production of protein within the CSF and/or obstruction of the flow and absorption of CSF. In a recent study, the most common pathologies associated with ACD were:
    - Cranial nerve neuropathy.
    - Brain tumours.
    - Idiopathic vestibular disease.
    - Brain vascular disease.

Increased cellularity

- The presence of increased numbers of nucleated cells in the CSF, above the reference interval, is usually addressed with the term *pleocytosis* (from Greek *pleoion*, 'more').
- The reference interval for the TNCC usually depends on the method of analysis used and can vary slightly in each laboratory.
- Several studies are present in veterinary literature that provide reference intervals in dogs and cats, but often these are derived from low numbers of subjects or unstated sources. These varied from a maximum of <6 cells/µl in dogs and 8 cell/µl in cats to a minimum of 0–2 cells/µl (manual methods). Frequently, a cutoff value of <5 cells/µl is adopted.
- Pleocytosis can be graded as:
    - Mild: 6-50 cells/uL in dogs and cats
    - Moderate:
        - 51–200 cells/µl: dogs.
        - 51–1000 cells/µl: cats.
    - Marked:
        - >200 cells/µl: dogs.
        - >1000 cells/µl: cats.

Main causes of pleocytosis include:

- Inflammation.
- Reactive changes.
- Neoplasia.

Abnormal leucocyte differential cell count

- It can reflect an underlying CNS pathology, also in absence of pleocytosis.
- An increased percentage of neutrophils in CSFs without increased TNCC has been associated with intervertebral disc disease, cerebrovascular accident, vertebral fractures and fibrocartilaginous thromboembolism. Attention should be paid to haemodiluted samples to avoid overinterpreting the presence of neutrophils (which could be blood-derived).
- In absence of blood contamination, a percentage of neutrophils >10–20% is considered unusual.

Presence of atypical cells

- Atypical cells are intended as those cells that are not commonly encountered in CSF of healthy dogs and cats. These may include:
  - Reactive or inflammatory cells: e.g. medium-large lymphoid cells (mixed morphology), plasma cells, eosinophils, macrophages.
  - Neoplastic cells: primary CNS neoplasms or metastatic tumours.

Presence of infectious agents

- Infectious agents that can be found in CSF of dogs and cats include viruses, bacteria, protozoa, algae and fungi.

Further reading

Di Terlizzi, R. and Platt, S.R. (2009) The function, composition and analysis of cerebrospinal fluid in companion animals: part II – analysis. *Veterinary Journal* 180(1), 15–32.

Suñol, A., Garcia-Pertierra, S. and Faller, K.M.E. (2021) Cerebrospinal fluid analysis in dogs: main patterns and prevalence of albuminocytological dissociation. *Veterinary Record* 188(5), e27.

5.7 Inflammatory CNS Disease

Inflammatory disease of the central nervous system may be caused by infectious agents (e.g. bacteria, viruses, protozoa, fungi, etc.) or have a non-infectious aetiology. Non-infectious causes are more common in dogs and are often immune mediated in origin.

5.7.1 Non-infectious CNS inflammatory diseases

Non-infectious inflammatory CNS diseases in dogs can have different anatomic localizations:

- Meninges and associated arteries: steroid-responsive meningitis arteritis (SRMA).
- Brain parenchyma: e.g. granulomatous meningoencephalitis (GME) and necrotizing encephalitis (NE), such as meningoencephalitis (NME) and necrotizing leucoencephalitis (NLE).

> **Pearl and Pitfalls**
>
> An accurate distinction between different non-infectious inflammatory pathologies affecting the brain parenchyma (GME and NE) requires post-mortem histopathology. Due to this, the broader term *meningoencephalitis of unknown origin* (MUO) is more commonly used in the clinical setting.

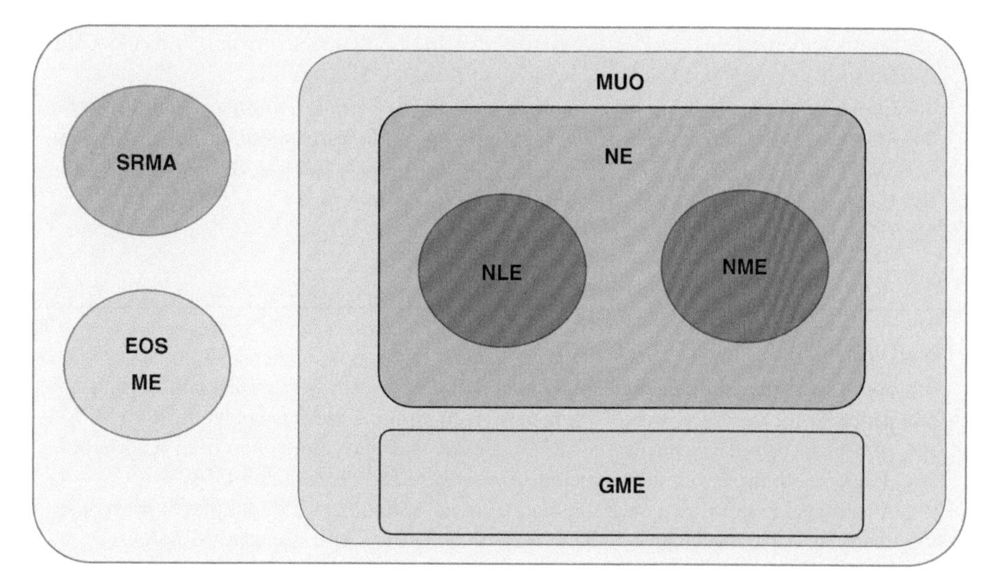

Fig. 5.6. Non-infectious CNS diseases. MUO: meningoencephalitis of unknown origin; NE: necrotizing encephalitis; meningoencephalitis; necrotizing leucoencephalitis; SRMA: steroid-responsive meningitis arteritis; EOS ME: eosinophilic meningoencephalitis.

5.7.1.1 Neutrophilic pleocytosis

Steroid-responsive meningitis arteritis (dog)

Immune-mediated disease affecting the leptomeninges and associated arteries. It is also known as Beagle pain syndrome, aseptic suppurative meningitis and necrotizing vasculitis.

Clinical features

- Both acute and chronic forms have been described.
- Age: most common in young dogs (6–18 months), but the age range extends from 4 months to 7 years.
- Aetiology: uncertain but with an immune-mediated pathophysiology. No environmental, infectious or neoplastic triggers have been identified to date.
- Most common clinical signs in the acute form include stiff and painful gait, cervical rigidity and lowered head carriage, hyperaesthesia along the spinal cord, pyrexia, lethargy and anorexia.
- In the chronic form, repeated episodes of neck pain may be present. Additionally, clinical signs associated to parenchymal involvement may occur, such as ataxia, paresis, tetraparesis and paraplegia.
- The ante-mortem diagnosis is based on a combination of clinical presentation, laboratory and imaging findings, exclusion of other diseases and response to immunosuppressive treatment (corticosteroids).
- The prognosis is guarded to favourable, especially in patients that are treated in the early stages.
- Monitoring of the progression or relapse of the disease may be achieved by measuring serum acute proteins, such as C-reactive protein (CRP) and serum amyloid A (SAA), with the advantage of being less invasive tests than CSF sampling.
- Over-represented canine breeds: Boxers, Beagles, Bernese Mountain Dogs, Nova Scotia Duck Tolling Retrievers, Weimaraners and Wirehaired Pointing Griffon (North America). In most recent studies, also Border Collie, Jack Russell Terrier and Whippet have shown increased odds of developing SRMA.

Pearl and Pitfalls

- Some dogs with immune mediate polyarthritis may present with similar clinical signs as patients with SRMA. Up to 46% of patients with immune-mediated polyarthritis (IMPA) and spinal pain have concurrent SRMA. Breeds that have more often been reported to develop both these pathologies include Akitas and Bernese Mountain Dogs.
- A recent study shows that analysing both cisternal and lumbar CSF samples improves the chance of detecting a high TNCC when evaluating dogs with suspected SRMA.

Cytological features

- Cellularity:
  - Acute form: marked pleocytosis.
  - Chronic form: mild-moderate pleocytosis.
- Protein concentration:
  - Acute form: increased.
  - Chronic form: normal to mildly increased.
- Background: clear with variable numbers of red blood cells.
- Acute form: characterized by numerous non-degenerate neutrophils (up to 75–100%). Low numbers of large mononuclear cells, lymphocytes and plasma cells may also be seen.
- Chronic form: mixed pleocytosis. This is characterized by a lower proportion of neutrophils and a higher percentage of large mononuclear cells and lymphocytes.

Differential diagnoses

- Bacterial and fungal neutrophilic meningitis
- Trauma
- Post-myelographic reactions
- Necrosis
- Underlying neoplasia

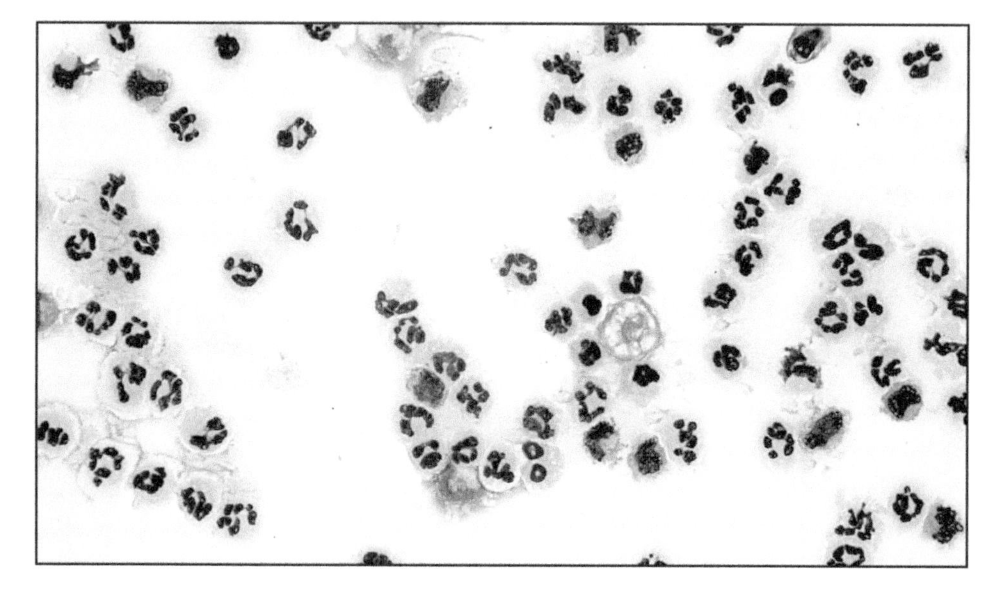

Fig. 5.7. Dog. CSF. Cytospin preparation. SRMA. Predominance of non-degenerate neutrophils. Extracellular myelin is also present. Wright-Giemsa.

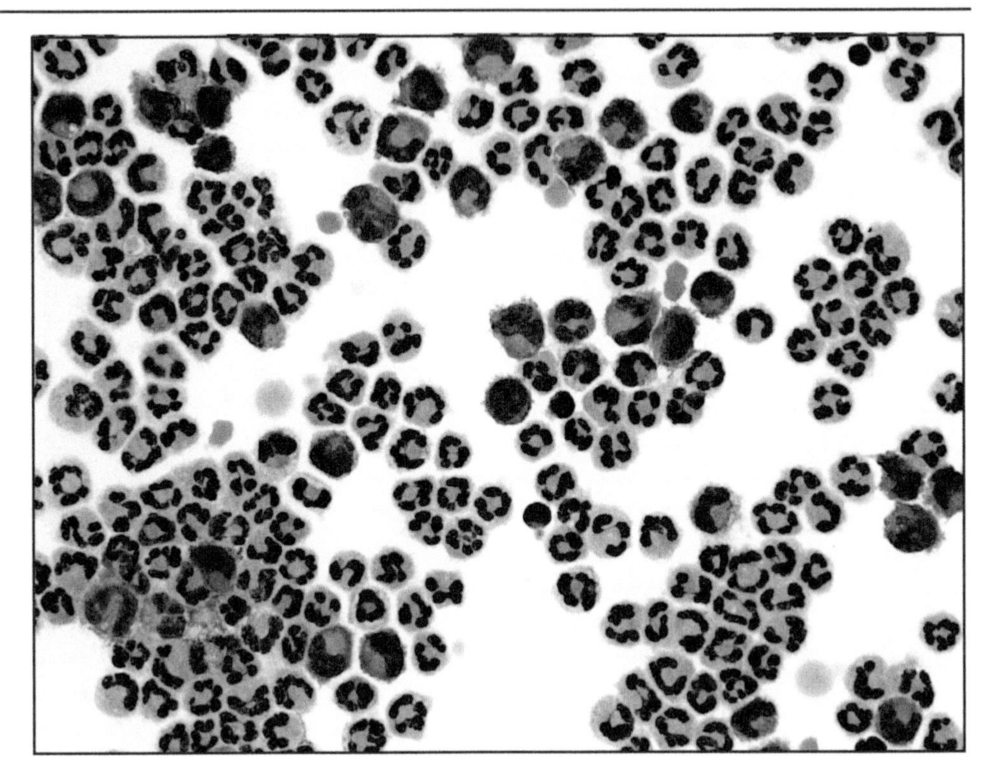

Fig. 5.8. Dog. CSF. Cytospin preparation. More chronic SRMA. Predominance of non-degenerate neutrophils with moderate numbers of monocytoid cells. Wright-Giemsa.

Further reading

Carletti, B.E., De Decker, S., Rose, J., Sanchez-Masian, D., Bersan, E. *et al.* (2019) Evaluation of concurrent analysis of cerebrospinal fluid samples collected from the cerebellomedullary cistern and lumbar subarachnoid space for the diagnosis of steroid-responsive meningitis arteritis in dogs. *Journal of American Veterinary Medicine Association* 255(9), 1035–1038.

5.7.1.2 *Mixed mononuclear pleocytosis*

Granulomatous meningoencephalitis

Idiopathic inflammatory disease of the central nervous system characterized by focal or disseminated granulomatous lesions within the brain and/or spinal cord.

Clinical features

- The clinical signs most typically reflect the localization of the disease, rather than being specific of this disease.
- Age:
  - Dogs: young to middle-aged. Mean age is 5 years, ranging from 6 months to 12 years.
  - Cats: median age 9.4 years old, ranging from 10 months to 12 years.
- Sex: in dogs, both males and females can be affected but females are over-represented. No sex predisposition has been observed in cats.
- In dogs, three forms have been described:
  - Disseminated or multifocal: lesions are localized in two or more areas including the cerebrum, brainstem, cerebellum, spinal cord, meninges and optic nerves. It accounts for approximately 50% of the cases of GME. The clinical signs depend on the area involved. The onset of the disease is usually acute.
  - Focal: limited to one location in the nervous system. It also accounts for approximately 50% of the cases of GME. It seems to have a slower onset and is characterized by signs attributable to a single space-occupying lesion. Most common reported signs reflect lesions within the cerebrum and brainstem.
  - Ocular: uncommon form characterized by lesions in the optic nerves and optic chiasm.
- Lesions usually occur within the white matter and consist of dense aggregates of inflammatory cells arranged in whorling patterns around blood vessels. The inflammatory cells include lymphocytes, monocytoid cells and macrophages, multinucleated giant inflammatory cells, plasma cells and lower numbers of neutrophils.
- Pathogenesis: still unknown, but hypotheses are as follows:
  - Infectious: suggested by some authors, but never been proved.
  - Immune mediated.
  - Neoplastic.
- In general, clinical signs in dogs may include seizures, ataxia, incoordination, falling, cervical hyperesthesia, head tilt, facial and/or trigeminal paralysis, nystagmus, circling, depression, visual deficits, occasionally pyrexia, etc.
- In cats, clinical signs usually have an acute onset. Systemic signs include obtunded mental status, anorexia and pyrexia. Neurological signs include ataxia, paresis with decreased postural reactions, spinal hyperesthesia, generalized or partial seizures, nystagmus, etc.
- The ante-mortem diagnosis is based on a combination of signalment, clinical signs, clinical course, laboratory results and imaging findings. The most useful diagnostic test is CSF analysis.
- The prognosis for permanent recovery is poor in dogs, while in cats it appears to be good with immunomodulatory therapy.
- Over-represented canine breeds: small breeds dogs such as Terriers, Poodles and Toy breeds.

Cytological features

- Cellularity: variable degree of pleocytosis. Occasionally, the cellularity may not be increased.
- Protein concentration: variably increased.
- Total cell count and protein concentrations in patients with GME are usually higher in cisternal samples than in lumbar taps.
- Background: clear with variable numbers of red blood cells.
- Cells are predominantly mixed mononuclear cells including monocytoid cells, foamy macrophages and small lymphocytes. Reactive lymphocytes and plasma cells may also be present. Macrophages may occasionally display leucophagia.
- Neutrophils are usually present in lower numbers (1–20%) although, in some cases, higher numbers may be observed.

Differential diagnoses

- Chronic bacterial meningitis treated with antibiotics
- Fungal infections
- Protozoal disease
- Algal infection
- Ehrlichiosis
- Infarction and necrosis
- Underlying neoplasia

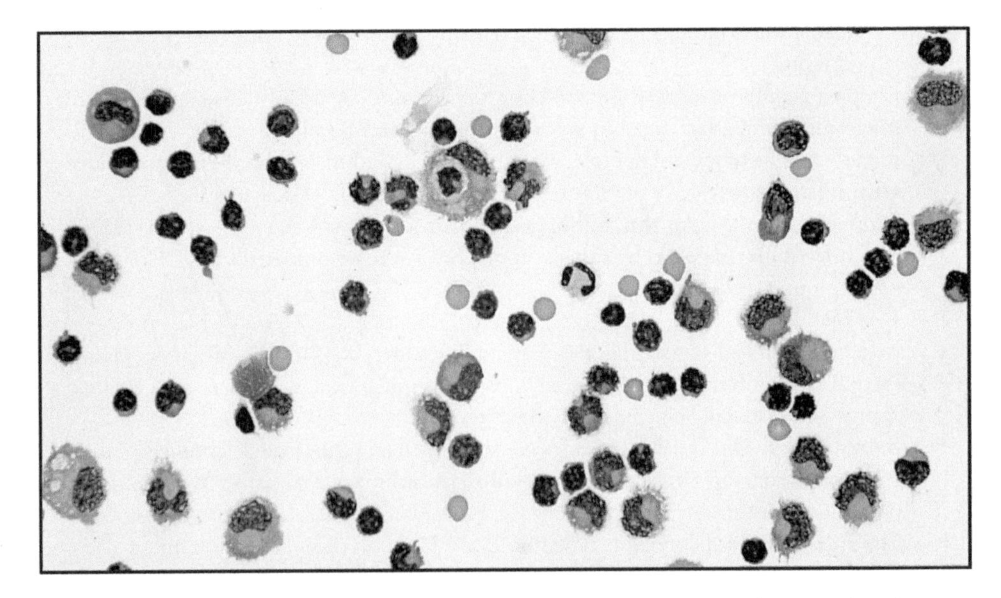

Fig. 5.9. Dog. CSF. Cytospin preparation. Granulomatous meningoencephalitis, mixed mononuclear pleocytosis with predominance of monocytoid cells and lower numbers of small lymphocytes. Leucophagia is observed. Wright-Giemsa.

5.7.1.3 *Lymphocytic pleocytosis*

Necrotizing encephalitis (dogs)

Canine necrotizing encephalitis is an inflammatory disease of unknown aetiology, characterized by fatal outcome. It was previously known as 'Pug dog encephalitis'.

Clinical features

- Rapidly progressive inflammatory disease most commonly occurring in small pure-bred, young dogs.
- Characterized by extensive bilateral asymmetric cerebral necrosis and non-suppurative inflammation, which can involve the following:
  - Cerebral cortex and leptomeninges (NME).
  - Cerebral white matter (NLE).
- Age: ranges from 6 months to 7 years of age but most commonly occurs in younger dogs with a mean age of 2.5 years.
- The aetiology is poorly understood. Several causes have been postulated (e.g. viral and neoplastic), but none have been confirmed. An auto-immune disease appears more likely.
- The clinical signs refer to the cortical disease and include generalized seizures, lethargy, ataxia and progression to coma. Specifically:
  - NME: usually manifests with forebrain signs including seizures, lethargy, anorexia, central blindness, circling and head-pressing. Cervical spinal hyperesthesia may be present, depending on the extent of leptomeningitis.
  - NLE: visual loss, seizures and central vestibular signs reflecting forebrain and brainstem involvement.
- Three histopathologic patterns of NME have been described in literature:
  - Mild inflammatory cell infiltration: acute phase.
  - Moderate malacic changes and intense inflammatory reactions, especially in the leptomeninges: subacute phase.
  - Extensive malacia: chronic phase.
- Over-represented breeds:
  - NME: Pugs, Maltese, Chihuahua, Pekingese, Shih Tzu, West Highland White Terriers, Papillons, Coton de Tulears, Brussels Griffons.
  - NLE: Yorkshire Terriers, French Bulldogs.

Cytological features

- Cellularity: variable degree of pleocytosis.
- Protein concentration: variably increased.
- Background: clear with variable numbers of red blood cells.
- The pleocytosis is mononuclear and most commonly consists of a majority of small lymphocytes (>80%) with lower numbers of monocytoid cells.
- Mixed pleocytosis may be observed in some cases.

Differential diagnoses

- Viral diseases: e.g. canine distemper virus (CDV)
- Ehrlichiosis and protozoal disease
- Rarely chronic bacterial meningitis following antibiotic therapy
- Lymphoma

Pearls and Pitfalls

NME and NLE are inflammatory necrotizing diseases whose nomenclature derives from the affected region of the brain. However, they are characterized by similar clinical signs, signalment and neuropathology. For this reason, the more inclusive term NE (which includes both NME and NLE) is preferred for ante-mortem diagnosis.

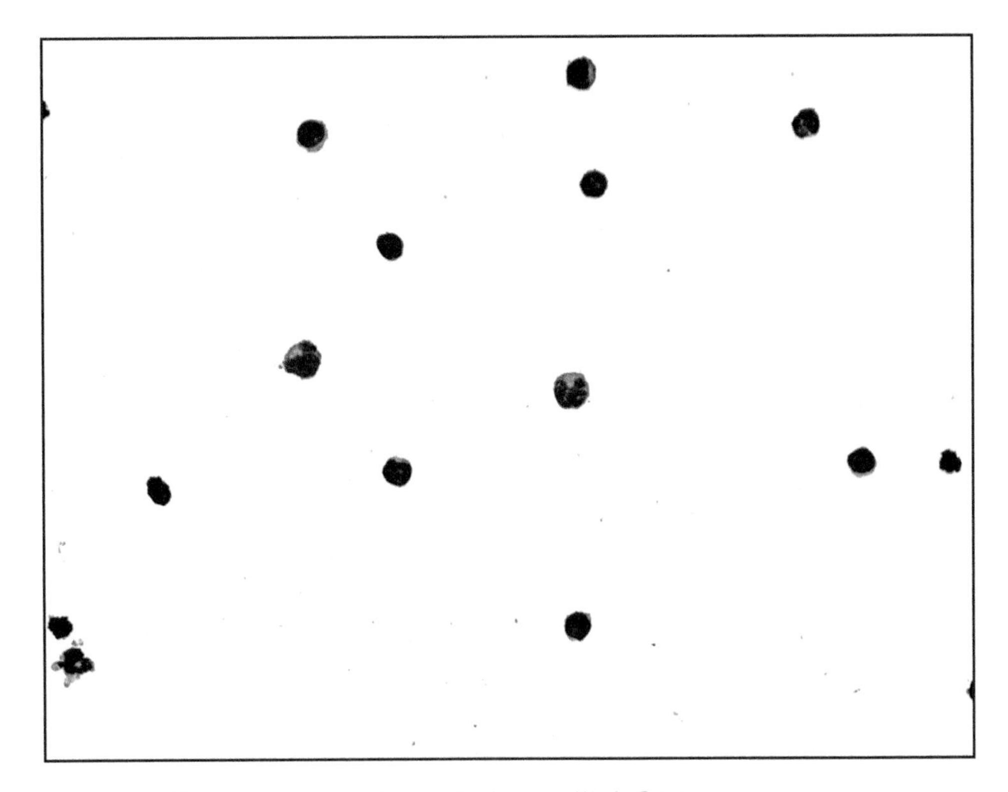

Fig. 5.10. Dog. CSF. Cytospin preparation. Lymphocytic pleocytosis. Wright-Giemsa.

5.7.1.4 *Eosinophilic pleocytosis*

Eosinophilic meningoencephalitis

Eosinophilic meningoencephalitis is a rare disease of unknown origin characterized by an eosinophilic pleocytosis. It can be referred to as eosinophilic meningoencephalitis of unknown origin (eosinophilic MUO) and steroid-responsive meningoencephalitis.

Clinical features

- Rare condition reported in dogs and, less frequently, in cats.
- Age: usually young dogs.
- The underlying aetiology is unknown, but an immune-mediated disorder appears likely.
- The clinical signs often reflect the anatomical distribution of the inflammatory lesions:
  - Diffuse forebrain involvement: ataxia, visual and proprioceptive deficits, cervical hyperaesthesia, mentation changes and convulsions.
  - Central vestibular lesions: head tilt, mentation changes, nystagmus and vestibular ataxia.
- Peripheral eosinophilia may be present.
- There is usually a good response to corticosteroid treatment.
- Over-represented canine breeds: large breeds are most commonly affected and breeds such as Rottweiler and Golden Retriever might be predisposed.

Cytological features

- Cellularity: variable degree of pleocytosis often marked.
- Protein concentration: variably increased.
- Background: clear with variable numbers of red blood cells.
- CSF cytology is characterized by numerous eosinophils (>20% by some sources) and low numbers of other inflammatory cells.

Differential diagnoses

- Protozoal disease: e.g. toxoplasmosis and neosporosis
- Bacterial infection: e.g. ehrlichiosis
- Fungal disease: e.g. cryptococcosis
- Parasitic infections: e.g. *Angiostrongylus vasorum*
- Algal disease: protothecosis

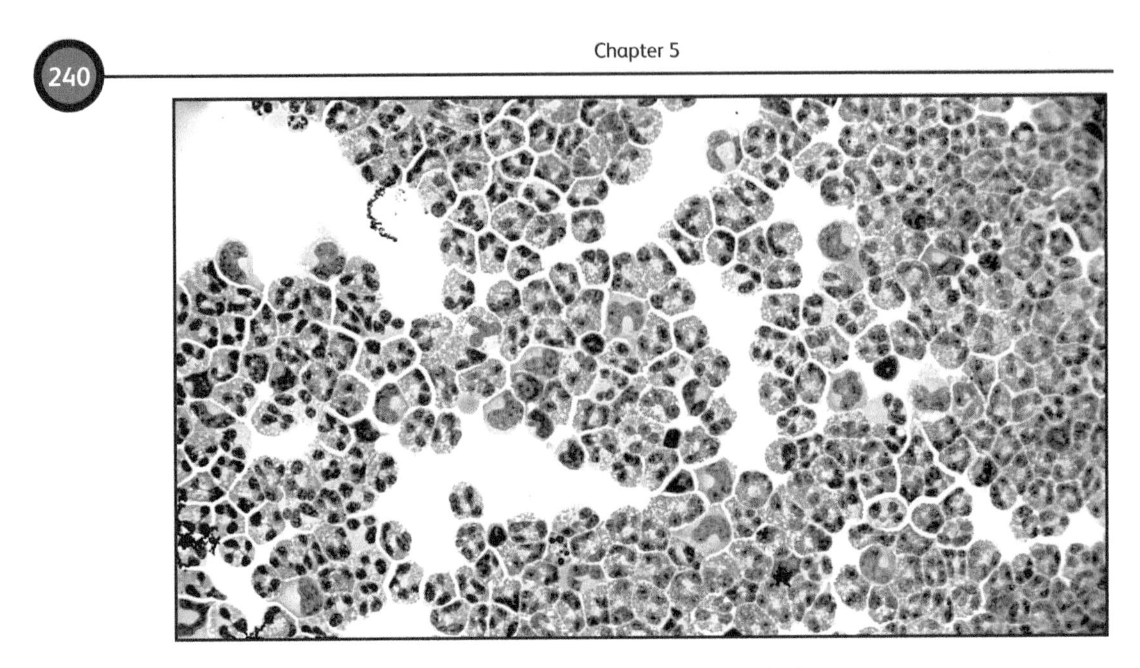

Fig. 5.11. Dog. CSF. Cytospin preparation. Eosinophilic pleocytosis. Wright-Giemsa.

5.7.2 Infectious CNS inflammatory diseases

Infectious agents that can cause CNS inflammation include viruses, bacteria, protozoa, rickettsia, fungi and algae.

5.7.2.1 Viral diseases of the CNS

- Different viruses can cause CNS disease in dogs and cats, but those most commonly encountered in clinical practice include canine distemper virus (CDV), feline infectious peritonitis (FIP) and feline immunodeficiency virus (FIV).
- Often associated with a lymphocytic pleocytosis, except for FIP which is more often associated with a neutrophilic inflammation.

Canine distemper encephalomyelitis

- Caused by a Paramyxoviridae, genus Morbillivirus: CDV.
- Relatively common CNS disorder, especially in non-vaccinated young dogs.
- Neurological signs are variable and depend if the disease has a multifocal or localized distribution. They include generalized seizures, depression, disorientation, head tilt, nystagmus, hypermetria, etc.
- Clinical signs also depend on the age and immune status of the patient. Only a subpopulation of infected patients develops neurological signs, which tend to occur 1–6 weeks after acute illness, but can also occur after subclinical infection. They can be associated with more systemic clinical signs, especially in young dogs. These include GI and respiratory signs and hyperkeratosis of footpads.

Cytological features

- Cellularity: usually mildly to moderately increased.
- Background: variably haemodiluted due to iatrogenic haemorrhage.
- As for most viral diseases affecting the CNS, a mild lymphocytic pleocytosis can be observed in dogs affected by CDV. An increased number of macrophages may also be observed.
- Rarely, viral inclusions can be found within leucocytes or erythrocytes. They appear as small round basophilic structures within the cytoplasm of the cells.

Differential diagnoses

- Necrotizing encephalitis
- Protozoal disease and ehrlichiosis

Pearls and Pitfalls

Distemper viral inclusions stain more darkly and are more often visible with Diff-Quik and Hemacolor, as compared to Wright's stain. This may facilitate their detection.

Feline infectious peritonitis

FIP is the most common cause of pleocytosis in cats.

- Caused by feline coronavirus (FCoV).
- Cats with FIP may develop neurological clinical signs (approximately 12%). Clinical signs relate to the area of the CNS that is affected. They commonly include ataxia, nystagmus and seizures. With meningitis, signs may include incoordination, hyperesthesia, behavioural changes, cranial nerve defects and fever.
- Ocular disease often accompanies the neurological signs. These often manifest with inflammation of the anterior uveal tract (ciliary body and iris). Monolateral or bilateral, partial or complete discolouration of the iris can be observed. FIP can also cause cuffing of the retinal vasculature visible on examination of the fundus.

Cytological features

- Cellularity: moderately increased (50–500 cells/µl).
- Protein concentration: high (usually >2 g/l).
- Background: variably haemodiluted due to iatrogenic haemorrhage.
- The pleocytosis can be mixed, but it is more frequently neutrophilic (>50% of neutrophils). Neutrophils are non-degenerate.
- CSF analysis can be unremarkable in some cats with FIP or show only elevated protein concentration.
- Immunostaining of FCoV antigen: detection of a large amount of viral antigen within macrophages (cytology or histopathology samples) indicates high viral replication in these cells. It is highly specific and is considered the gold standard for the diagnosis of FIP. Negative results do not exclude the disease. In particular, the sensitivity of FCoV immunostaining in fluids is reported to vary between 57% and 100%.
- Fluid FCoV PCR: this may be used to confirm FCoV as the underlying cause of the clinical signs. However, less virulent FCoV can occasionally spread systemically in cats without FIP. Therefore, this test is not necessarily specific for a diagnosis of FIP, although it is highly sensitive. Detection of higher viral loads by real-time RT-qPCR increases the probability of FIP.

Differential diagnoses

- Bacterial meningitis
- Protozoal disease
- Necrosis
- Underlying neoplasia

Further reading

Thayer, V., Gogolski, S., Felten, S., Hartmann, K., Kennedy, M. *et al.* (2022) 2022 AAFP/EveryCat feline infectious peritonitis diagnosis guidelines. *Journal of Feline Medicine and Surgery* 24(9), 905–933.

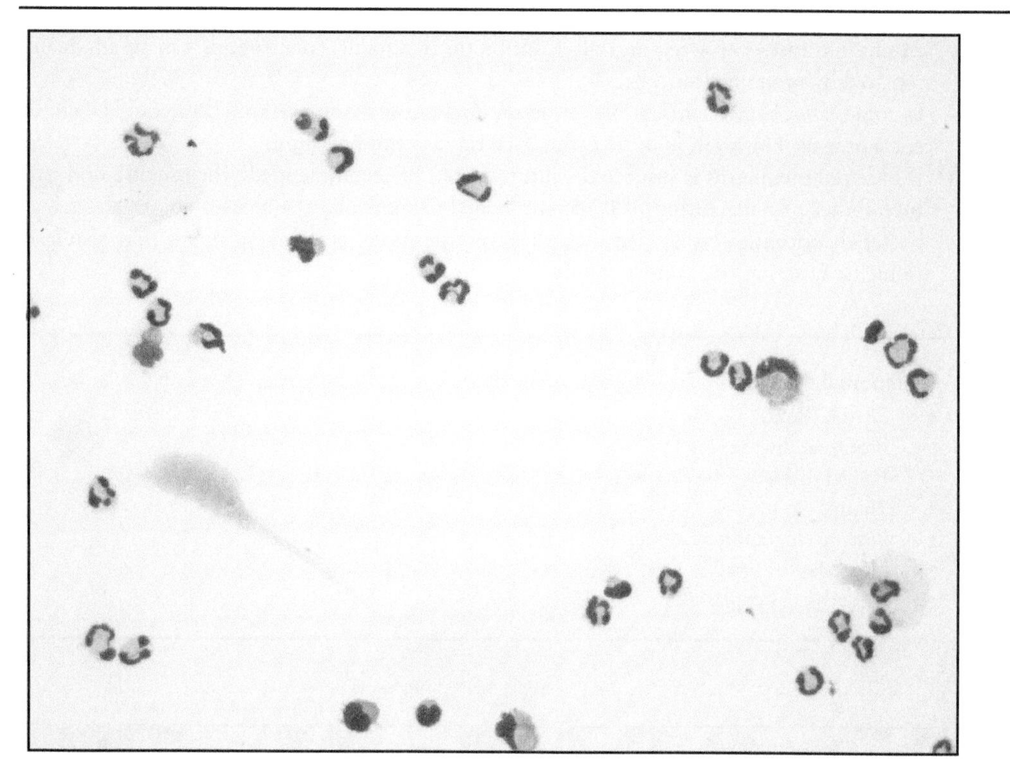

Fig. 5.12. Cat. CSF. Cytospin preparation. FIP, neutrophilic pleocytosis. Wright-Giemsa. (*Courtesy of Laura Pintore.*)

5.7.2.2 Bacterial meningitis

- Bacterial meningitis is a rare condition described in dogs and cats.
- Age: animals of any age can be affected, although adult patients are predisposed (dogs).
- Pathogenesis:
  - Haematogenous spread from a distant inflammatory focus (e.g. vegetative endocarditis, urinary tract infection and splenic or pulmonary abscess).
  - Contiguity: direct extension from ears, sinuses, eyes.
  - Trauma: e.g. bite wound.
  - Iatrogenic: e.g. via spinal needle.
- Clinical signs usually have an acute onset. Common neurological signs are hyperesthesia, fever, cervical pain and rigidity, seizures, vomiting (due to increased intracranial pressure or direct effect on vomit centre).
- Examples of aetiologic agents cultured in CSF include: *Pasteurella* spp., *Staphylococcus aureus*, *Actinomyces* spp., *Nocardia* spp., *Escherichia coli*, *Streptococcus* spp.

Cytological features

- Cellularity: high to very high (500 cells/μl to >1000 cells/μl).
- Protein concentration: increased.
- Background: variably haemodiluted due to iatrogenic haemorrhage.
- The pleocytosis in subjects with bacterial meningitis is typically neutrophilic, especially in the acute phase. Neutrophils may not be degenerate or could show variable degrees of karyolysis.

- In chronic cases (>1 week and after antibiotic treatment), neutrophils can be gradually replaced by mononuclear cells.
- In some cases, bacteria are readily found on microscopic examination. They could be either cocci or rods. However, in other cases, bacteria may not be found.
- If bacterial meningitis is suspected, culture would be recommended. The use of blood culture bottles or nutrient broths is recommended to maximize the recovery of organisms, as bacterial concentration is often low. However, the use of enrichment media may also lead to higher false-positive culture results.

Differential diagnoses

- SRMA (dogs)
- Protozoal disease (cats)
- Fungal disease
- Trauma
- Post-myelographic reactions
- Necrosis
- Underlying neoplasia

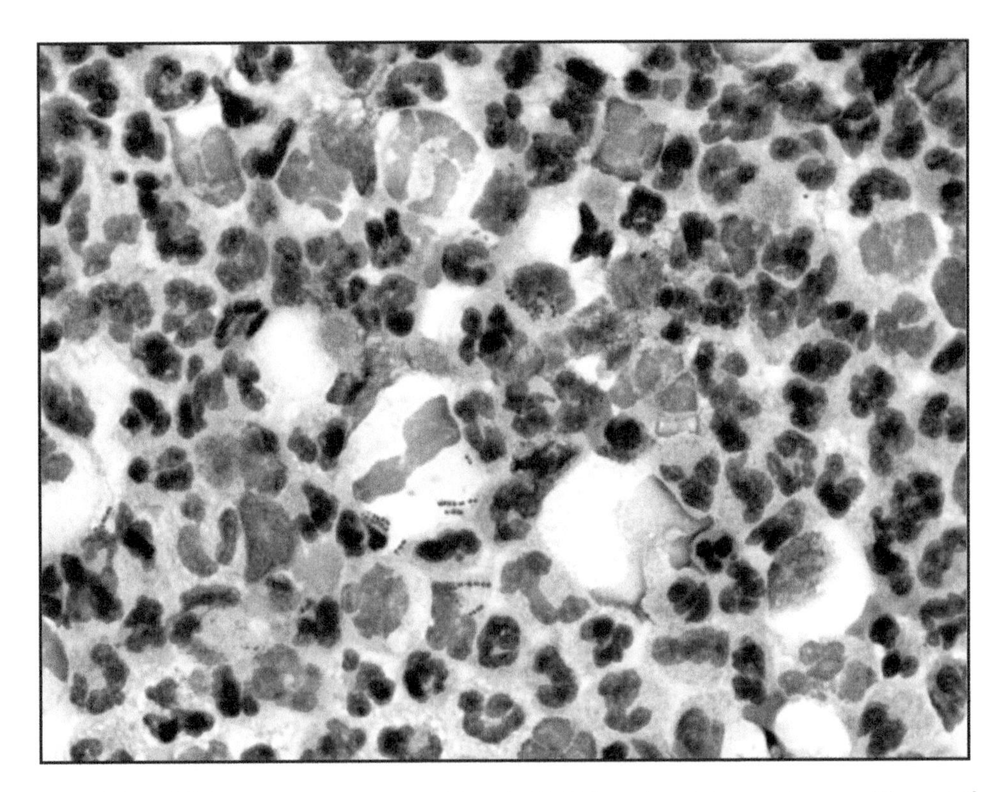

Fig. 5.13. Dog. CSF. Cytospin preparation, bacterial meningitis, high numbers of degenerate neutrophils, some of which contain phagocytosed bacteria. Wright-Giemsa.

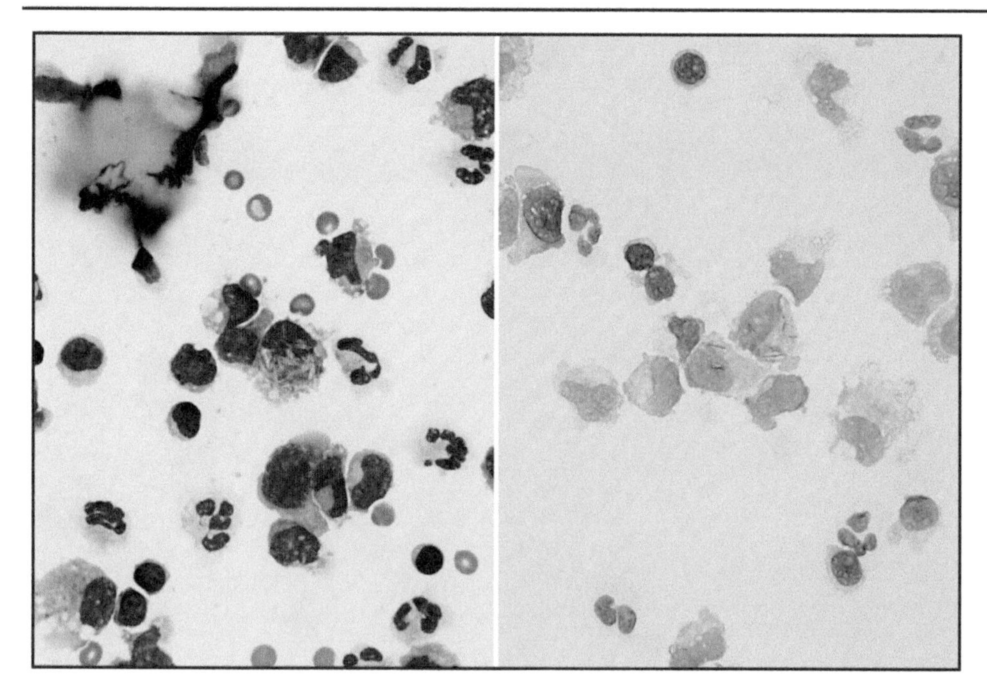

Fig. 5.14. Dog. CSF. Cytospin preparation, bacterial infection caused by *Mycobacterium* spp.. (Left) Wright-Giemsa; (right) Acid-Fast. (*Courtesy of Angela Royal.*)

5.7.2.3 Fungal diseases of the CNS

- Fungal infections of the CNS can occur in both dogs and cats, causing a granulomatous meningoencephalitis.
- CNS fungal diseases described in dogs and cats include cryptococcosis (cats > dogs), blastomycosis, coccidiomycosis (dogs > cats), histoplasmosis, phaeohyphomycosis, aspergillosis and fusariosis.
- Some of these agents are ubiquitous; others are linked to specific geographic areas.
- Immunosuppressed patients (e.g. concurrent underlying disease, immunosuppressive therapy, chemotherapy) are more susceptible.
- Clinical signs may be acute or chronic and reflect either localized or, more frequently, multifocal changes. They are variable and include seizures, depression, circling, ataxia, disorientation, pelvic limb paresis, paraplegia, anisocoria, mydriasis, blindness and cranial nerves deficit.
- Other organ systems can be involved and concurrent respiratory and ocular disease is not uncommon.

Cytological features

- Cellularity: most frequently increased. In a small percentage of cases with CNS cryptococcosis, the TNCC was reported to be within the reference interval.
- Protein concentration: usually increased.
- Background: variably haemodiluted due to iatrogenic haemorrhage.
- The type of pleocytosis can be variable: neutrophilic, eosinophilic, mononuclear or mixed. Low numbers of plasma cells and mast cells can be found in some cases.
- Fungal elements may or may not be found on CSF microscopic examination.

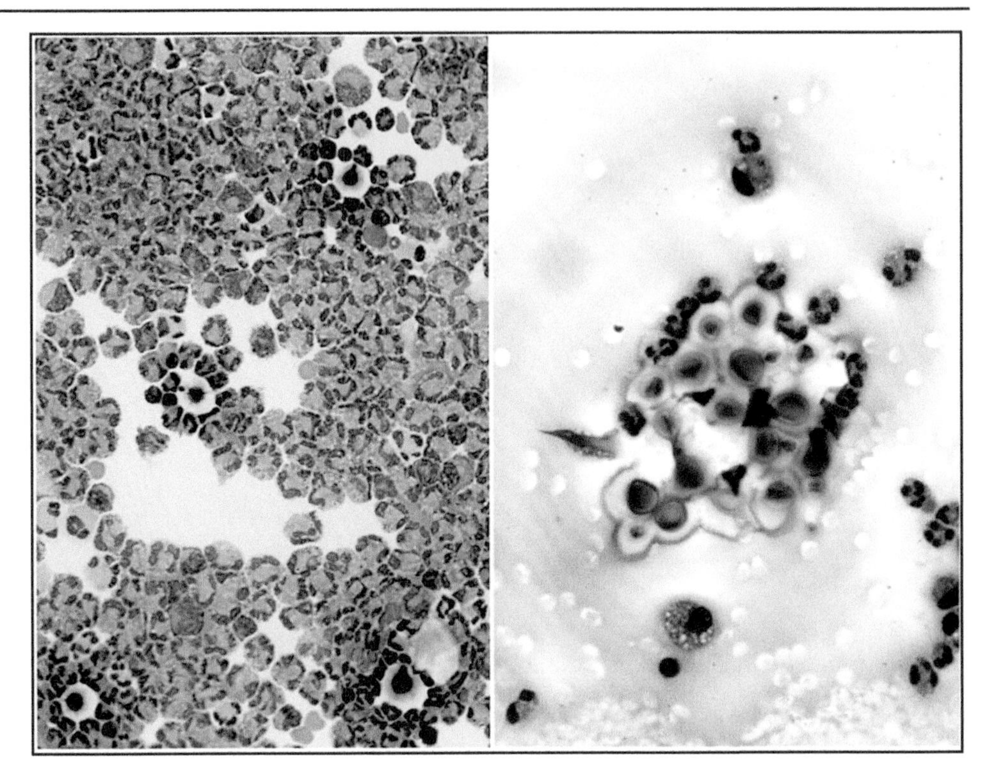

Fig. 5.15. Dog. CSF. Cytospin preparation. CNS cryptococcosis, fungal elements are seen among numerous eosinophils. Wright-Giemsa. (Left: *courtesy of Alice Pastorello.*)

5.7.2.4 Prothotecosis (algal disease)

- *Prototheca* is a ubiquitous algae with worldwide distribution.
- Clinically significant disease is relatively rare in dogs and cats.
- The clinical manifestation depends on the species infected:
  - Cats: only cutaneous forms have been reported.
  - Dogs: often develop disseminated infections. Gastroenteric signs are the most common, followed by the neurological signs. Skin lesion may also be present. Rarely, only the neurological manifestation has been described.

Cytological features

- Cellularity: most frequently high.
- Background: variably haemodiluted due to iatrogenic haemorrhage.
- The pleocytosis is often eosinophilic, with a percentage of eosinophils often ≥50%. Other inflammatory cells that might be present consist of large mononuclear cells, lymphocytes (including large granular lymphocytes) and neutrophils.
- Infectious agents have rarely been observed on CSF microscopic examination.
- Organisms vary in size, depending on the species and stage of development. They range from 1.3 μm to 13.4 μm in diameter and from 1.3 μm to 16.1 μm in length. They have thin non-staining cell walls, basophilic granular cytoplasm and small centrally placed nuclei.

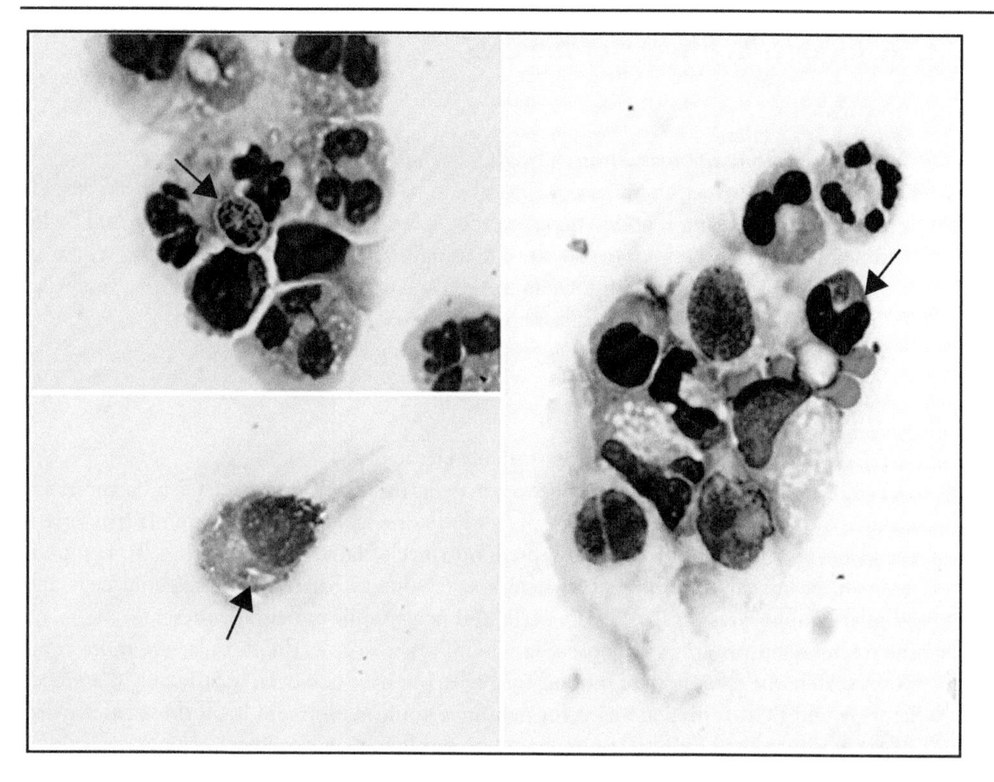

Fig. 5.16. Dog, CSF. Cytospin preparation. (Top left) Prototechosis. (*Courtesy of L.V. Lane*); (Bottom left) Neospora – tachyzoite seen within the inflammatory cells (*Courtesy of Alice Pastorello*); (Right) Ehrlichiosis, Morula seen within a monocytosis cell. (*Courtesy of Robert Lukacs.*)

5.7.2.5 Protozoal encephalitis/encephalomyelitis

- Caused by *Toxoplasma* (dogs and cats), *Neospora* (dogs) or *Sarcocystis* (rare in dogs and cats).
- Most frequent in young or adult immunocompromised animals. Co-infections with CDV and *Ehrlichia* (dogs) or FIP (cats) are not uncommon.
- Clinical signs depend on the area of the CNS that is affected. These may include seizures, behavioural changes, cranial nerve deficits, diffuse neuromuscular disease. A progressive cerebellar ataxia has been described in adult dogs with neosporosis.

Cytological features

- Cellularity and protein concentration: can be variably increased.
- Background: variably haemodiluted due to iatrogenic haemorrhage. In case of true haemorrhage, xanthochromia of the CSF supernatant might be present.
- Pleocytosis is often mononuclear or mixed, especially in dogs. An eosinophilic pleocytosis has been also described in some dogs with protozoal disease. Cats may mount a neutrophilic inflammation.
- The infectious agents can rarely be found in the CSF within leucocytes.
- The organisms are usually crescent- or banana-shaped with a small purple nucleus and clear or pale basophilic cytoplasm.

5.7.2.6 Rickettsial disease of the CNS

Canine monocytic ehrlichiosis

- Caused by *Ehrlichia canis* transmitted by *Rhipicephalus sanguineus.*
- The disease manifests with a variety of clinical and haematological signs and can affect multiple organs, such as lymph nodes, bone marrow, spleen, liver, ophthalmic system and CNS.
- Neurological clinical signs are the result of meningitis and/or meningeal bleeding. Signs of meningitis include seizures, stupor, ataxia, vestibular dysfunction, anisocoria, cerebellar dysfunction and generalized or localized hyperesthesia.
- *E. canis* often causes a lymphoplasmacytic leptomeningitis.

Cytological features

- Cellularity and protein concentration: variably elevated.
- Background: variably haemodiluted due to iatrogenic haemorrhage or true CNS haemorrhage secondary to thrombocytopenia. In case of true haemorrhage, CSF xanthochromia is observed.
- The pleocytosis is often mixed, with a predominance of large mononuclear cells. Lymphocytes can be mixed including small lymphocytes, intermediate/large lymphoid cells and granular lymphocytes (LGLs). Plasma cells and neutrophils can also be present.
- The microorganisms are rarely observed on CSF microscopy. The morulae are more commonly seen in the cytoplasm of monocytoid cells, but have also been occasionally described.
- Serology and PCR testing are used for definitive confirmation and in all those cases when infection is suspected but infectious agents are not found on cytology.

Further reading

Aroch, I., Baneth, G., Salant, H., Nachum-Biala, Y., Berkowitz, A. *et al.* (2018) Neospora caninum and Ehrlichia *canis* co-infection in a dog with meningoencephalitis. *Veterinary Clinical Pathology* 47(2), 289–293.

Cardy, T.J.A. and Cornelis, I. (2018) Clinical presentation and magnetic resonance imaging findings in 11 dogs with eosinophilic meningoencephalitis of unknown aetiology. *Journal of Small Animal Practice* 59(7), 422–431.

Coates, J.R. and Jeffery, N.D. (2014) Perspectives on meningoencephalomyelitis of unknown origin. *Veterinary Clinics of North America: Small Animal Practice* 44(6), 1157–1185.

Di Terlizzi, R. and Platt, S.R. (2009) The function, composition and analysis of cerebrospinal fluid in companion animals: part II – analysis. *Veterinary Journal* 180(1), 15–32.

Negrin, A., Spencer, S. and Cherubini, G.B. (2017) Feline meningoencephalomyelitis of unknown origin: a retrospective analysis of 16 cases. *Canadian Veterinary Journal* 58(10), 1073–1080.

Windsor, R.C., Sturges, B.K., Vernau, K.M. and Vernau, W. (2009) Cerebrospinal fluid eosinophilia in dogs. *Journal of Veterinary Internal Medicine* 23(2), 275–281.

Table 5.1. Differential diagnoses for different cytological patterns.

Neutrophilic pleocytosis	**Non-infectious** SRMA Underlying neoplasia Trauma Post-myelographic reactions Necrosis **Infectious** Bacterial infection FIP (cats) Protozoal disease (cats. Can also be mixed) Fungal disease (most frequently mixed)
Mixed mononuclear pleocytosis	**Non-infectious** GME Infarction and necrosis Underlying neoplasia **Infectious** Chronic bacterial infection post-antibiotic therapy Protozoal disease Fungal infection Ehrlichiosis Algal infection (e.g. protothecosis)
Lymphocytic pleocytosis	**Non-infectious** NE (dogs) (small cell) lymphoma (cats) **Infectious** Viral diseases: e.g. CDV Ehrlichiosis Protozoal disease Rarely chronic bacterial meningitis post-antibiotic therapy
Eosinophilic pleocytosis	**Non-infectious** Eosinophilic MUO/SRMA **Infectious** Protothecosis Fungal infection Protozoal disease (dogs. Most frequently mixed) Migrating helminths

5.8 Lysosomal Storage Disease

Lysosomal storage diseases (LSDs) are a heterogeneous group of inherited metabolic disorders caused by a defect in lysosomal function that leads to the accumulation of substrates in excess in various organs' cells, including the CNS.

Pathophysiology

- Most commonly autosomal recessive (except for MPS II that is X-linked).
- Caused by the deficiency of one or more enzymes within the lysosomes or by the deficiency of an activating protein or co-factor necessary for enzyme activity, resulting in the reduction or elimination of the catalytic activity of that particular enzyme. This causes the accumulation within the lysosome of the substrate of that enzyme and subsequent cell swelling.
- Historically, the clinical manifestations of LSDs have been considered as direct consequences of the storage of inert substrates in tissues.
- Recent studies are highlighting a more complex mechanism of the disease associated with LSDs, including altered autophagy and accumulation of autophagic substrates, dysregulation of signaling pathways and activation of inflammation, mitochondrial dysfunction, abnormalities of calcium homeostasis and oxidative stress.
- LDSs can be subclassified based on the metabolic pathway affected and type of storage found. Most common subgroups described in dogs and cats include as follows:
  - Glycoproteinoses.
  - Sphingolipidoses.
  - Oligosaccharidoses.
  - Mucopolysaccharidoses.
  - Proteinoses.
- Some of the LSDs affect only the CNS; others may involve other organs causing organomegaly or musculoskeletal abnormalities.
- The accumulation of material can microscopically present as vacuoles or granules.

Clinical features

- LSDs are chronic and progressive disorders.
- Age: often young animals are affected (1–2 years). The age of onset of the clinical signs can depend on the severity and mechanism of the underlying mutation.
- Clinical signs start developing when the accumulated material interferes with cell function.
- Most of LSDs can be divided into:
  - LSDs with CNS clinical signs.
  - LSDs without CNS clinical signs.
- The clinical signs depend on the specific disorder, but often include behavioural changes, ataxia, blindness, dementia and seizures.
- Often, the neuronal storage diseases begin with cerebellar or cerebellovestibular signs, such as tremor, ataxia, dysmetria and nystagmus with progression to paresis and paralysis.
- Sex: no gender predisposition is described.
- When LSD is suspected clinically, the diagnosis is reached by confirmation of the metabolic anomaly by genetic testing, by confirming the presence of substrate accumulation on tissue biopsy (muscle, brain, nerves) or less frequently by haematology/cytology.
- Over-represented breeds: there are reported breed predispositions for most of the lysosomal storage diseases. However, these disorders may occur in any breed, and new mutations can be identified at any time.

Cytological features

- Cellularity and protein concentration are generally within reference intervals.
- Background: clear. Iatrogenic haemodilution is possible.
- In some LSDs but not all, the leucocytes present in the CSF could be vacuolated or may contain purple granules representing the storage material.
- When suspected clinically, blood-film examination for screening for abnormal leucocyte granulation and vacuolation is a helpful addition to CSF analysis.

Pearls and Pitfalls

Although the excess of substrates may be present in all cells with lysosomes, not all cells will be vacuolated or granulated.

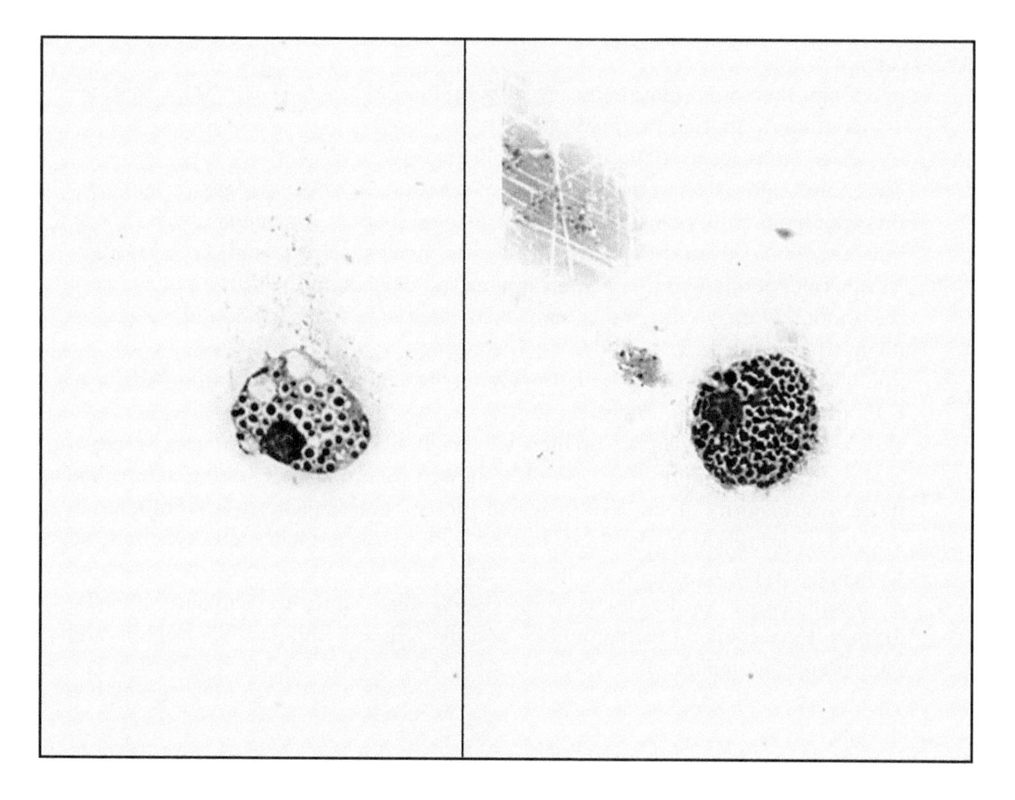

Fig. 5.17. Dog. CSF. Cytospin preparation. Lysosomal storage disease. (Left: *courtesy of Taryn Sibley*; right: *courtesy of Reema Patel.*)

Further reading

Skelly, B.J. and Franklin, R.J. (2002) Recognition and diagnosis of lysosomal storage diseases in the cat and dog. *Journal of Veterinary Internal Medicine* 16(2), 133–141.

5.9 Neoplasms

Tumours affecting the CNS could be primary or metastatic.

5.9.1 Primary CNS neoplasia

Clinical features

- Dogs: approximately 90% of the primary brain tumours encountered in clinical practice include meningiomas, gliomas (astrocytomas, glioblastomas, ependymomas and oligodendrogliomas) and choroid plexus neoplasms. Other tumours such as medulloblastoma have also been reported but are extremely rare.
- Cats: the most common primary CNS neoplasm is meningioma (59% of total brain tumours).
- Other tumours that may arise primarily in the CSF or be part of a more systemic disease (disseminated) are lymphoma and histiocytic sarcoma (HS).
- Age:
    - Dogs: they can occur at any age, although middle-aged to older dogs are more commonly affected (>5 years old).
    - Cats: mean age for brain tumours is 11 years old.
- The clinical signs relate to the mass effect of the tumour, which may invade and compress the brain tissue, causing secondary changes such as intracranial haemorrhage, inflammation, oedema and obstructive hydrocephalus. Seizures and central vestibular signs are the most common clinical signs and depend on the neurolocalization of the tumour. Non-specific clinical signs such as lethargy, inappetence and weight loss might be also observed.
- The diagnosis of brain tumour is usually reached by advanced imaging (MRI and CT), histopathology and necroscopy.
- CSF analysis is often used as a preliminary test. Based on two retrospective studies of canine primary brain tumours, over 90% showed abnormal CSF findings consisting, in the vast majority of cases, of increased protein and/or pleocytosis. Tumour cells only rarely exfoliated in the fluid, making CSF cytology highly sensitive for CNS pathology but poorly specific for neoplasia.
- Over-represented breeds: Golden Retrievers, Boxers, Miniature Schnauzer and Rat Terriers (intracranial meningiomas); Boston Terriers, Bullmastiffs, English and French bulldogs (gliomas).

Cytological features

- Neoplastic cells of primary CNS tumours are rarely encountered in CSF cytology. This depends on the location of the neoplasm and its access to the ventricle system.
- Only the primary brain tumours that have been reported to have exfoliated in CSF samples are described below. For detailed cytological description of primary neoplasms observed on tissue imprint of the primary mass, the reader can refer to other textbooks.

Choroid plexus papilloma/carcinoma

Clinical features

- In dogs, choroid plexus tumours account for approximately 10% of all primary intracranial CNS neoplasms and could be papillomas (CPPs) or carcinomas (CPCs).
- Age: middle-age dogs (mean: 6 years old).
- They arise from the epithelium lining the choroid plexus and are generally found in the lateral, third or fourth ventricles or lateral apertures.
- Approximately 50% of CPCs can be associated with distant metastases to the subarachnoid space, but extraneural metastases are not reported.
- A definitive diagnosis is usually reached with histopathology.

Cytological features

- Cellularity: variably increased with a mixed but mostly large mononuclear pleocytosis.
- Protein concentration: increased. In one study on choroid plexus tumours, it was found that carcinomas had a higher protein concentration than papillomas and that a value >8 g/l was exclusively associated with a diagnosis of carcinoma.
- When present, pleocytosis is often mixed. Neoplastic cells rarely exfoliate in CSF. When they do, they can be found in variably sized, cohesive clusters and rafts (up to >200 cells per cluster). Cells have round-to-oval nuclei with moderately coarse chromatin and a single, irregularly shaped nucleolus. The cytoplasm is small in amount, slightly granular, basophilic and often vacuolated. In carcinomas, moderate to marked anisokaryosis and anisocytosis may be observed and mitoses can be found.

Differential diagnoses

- Metastatic carcinoma
- Ependymoma
- Meningioma

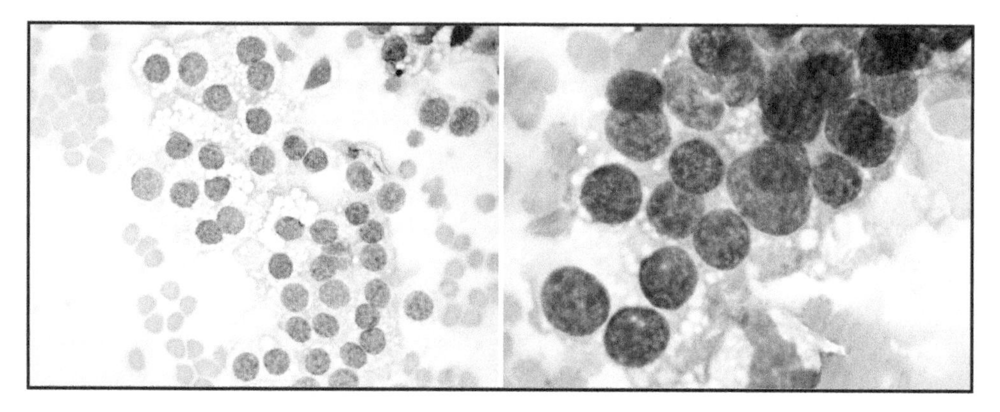

Fig. 5.18. Dog. CSF. Cytospin preparation. Choroid plexus carcinoma. The neoplastic cells have exfoliated in cohesive clusters. Wright-Giemsa. (*Courtesy of Alice Pastorello.*)

Further reading

Pastorello, A., Constantino-Casas, F. and Archer, J. (2010) Choroid plexus carcinoma cells in the cerebrospinal fluid of a Staffordshire Bull Terrier. *Veterinary Clinical Pathology* 39(4), 505–510.
Westworth, D.R., Dickinson, P.J., Vernau, W., Johnson, E.G., Bollen, A.W. *et al.* (2008) Choroid plexus tumors in 56 dogs (1985–2007). *Journal of Internal Veterinary Medicine* 22(5), 1157–1165.

Lymphoma

Clinical features

- In dogs, primary CNS lymphomas are rare, accounting for approximately 3% of all CNS lymphomas.
- CNS lymphoma can present as a solitary intraparenchymal mass or as a diffuse infiltrate of the brain.
- In cats, approximately 35% of all CNS lymphomas are primary.
- In dogs and cats, approximately 80% of CNS lymphomas have a B-cell immunophenotye and the remaining 20% a T-cell lineage. Null-immunophenotype lymphomas are rare and could be NK.
- The diagnosis of primary CNS lymphoma requires a rigorous exclusion of extraneural lesions of lymphoma.

Cytological features

- Cellularity: variably increased.
- Background: variably haemodiluted.
- The cell morphology mirrors that seen in lymphomas arising in other locations. Lymphoid cells are monomorphic and usually large. Nuclei are medium-large, round and eccentric. They have finely stippled chromatin and one to multiple, variably prominent nucleoli may be seen. The cytoplasm is scant to moderate, variably basophilic. Depending on the subtype, azurophilic granules may be observed in the cytoplasm (LGL lymphomas). Mitoses can be seen.
- In cats, small cell primary CNS lymphomas have also been described in the literature.
- Mixed pleocytosis can also be present. Rarely, an eosinophilic paraneoplastic CNS inflammation has been described associated with a T-cell immunophenotype.
- When lymphoma is suspected cytologically, clonality testing (PARR) on the CSF sample can be used to confirm the diagnosis.

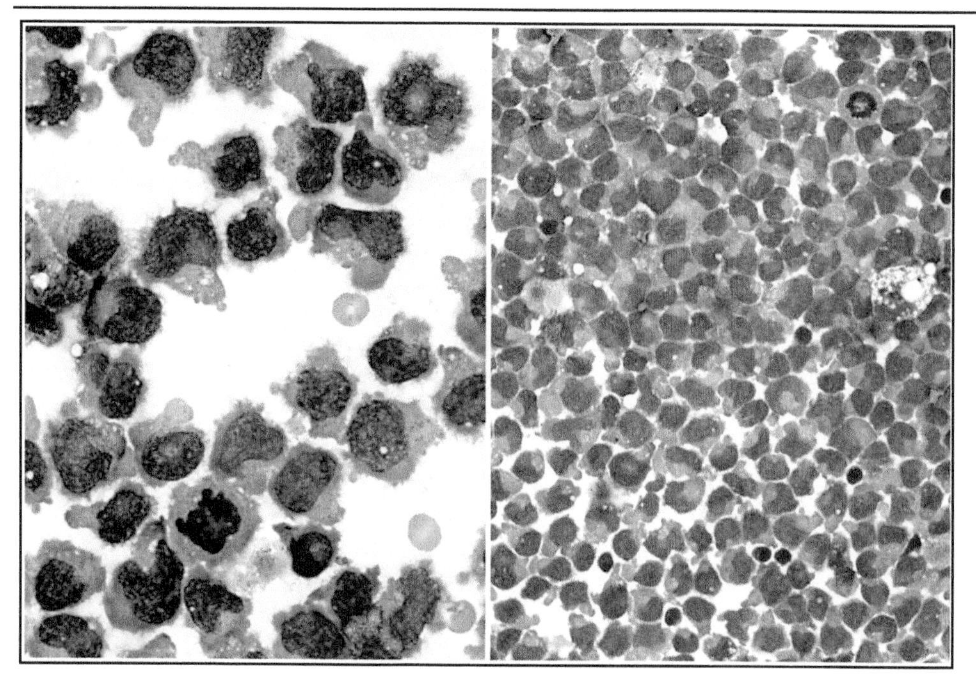

Fig. 5.19. Dog. CSF. Cytospin preparation. Lymphoma, numerous monomorphic large lymphoid cells are seen. Cells in the left picture contain azurophilic granules. Wright-Giemsa.

Further reading

Troxel, M.T., Vite, C.H., Van Winkle, T.J., Newton, A.L., Tiches, D. *et al.* (2003) Feline intracranial neoplasia: retrospective review of 160 cases (1985–2001). *Journal of Veterinary Internal Medicine* 17(6), 850–859.

Histiocytic sarcoma

Clinical features

- Tumour arising from the interstitial dendritic cells. It can present as a localized form or as a diffuse disease affecting multiple organs.
- Primary CNS HS sarcoma is uncommon, with an incidence of approximately 2.2% of all primary CNS tumours in dogs.
- Primary CNS HS more commonly arises in the brain and less frequently in the spinal cord.
- Age: mean of 8 years old.
- Over-represented breeds: including primary CNS and disseminated HS, Bernese Mountain dogs, Golden Retrievers, Rottweilers, Shetland Sheepdogs and Corgis are most represented. Of these, Corgis and Shetland Sheepdogs more commonly have primary CNS HS, whereas Rottweilers seem to exclusively develop disseminated CNS HS.

Cytological features

- Cellularity and protein concentration: variably increased. In a study in dogs with HS affecting the CNS, patient with primary HS had a higher TNCC (median 170 cells/μl) compared with dogs with disseminated disease (median 4 cells/μl). Similarly, the protein concentration was higher in dogs with primary rather than disseminated HS.
- Background: variably haemodiluted.
- In the same study, neoplastic cells were found in the CSF of approximately 52% of the cases. The neoplastic cells are similar to those seen in other locations. They exfoliate individually and are round to plump-oval. Multinucleation can be observed and anisokaryosis and anisocytosis may be marked. Nuclei are usually paracentral, large, round-to-oval and may contain prominent nucleoli. The cytoplasm is moderate in amount, pale to moderately basophilic and may contain small vacuoles. Mitoses can be found.

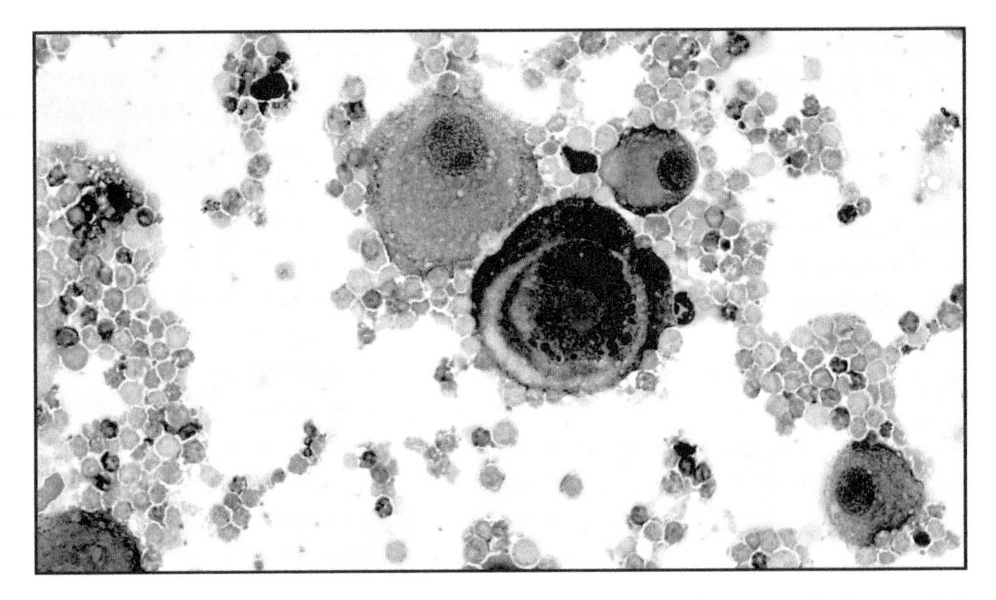

Fig. 5.20. Dog. CSF. Cytospin preparation. Primary HS, confirmed on necroscopy. Large atypical cells are seen individually. Cannibalism is shown by one of the cells. Wright-Giemsa.

Further reading

Toyoda, I., Vernau, W., Sturges, B.K., Vernau, K.M., Rossmeisl, J. *et al.* (2020) Clinicopathological characteristics of histiocytic sarcoma affecting the central nervous system in dogs. *Journal of Veterinary Internal Medicine* 34(2), 828–837.

5.9.2 Secondary CNS neoplasia

Non-primary CNS neoplasms include metastatic carcinomas, melanomas, disseminated lymphomas and HSs.

Cytological features

- Cellularity and protein concentration: variable often increased.
- Background: variably haemodiluted.
- Concurrent inflammatory pleocytosis may be present or absent.
- Carcinoma: metastatic carcinomas to the CNS are most frequently mammary in origin. The neoplastic cells often exfoliate individually. Cells are large, pleomorphic, ranging from round to polygonal. They have a moderate amount of lightly granular basophilic cytoplasm and well-defined borders, which can appear fringed. Nuclei are usually round, central to paracentral and have granular chromatin and small round multiple nucleoli. Anisocytosis and anisokaryosis can be marked. Binucleated and trinucleated cells may be present and atypical mitotic figures are not uncommon.
- Lymphoma and HS: these tumours can occur in the CNS as part of a systemic/disseminated disease. The cytological findings in the CSF are similar to primary CNS lymphoma and HS (refer to previous section for morphological description).
- Melanoma: neoplastic cells rarely exfoliate in the CSF fluid. A mixed and variable pleocytosis may be present and fine melanin granules may occasionally be found free in the fluid or phagocytosed by the macrophages.

Pearls and Pitfalls

The morphology of the metastatic cells that exfoliate in the CSF not always mirrors that of the primary tumour and frequently the identification of their lineage might be difficult. In those cases, immunocytochemistry might help in the diagnosis.

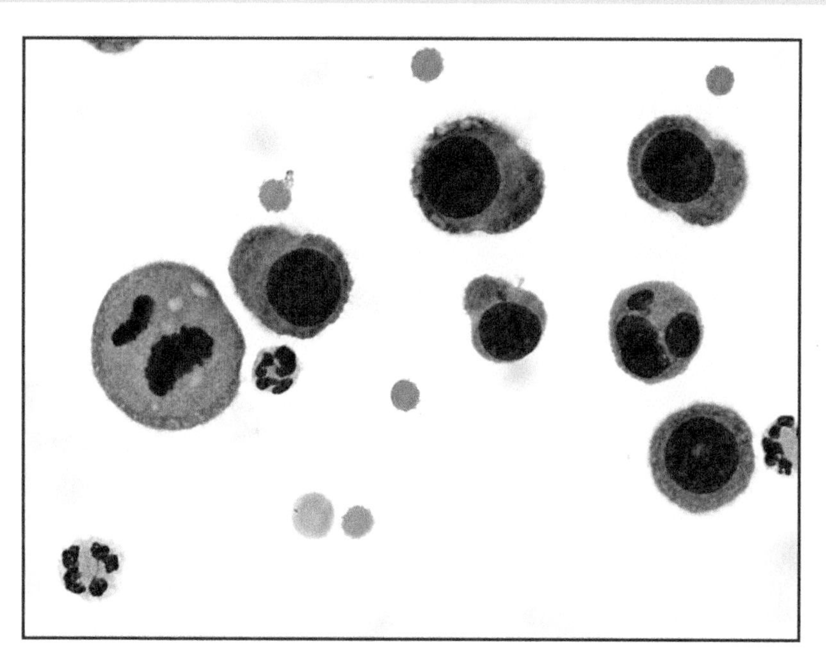

Fig. 5.21. Dog. CSF. Cytospin preparation. Metastatic mammary carcinoma. The neoplastic epithelial cells have exfoliated individually. A mitotic figure is seen on the left. Wright-Giemsa.

6 Aqueous and Vitreous Humour

6.1 Anatomy and Physiology

The aqueous humour is a clear watery fluid secreted from the vascular sinuses of the ciliary body. It flows from the posterior chamber through the pupil, into the anterior chamber, which is filled with this fluid. From there, it flows out through the trabecular meshwork and is then absorbed into the episcleral veins. It is largely composed of water and contains amino acids, electrolytes, carbohydrates, glutathione, urea, oxygen and carbon dioxide.

Aqueous humour is an important component of the eye's optical system and has several functions:

- Provides nutrition to ocular structures.
- Removes excretory products of metabolism.
- Transports neurotransmitters.
- Stabilizes the ocular structures guaranteeing the homeostasis of ocular tissues.
- Allows inflammatory cells and mediators to circulate in the eye in pathological conditions.

The vitreous humour is a clear jelly-like fluid that fills the space between the lens and the retina (also called vitreous or posterior chamber). It is produced by cells in the ciliary body. It is mainly composed of water; it also contains collagen and hyaluronic acid, which provides its characteristic gelatinous consistency. Along with maintaining the shape of the eye, the vitreous helps to absorb shocks to the eye and keeps the retina properly connected to the back wall of the eye.

6.2 Sampling Techniques

Indications

Aqueocentesis may help in diagnosing the presence of inflammation, infection or neoplastic disease of the anterior chamber of the eye. Vitreous aspiration is very rarely performed.

Materials

- Disinfectant and sterile gloves.
- Syringe: preferably 0.5–2.5 ml depending on the size of the patient.
- Needles: 25–30 G for aqueocentesis. The smaller is the needle, the lower is the risk of uveitis. For the vitreous aspiration, 18–22 G needles may also be used.
- Tubes:
  - EDTA tube for cytology.
  - Plain tube for total protein measurement and microbiology.
- Glass slides.

DOI: 10.1079/9781789247787.0006

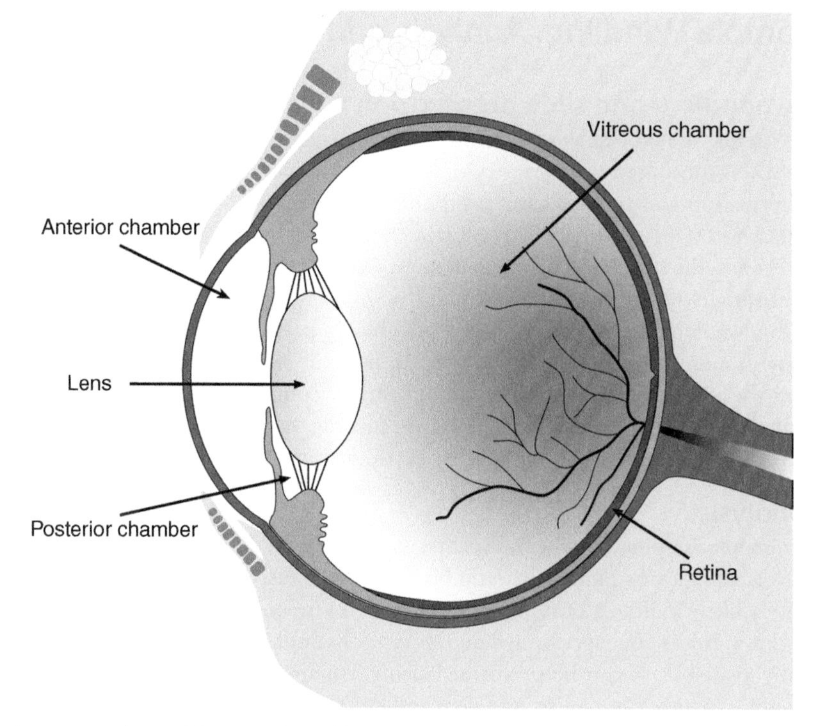

Fig. 6.1. Anatomy of the eye. (*Courtesy of Nic Ilchyshyn.*)

Technique

General indications are listed below:

- General anaesthesia (select a protocol that keeps the eye in central position and avoid downward eye positioning).
- Stabilize the adjacent bulbar conjunctiva with fixation forceps.
- For aqueous humour collection, identify limbal entry and insert the needle horizontally. Redirect the needle orthogonally and directed to the anterior chamber. The change in the direction of needle reduces the risk of fluid leakage at the end of the procedure when the needle is extracted.
- For vitreous humour collection, prefer a peri-limbar entry as needle should be behind the lens to reach the posterior chamber.
- Aspirate small amounts of aqueous or vitreous humour fluid, generally 0.1–0.2 ml per eye.
- Hold the conjunctiva securely with a conjunctival clamp for a few seconds to avoid fluid leakage.

Complications

- Aqueocentesis: uveitis, endophthalmitis, trauma to iris or lens, retinal detachment and blood pressure imbalances.
- Vitreous aspiration: complications are higher; hence, this procedure is rarely performed. They include uveitis, local haemorrhage, inflammation and retinal/lens-induced lesions.

6.3 Sample Handling, Analysis and Slide Preparation

Sample handling and slide preparation

- Fluid sample should be collected in the following tubes:
  - EDTA tube: used mainly for cytology preparations. The anticoagulant avoids clotting formation and preserves cell morphology. It can also be used for polymerase chain reaction (PCR) testing when required.
  - Plain sterile tube: used for measurement of total protein. It is also used for culture and sensitivity testing, when required.
- The fluid should be analysed as soon as possible, in particular the aqueous humour due to the low amount of protein, which may result in rapid *in vitro* disintegration of cells.
- Given the low cellularity of this type of sample, concentrated preparations are usually required and may be obtained by standard centrifugation at low speed and preparation of direct smears of the sediment or by cytocentrifugation.

Fluid analysis

- Macroscopic examination: the fluid is first grossly evaluated for colour, turbidity and viscosity. Normal aqueous humour should be clear and transparent. Increased viscosity and/or turbidity likely indicates a pathological condition. Vitreous humour is clear and viscous.
- Cell count: this is rarely performed on this type of sample due to the small amounts of fluid usually available. It can be performed using a manual counting chamber. In a study, unmodified aqueous humours from dogs and cats showed a mean direct cell count of 8 cells/μl (range 0–38 cells/μl) and 2 cells/μl (range 0–15 cells/μl), respectively.
- Total protein: given the very low amount of protein commonly present in aqueous humour, this should be measured by micro techniques only, similar to those used for cerebrospinal fluid. In unmodified aqueous humour from dogs and cats, the mean protein concentration is 0.36 g/l (range 0.21-.065 g/l) and 0.43 g/l (range 0.22-0.75 g/l), respectively. Excess EDTA may produce spuriously high results.

Pearls and Pitfalls

- Since the amount of fluid collected is generally very low, often only a single tube can be partially filled, and this can be either EDTA or plain. If EDTA tube is used, a paediatric version (0.5 ml) is preferred to reduce the risk of excessive anticoagulant effects on small volumes.
- According to some studies, vitreous humour testing is more likely to yield a diagnosis of endophthalmitis than aqueous humour, in particular in infectious forms.

6.4 Normal Aqueous and Vitreous Body Humour Cytology

Aqueous humour

- Cellularity: generally very low.
- Background: usually clear to lightly basophilic. Red blood cells should be absent.

- Nucleated cells: generally absent or very rare. They include scattered mononuclear cells, melanocytes and scattered degenerate/disrupted cells.

Vitreous humour

- Poorly described in the literature. It can be acellular, or it may contain rare erythrocytes. Melanin granules can be found free in the background or inside cells. The background is usually pale eosinophilic and granular.
- Lens and retinal cells may rarely be aspirated, together with rare fibrocytes and hyalocytes (type of histiocytes producing hyaluronic acid).

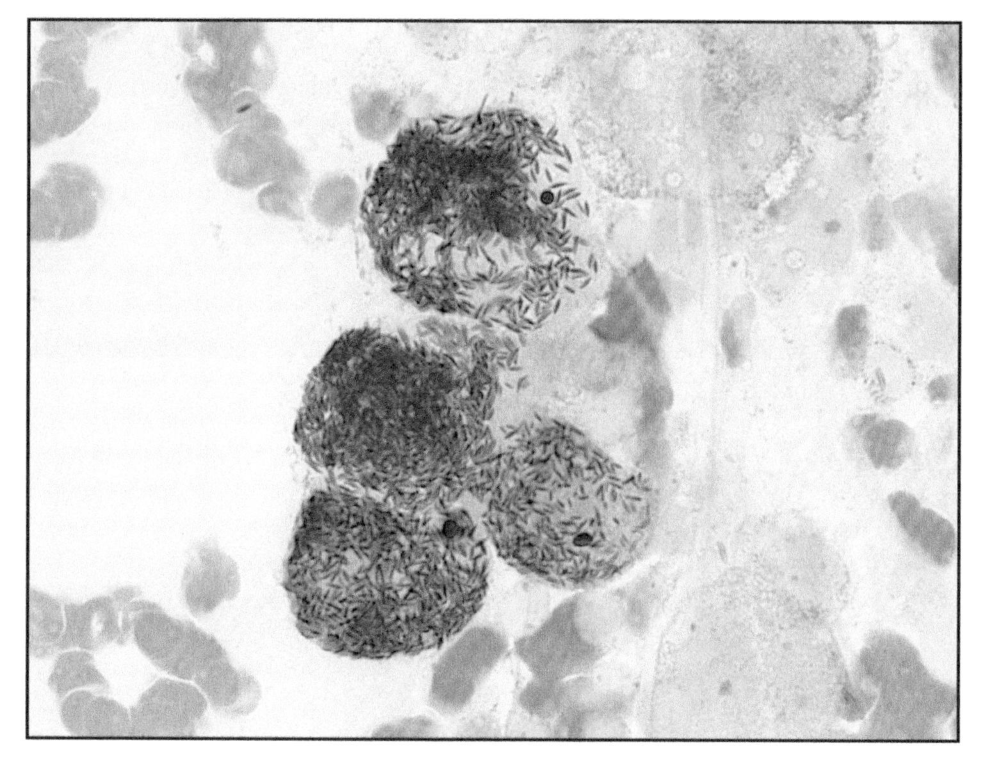

Fig. 6.2. Dog. Retinal pigmented epithelial cells (RPE). Wright-Giemsa. (*Courtesy of Anne Barger.*)

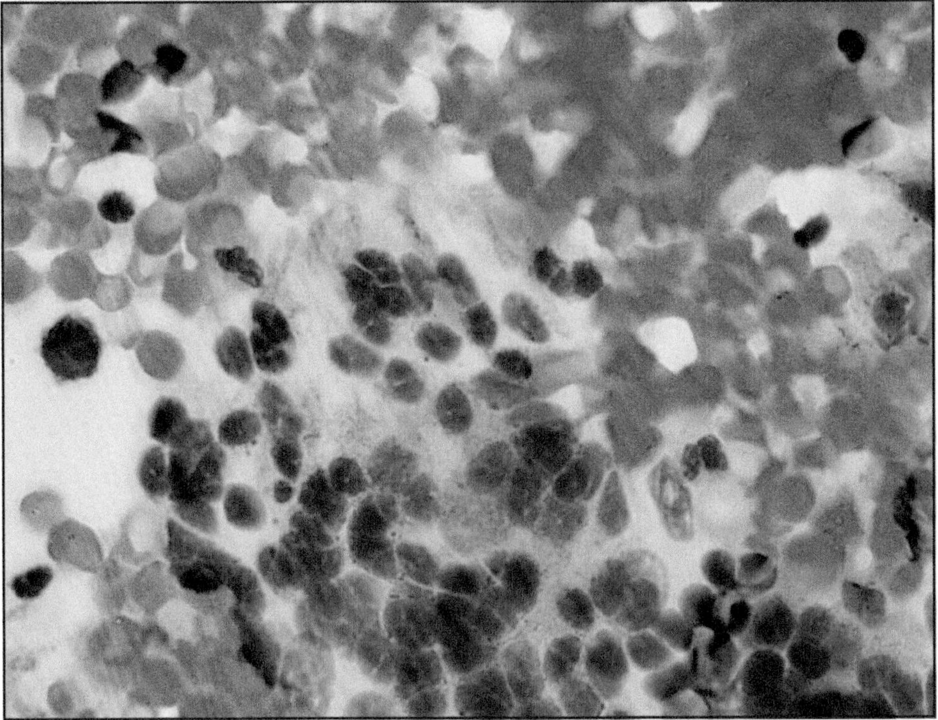

Fig. 6.3. Dog. Aggregate of photoreceptor cells. Wright-Giemsa. (*Courtesy of Anne Barger.*)

6.5 Inflammatory Diseases

Clinical features

- Uveitis is the inflammation of the uveal tract (iris, ciliary body and choroid). It can be anterior or posterior.
- It is the result of a disruption of the blood aqueous barrier, allowing inflammatory proteins and cells to access the aqueous humour. The term 'hypopyon' is used to describe an accumulation of leucocytes in the anterior chamber of the eye.
- In over half of the cases in both dogs and cats, uveitis is idiopathic. The diagnosis is based on a non specific or inconclusive aqueous humour cytology and an absence of specific abnormalities on bloodwork, imaging and infectious disease testing.
- 'Endophthalmitis' is a more generic term used to indicate inflammation of the tissues and/or fluids (aqueous and vitreous humours) within the eyeball.

Causes

- Trauma (e.g. foreign body).
- Immune-mediated conditions (e.g. lens-induced uveitis, immune-mediated vasculitis and uveodermatologic syndrome).
- Infectious:
  - Bacteria (e.g. *Brucella* spp., *Bartonella* spp. and *Leptospira* spp.).
  - Virus (e.g. canine adenovirus 1, feline infectious peritonitis [FIP]).
  - Fungi (*Blastomyces* spp., *Coccidioides* spp., *Histoplasma* spp., *Cryptococcus* spp., *Aspergillus* spp. and *Candida* spp.).
  - Protozoa (*Leishmania* spp., *Toxoplasma* spp., *Neospora* spp. and *Trypanosoma* spp.).
  - Rickettsia (*Ehrlichia* spp. and *Rickettia* spp.).
  - Algae (*Prototheca* spp.).
  - Parasites (e.g. nematodes and aberrant migration of *Cuterebra* spp.).
- Intraocular haemorrhage.
  - Metabolic disorders (e.g. diabetes mellitus and hyperlipidaemia).
  - Underlying neoplasia (e.g. lymphoma) or paraneoplastic.
  - Idiopathic.

Cytological features

- Cellularity and protein concentration: usually increased.
- Inflammatory cells are seen and may include neutrophils, lymphocytes, macrophages and/or eosinophils.
- Increased neutrophils are observed more often in septic and selected non-infectious uveitis (e.g. lens-induced uveitis and foreign body uveitis). Idiopathic forms are most often associated with mononuclear or mixed inflammation.
- Plasma cells may be present in chronic and immune-mediated processes.
- Phagocytosis of dark round granules (melanin) by neutrophils and macrophages may occur and may be secondary to damage to the ciliary body and/or iris.
- Infectious agents are rarely observed in cytology. On rare occasions, they may be observed without signs of inflammation.

- In protothecosis with ocular involvement, a proteinaceous background with variable numbers of degenerate neutrophils and extracellular/intracellular organisms has been described. Inflammation may be absent.
- In FIP infection, non-degenerate neutrophils predominate, along with lower percentages of macrophages and lymphocytes.

Pearls and Pitfalls

- Aqueous humour aspiration is rarely diagnostic for infectious aetiologies, but it can provide samples for ancillary testing (e.g. bacterial culture and PCR).
- A number of molecular and serologic assays have been used to test aqueous humour and are helpful in the diagnostic process. These include:
  - Tests to document intraocular production of specific antibodies directed against *Bartonella* sp., feline herpesvirus 1 and *Toxoplasma gondii* in some animals with uveitis.
  - PCR has been used to amplify *Bartonella* sp., *Toxoplasma gondii*, feline herpesvirus 1 DNA and for the detection of feline coronavirus (FCoV) RNA in cats with FIP infection.

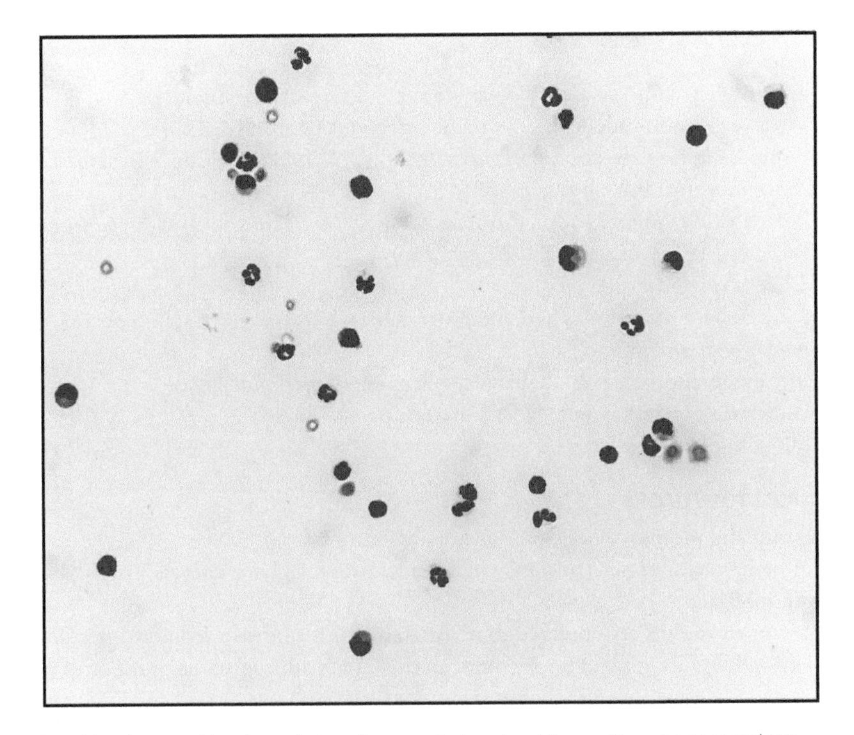

Fig. 6.4. Dog. Mixed uveitis. Mixed population of segmented neutrophils, small lymphocytes and rare macrophages. Quick Panoptic. (*Courtesy of Antonio Melendez Lazo.*)

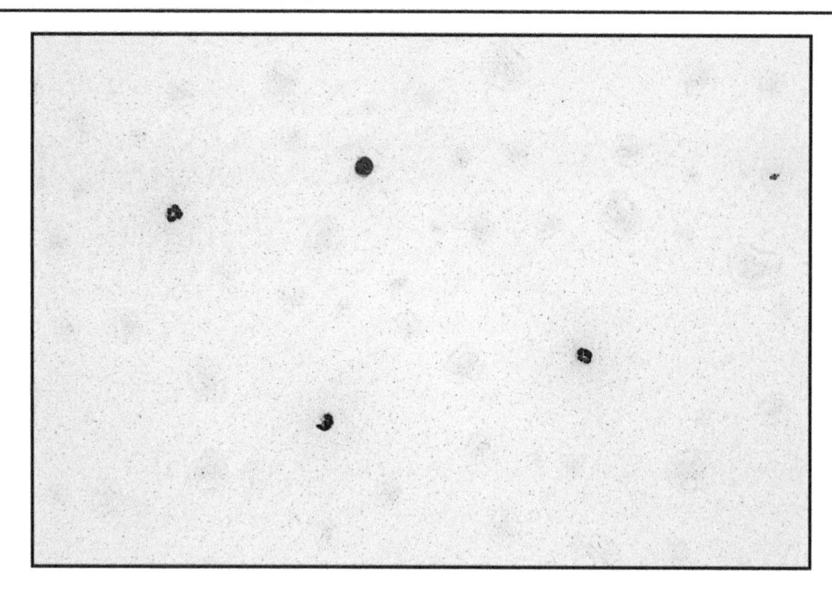

Fig. 6.5. Cat. Neutrophilic uveitis. caused by FIP infection. Wright-Giemsa. (*Courtesy of Ugo Bonfanti.*)

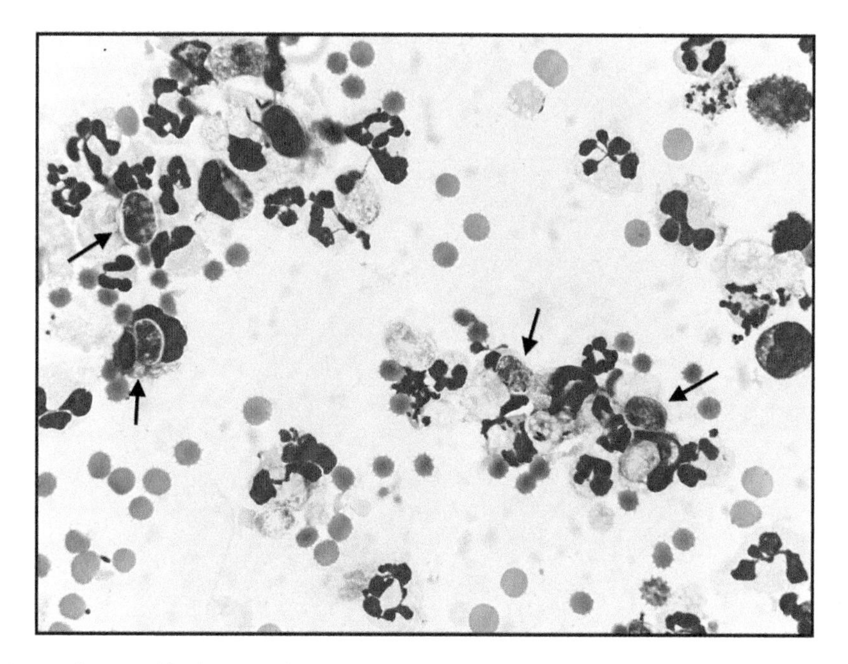

Fig. 6.6. Dog. Subretinal fluid, mixed inflammation and infection by *Prototheca* spp. Variably sized, round to oval clear structures with eosinophilic to basophilic stippling. These are noticed both free in the background and within the cytoplasm of leucocytes. Quick Panoptic. (*Courtesy of Antonio Melendez Lazo.*)

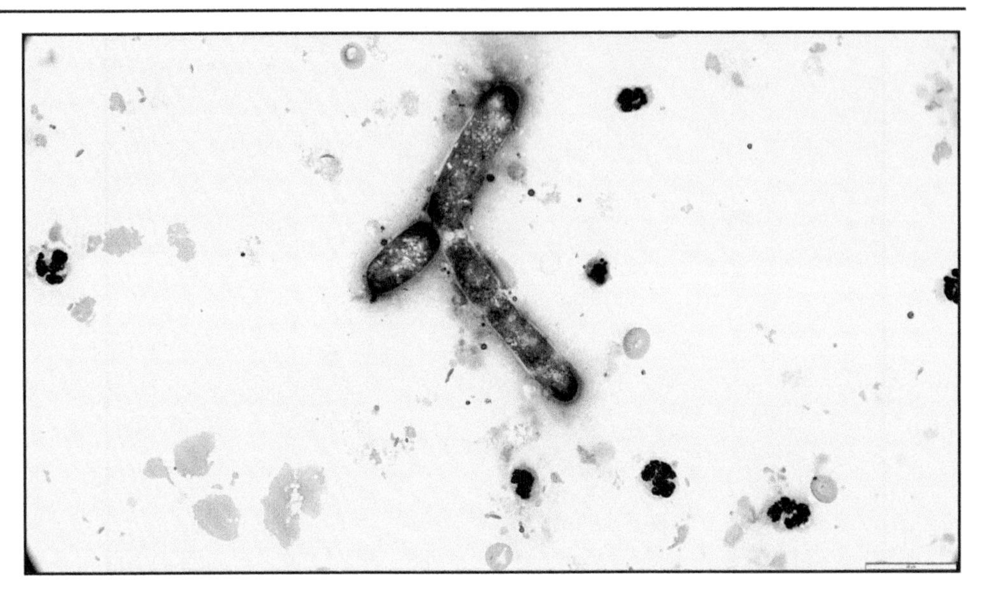

Fig. 6.7. Dog. Vitreous humour. Neutrophilic inflammation with fungal hyphae (Aspergillus sp). (*Courtesy of Christopher Lanier.*)

6.6 Non-inflammatory Diseases

6.6.1 Haemorrhage

Clinical features

- Escape of blood from a ruptured blood vessel. When it involves the anterior chamber, it is referred to as hyphaema. When present, the aqueous humour resembles blood.
- Causes include trauma, neoplasia, uveitis, hypertension and coagulopathies.

Cytological features

- Variable numbers of red blood cells and blood-derived leucocytes. Platelets are not seen unless it is a per-acute event.
- Macrophages containing phagocytosed erythrocytes (erythrophagocytosis) or products of red blood cell degradation, such as haemosiderin (haemosiderophages) and/or haematoid crystals may be seen.
- Haemorrhage may elicit an inflammatory response, mainly neutrophilic and/or macrophagic.

6.6.2 Other pathologic conditions

- Ocular melanosis: pathologic condition most commonly described in Cairn Terrier dogs, characterized by the bilateral expansion of pigmented cells in the anterior uveal structures. Rafts of pigmented cells may be found in the aqueous humour.
- Retinal detachment: often secondary to other disorders (e.g. uveitis, glaucoma), it may result in the presence of retinal cells in the aqueous humour. Photoreceptors and ganglion cells may also be seen. A mild neutrophilic inflammation may also be present and neutrophils are generally non degenerate.

6.7 Neoplasms

Clinical features

- Lymphoma is the most common neoplasm with ocular involvement that can be diagnosed via aqueous humour cytology. It could be primary (extra nodular form/ocular lymphoma) or it may be part of a systemic process.
- Other tumours that have been described exfoliating in the aqueous humour are melanoma and mast cell tumour.
- Primary ocular neoplasms are unlikely to be diagnosed by aqueous humour cytology. Very rare cases of carcinomas exfoliating in the aqueous humour have been described, including, more recently, a dog with iridociliary adenocarcinoma.
- Diagnosis of neoplasia by cytologic examination of vitreous humour in dogs has been poorly described. Vitreous tumours are rare and generally reflect the result of extension of uveal neoplasms. Rare cases of histiocytic sarcoma in dogs with free-floating cells in the vitreous have been reported.

Cytological features

- Lymphoma: monomorphic population of lymphoid cells, often large. Cell morphology may vary. Mitotic figures might be present.
- Mast cell tumour: evidence of mast cells with variable degree of granulation and morphological atypia. Concurrent increase of eosinophils may be observed.
- Melanoma: presence of melanocytes containing variable numbers of melanin granules and showing variable degree of atypia.
- (Iridociliary) carcinoma: cohesive clusters of cuboidal to polygonal epithelial cells showing variable degrees of cellular atypia. Variable numbers of leucocytes, in particular macrophages may be seen.

Pearls and Pitfalls

- Aqueous humour aspiration is particularly valuable for diagnosing neoplastic uveitis, particularly lymphoma and melanoma in both dogs and cats. The sensitivity of lymphoma diagnosis has been demonstrated to be reduced by prior administration of corticosteroids.

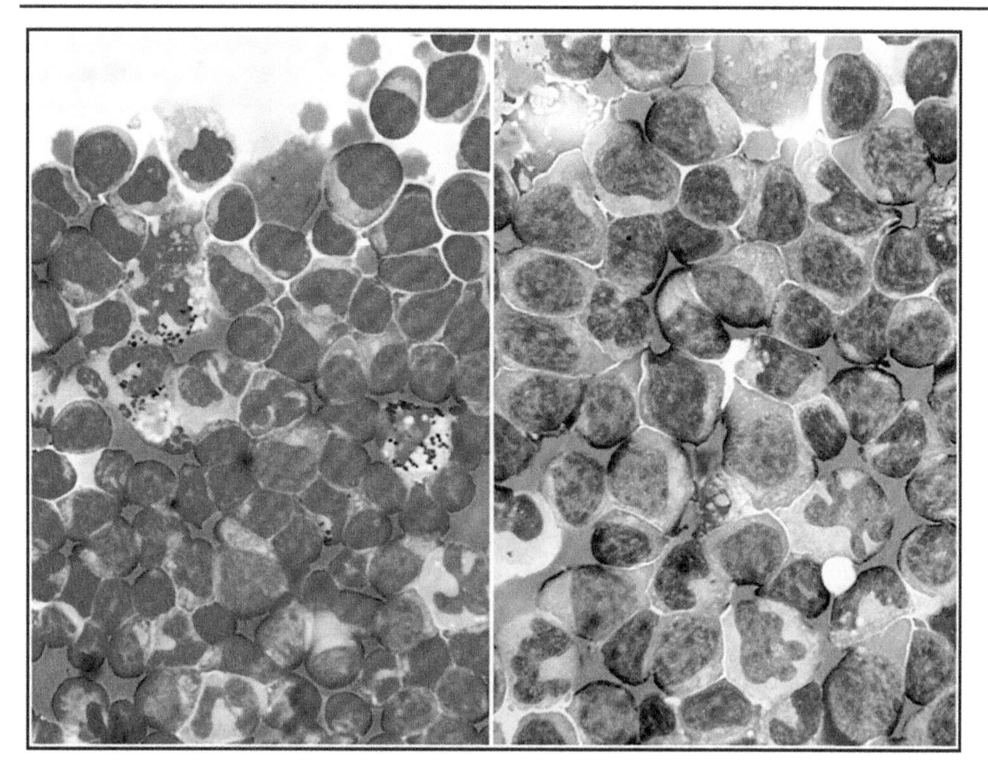

Fig. 6.8. Dog. Cytocentrifuge preparation of aqueous humour. Ocular lymphoma. Lymphoid cells are large with irregular nuclei and coarse granular chromatin. Scattered cells containing melanin pigment are seen. Wright-Giemsa.

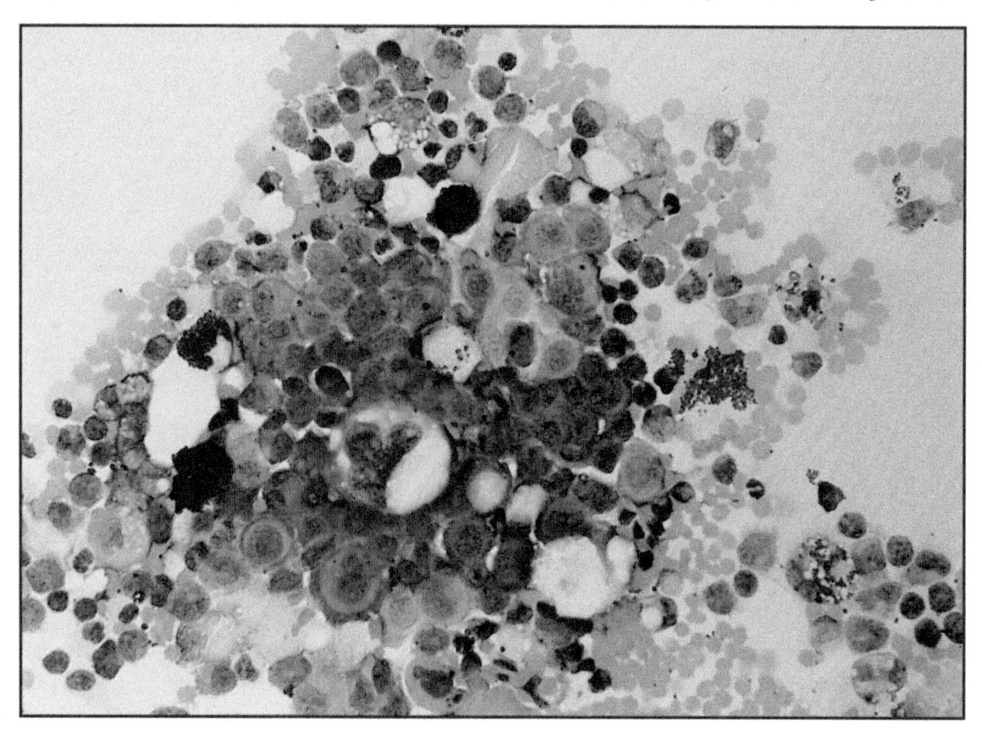

Fig. 6.9. Dog. Cytocentrifuge preparation of aqueous humour. Iridociliary carcinoma. Neoplastic epithelial cells arranged in clusters and showing signs of atypia, admixed with macrophages with melanin like material and small lymphocytes. Wright-Giemsa. (*Courtesy of Helena Ferreira.*)

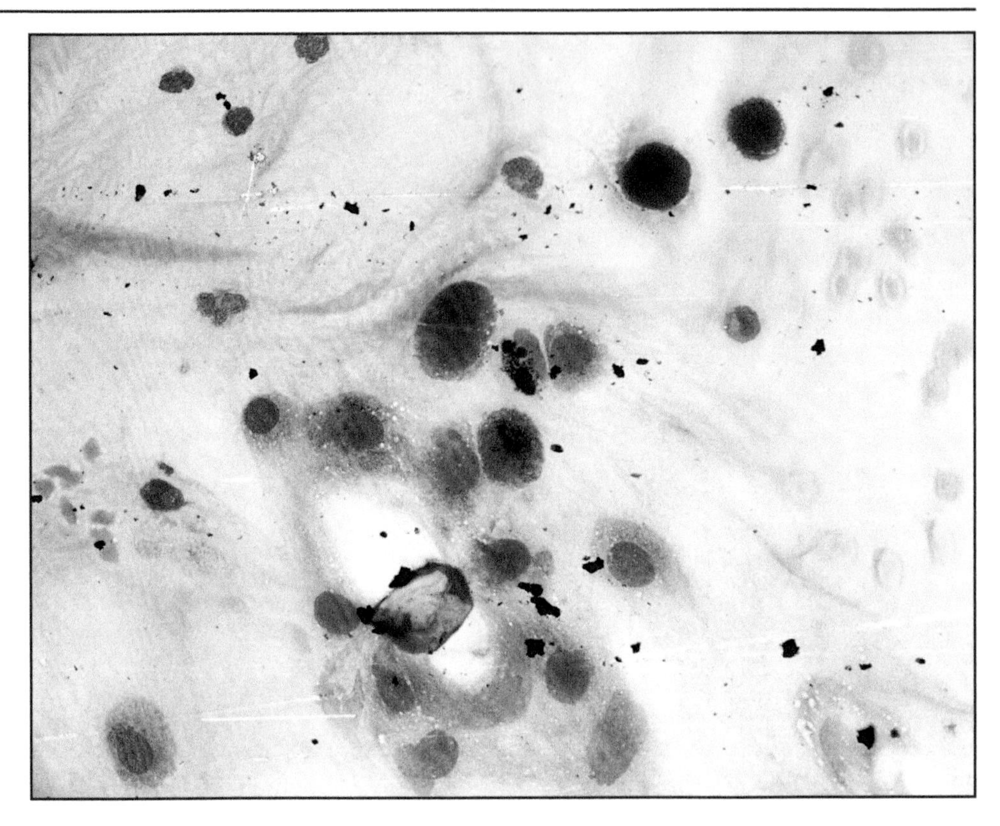

Fig. 6.10. Dog. Cytocentrifuge preparation of aqueous humour. Metastatic melanoma. Pleomorphic melanocytes containing ine melanin granules and exhibiting signs of atypia. Wright-Giemsa (*Courtesy of Nic Ilchyshyn.*)

Further reading

Ferreira, H., Scurrell, E., Bass, J. and Salmon, K. (2019) What is your diagnosis? Aqueous humor from a dog. *Veterinary Clinical Pathology* 48(3), 484–486.

Linn Pearl, R.N., Powell, R.M., Newman, H.A. and Gould, D.J. (2015) Validity of aqueocentesis as a component of anterior uveitis investigation in dogs and cats. *Veterinary Ophthalmology* 18(4), 326–334.

Swain, C.E., Pittaway, R., Ilchyshyn, N.P., Blacklock, B. and Stavinohova, R. (2020) Bilateral ocular metastatic melanoma of unknown primary (MUP) in a dog. *Veterinary Record Case Reports* 8(4).

Wiggans, K.T., Vernau, W., Lappin, M.R., Thomasy, S.M. and Maggs, D.J. (2014) Diagnostic utility of aqueocentesis and aqueous humor analysis in dogs and cats with anterior uveitis. *Veterinary Ophthalmology* 17(3), 212–220.

7 Bile Fluid

7.1 Anatomy and Physiology

Bile is a dark-green-to-yellowish-brown fluid produced by the liver, stored in the gallbladder and released through the bile duct system into the duodenum.

Bile fluid has several functions:

- Emulsify, solubilize the lipids present in the food and increase the surface area for the action of the enzyme pancreatic lipase.
- Help absorption of other substances, in particular vitamins.
- Excrete bilirubin (product of degradation of red blood cells) and other substances (e.g. metals).
- Carry excess of cholesterol out of the body.
- Neutralize excess stomach acid at the level of the duodenum.
- Stimulate intestinal peristalsis and act as lubricant.

7.2 Sampling Techniques

Indications

Cholecystocentesis may help in diagnosing diseases affecting the biliary tract, such as inflammation, cholelithiasis and mucocele. It has also been proven useful to monitor antimicrobial treatment.

Materials

- Disinfectant and sterile gloves.
- Syringe.
- Needle: 22 G.
- Tubes:
    - EDTA tube for cytology.
    - Plain tube for microbiology testing.
- Glass slides.

Technique

General indications are listed below:

- Ultrasonographic guidance.
- General anaesthesia.
- Allocate the patient in dorsal or lateral recumbency.
- Introduce the needle through the ventral aspect of the liver, until the gallbladder is reached.
- Aspirate the fluid until the gallbladder is flaccid, in order to minimize potential leakage (bile is very irritant).

DOI: 10.1079/9781789247787.0007

- Reevaluate the aspiration site for the evidence of free abdominal fluid.
- This procedure can also be performed intraoperatively during laparoscopy or laparotomy.

Complications

Leakage of bile into the abdominal cavity and gallbladder/bile duct rupture are rare events but have been described.

7.3 Sample Handling, Analysis and Slide Preparation

Sample handling

- Fluid sample should be collected and aliquoted in the following tubes:
  - EDTA tube: mainly used for cytology preparations. The anticoagulant avoids clott formation and preserves cell morphology.
  - Plain sterile tube: used for culture and sensitivity testing.

Fluid analysis

- Macroscopic evaluation: The fluid is first grossly evaluated for colour, turbidity and viscosity. In normal instances, bile fluid should be dark green and slightly viscous.
- Cytological examination: this is the only examination performed on this fluid, with culture and sensitivity testing. Cell count and protein measurement are not commonly performed, as not clinically relevant. Both direct and concentrated preparations are prepared. Slides could be stained with any type of Romanowsky stain.

7.4 Normal Bile Fluid Cytology

- Macroscopic appearance: dark-green-to-yellowish-brown and slightly viscous fluid.
- Cellularity: very low to acellular.
- Background: slightly basophilic and granular. It often contains amorphous material, sometimes with aggregates of unstained debris. Needle-shaped, golden-to-brown bilirubin crystals may be seen.
- Erythrocytes: generally absent.
- Nucleated cells: generally absent or very rare. Scattered hepatocytes, biliary epithelial cells or mesothelial cells may be seen due to sample contamination.

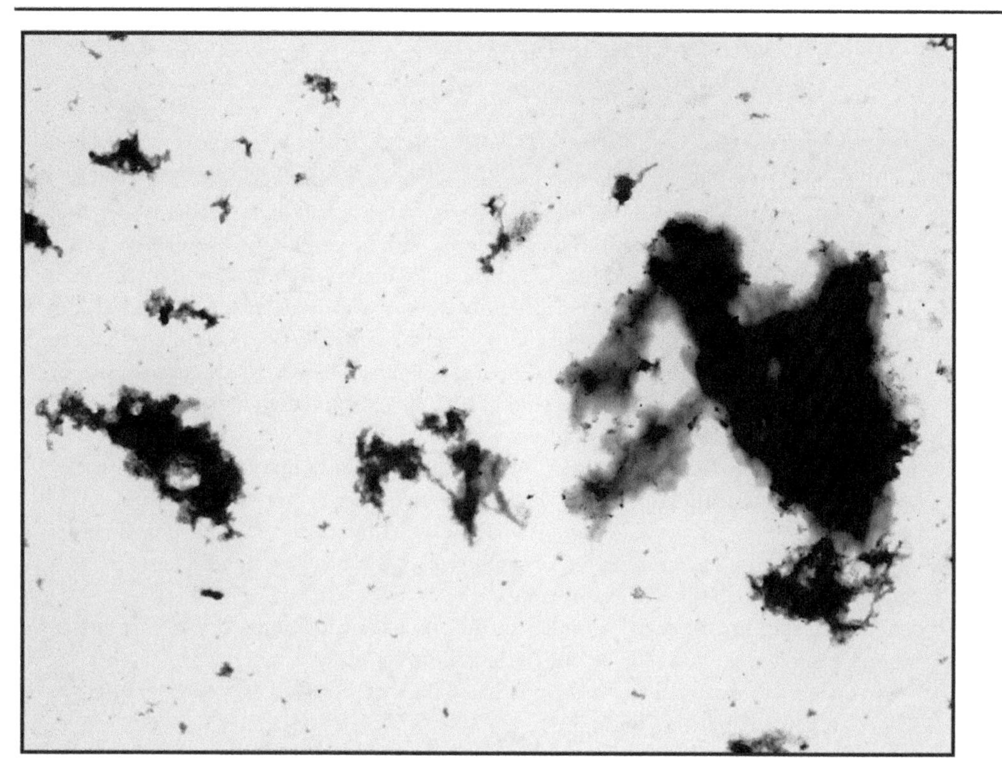

Fig. 7.1. Dog. Bile fluid. Amorphous basophilic material on the right side of the picture. Wright-Giemsa. (*Courtesy of Giulia Mangiagalli.*)

7.5 Inflammatory Diseases

Clinical features

- Inflammation can be due to either non-infectious or infectious causes.
- The presence of bacteria in the bile fluid is referred to as bactibilia. This is reported in up to 30% of bile samples from dogs and cats with hepatobiliary disorders.
- Commonly cultured bacteria include normal inhabitants of the gastrointestinal tract, such as *Escherichia coli* and other Enterobacterales, *Enterococcus* spp. and anaerobes predominantly including *Clostridium* spp. and *Bacteroides* spp. Ascending migration from the intestine has thus been accepted as the most plausible pathomechanism for bactibilia. However, experimental studies have also documented that haematogenous spread of bacteria from the portal vein is possible.
- Other organisms that are involved in hepatobiliary diseases but are not easily isolated on routine culture include *Leptospira* spp., *Borrelia burgdorferi*, *Ehrlichia* spp., *Rickettsia rickettsii*, *Toxoplasma gondii*, trematodes (cat) and cestodes. These infections are best identified by a combination of serological and molecular techniques (e.g. PCR or FISH), as well as faecal examination.
- The presence of bacteria (bactibilia) in the absence of inflammatory cells is not an uncommon event and may be due to the following causes:
  - Transient bacterial colonisation: bactibilia has been occasiobally reported in apparently healthy dogs.
  - Inflammation confined to the wall of the gallbladder without exfoliation of inflammatory cells in the bile.
  - Cell damage/destruction secondary to long standing suspension in bile.
- Therefore, the clinical significance of the finding is established by evaluating the overall clinical picture (e.g. concurrent hepatic and biliary tree pathology that can trigger opportunistic infection).

Causes

- Ascending migration from the intestinal lumen. This has been accepted as the most plausible pathomechanism.
- Haematogeneous spread of bacteria from the portal vein: demonstrated in experimental studies only.

Cytological features

- Inflammatory cells may be found in variable numbers, or might be absent. When present, they include neutrophils, lymphocytes and/or macrophages.
- Neutrophils may show signs of degeneration, in particular when associated with infection.
- Bacteria (rods and/or cocci) may be seen, often free in the background. Several studies have shown that bacteria are more often detected on bile cytology than inflammatory cells.
- Other infectious agents that have been described include *Cyniclomyces guttulatus* and *Isospora* spp. in dogs, and *Candida albicans* and egg fluke of *Platynosomum fastosum* in cats.

Pearls and Pitfalls

While cytology and culture often correlate for the presence of bacteria, the morphology of bacteria observed on cytology (cocci vs bacilli) not always correspond to the organism identified on microbiology. This may reflect a difference between the organisms identified on cytology and those isolated on culture. This has been hypothesized to relate to the presence of fastidious organisms or overgrowth by a dominant organism. Transient colonization rather than true infection is also possible in those cases.

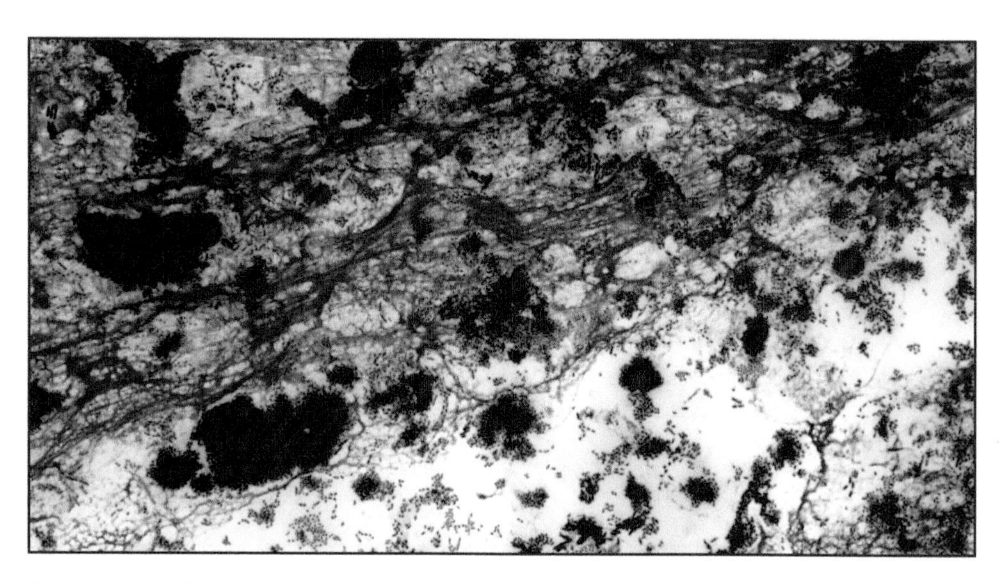

Fig. 7.2. Cat. Bile fluid. Bactibilia, large numbers of bacteria, mostly short rods, arranged in variably sized colonies and admixed with amorphous basophilic material. Wright-Giemsa. (*Courtesy of Giulia Mangiagalli.*)

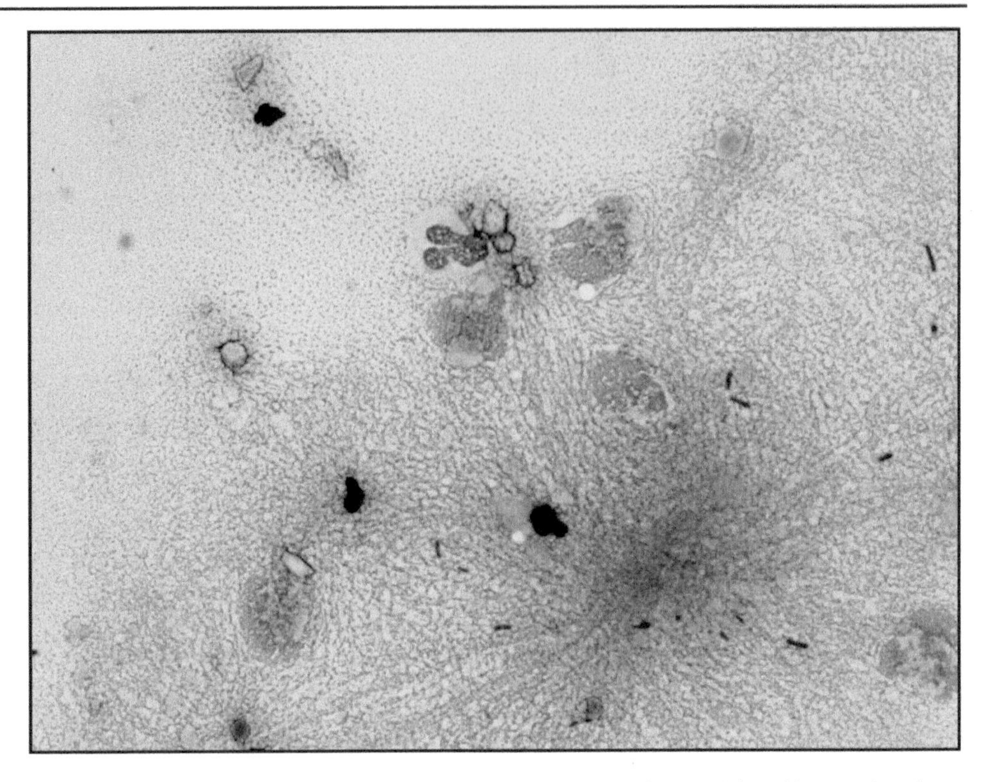

Fig. 7.3. Dog. Bile fluid. Septic neutrophilic inflammation, poorly preserved neutrophils and bacteria (cocci) on a granular basophilic background. Wright-Giemsa.

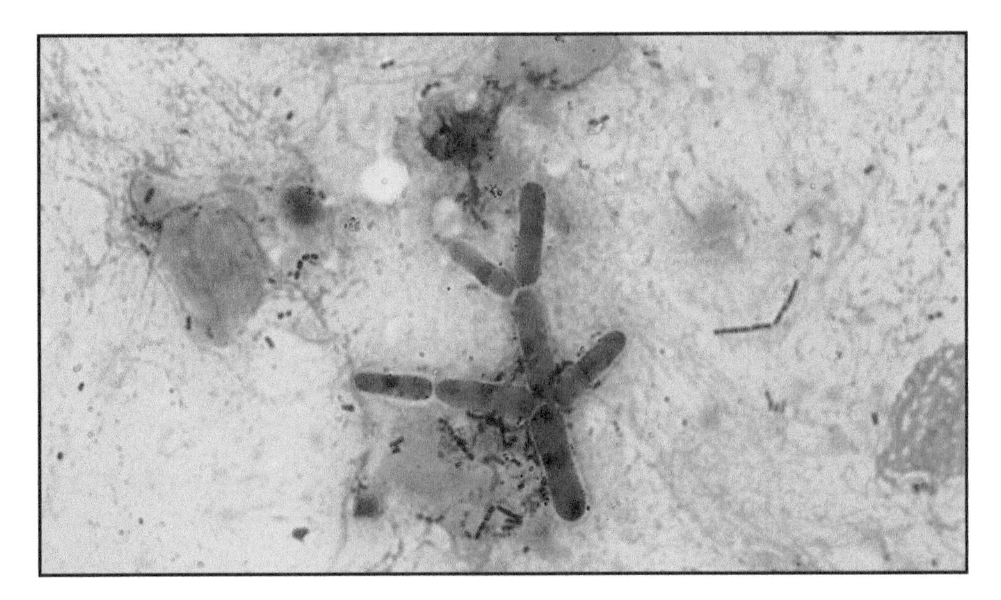

Fig. 7.4. Dog. Bile fluid. *Cynoclomyces guttulatus* and mixed bacteria. Wright-Giemsa.

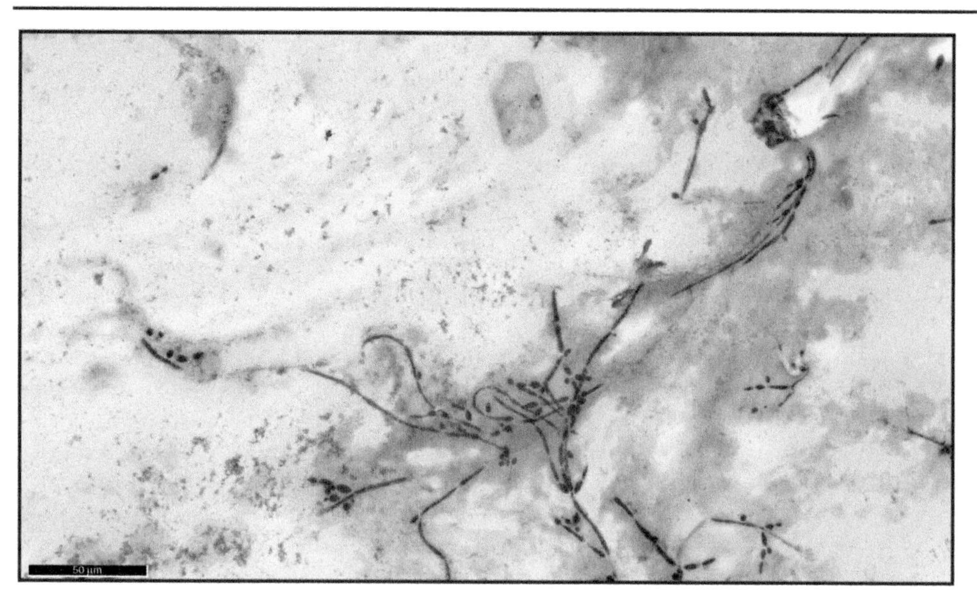

Fig. 7.5. Dog. Bile fluid. *Candida sp.* infection. Wright-Giemsa. (*Courtesy of Marta Costa.*)

7.6 Non-inflammatory Diseases

The conditions listed below are very unlikely to produce significant changes in bile cytology.

- Mucinous hyperplasia: it may be associated with the presence of very dense/viscous bile fluid, which is characterized on cytology by a basophilic and granular background forming variably sized lakes of amorphous material.
- Haemorrhage into the gallbladder lumen: characterized by the presence of erythrocytes and products of their degradation, including haemosiderin (haemosiderophages) and/or haematoidin crystals. Macrophages displaying erythrophagia can also be seen.
- Neoplasia: lymphoma has been described in a cat with extranodal B-cell lymphoma affecting both the urinary bladder and the gallbladder. Neoplastic cells were identified on bile fluid cytology.
- Cholelithiasis: can affect both dogs and cats. It is an uncommon and frequently incidental finding. Occasional incidental finding; occasionally, symptomatic cases may be associated with biliary duct obstruction, biliary peritonitis, emphysematous cholecystitis and acute cholecystitis. Most choleliths in dogs and cats contain calcium carbonate and calcium-bilirubinate pigments. Crystals of these types may also be seen in bile cytology.

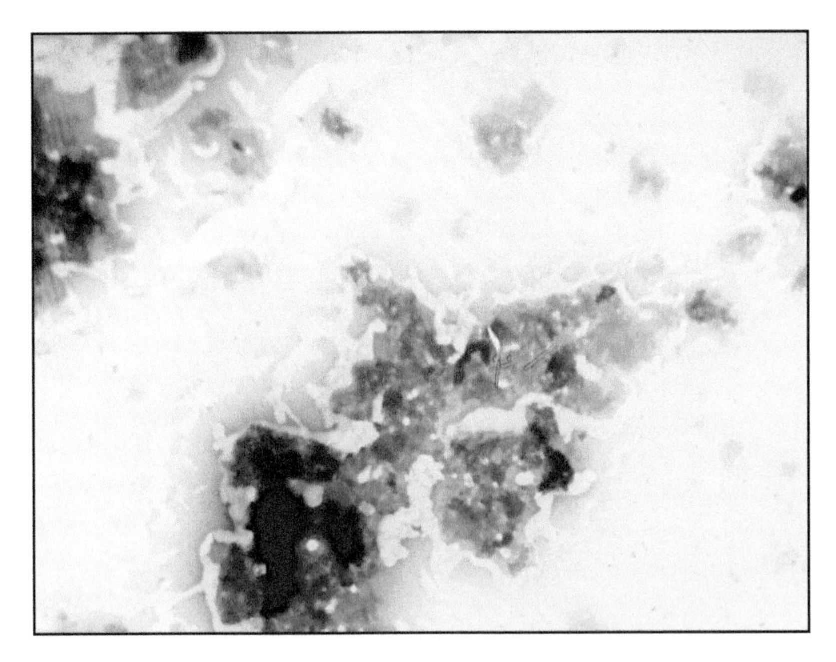

Fig. 7.6. Dog. Bile fluid. Bilirubin crystals. Quick Panoptic. (*Courtesy of Antonio Melendez Lazo.*)

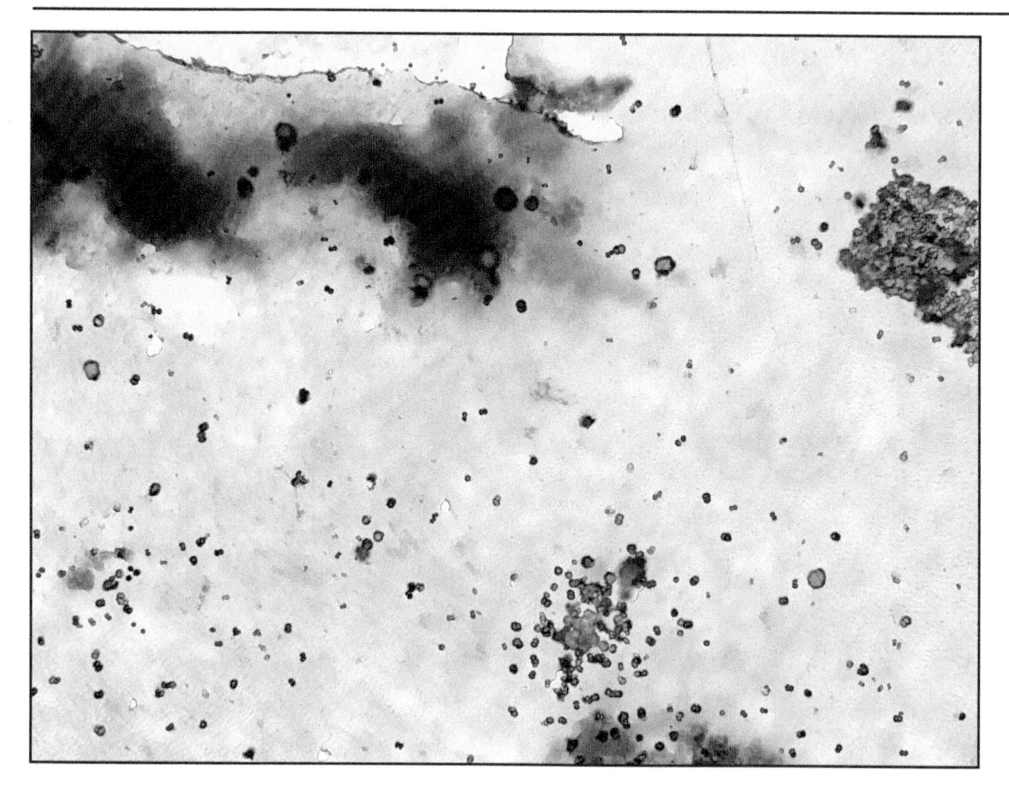

Fig. 7.7. Dog. Bile fluid. Calcium carbonate crystals. Quick Panoptic. (*Courtesy of Antonio Melendez Lazo.*)

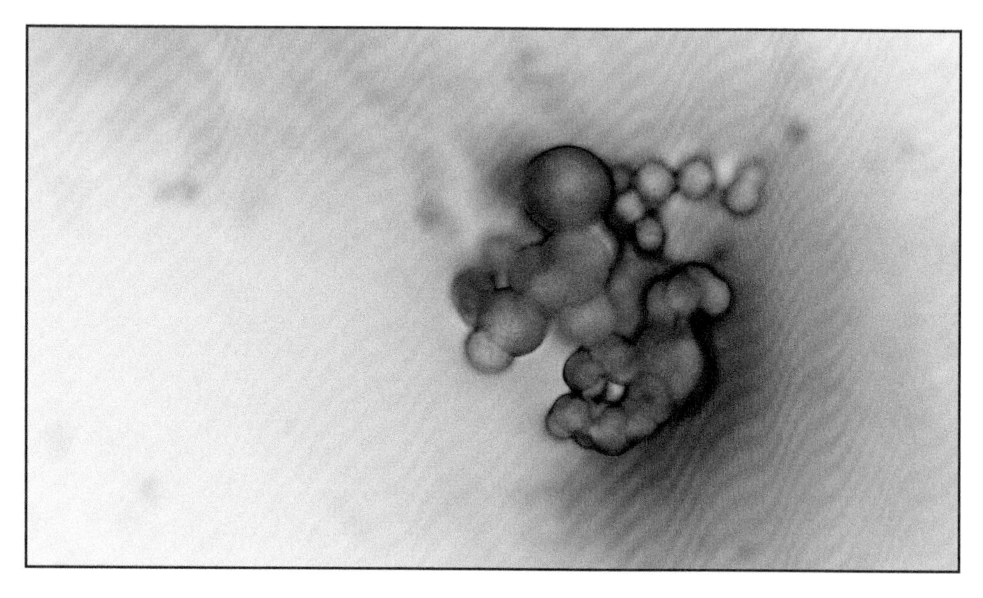

Fig. 7.8. Dog. Bile fluid. Gallbladder crystals. (*Courtesy of Christian Bédard.*)

Further reading

Geigy C.A., Dandrieux J., Miclard J. et al. (2010). Extranodal B-cell lymphoma in the urinary bladder with cytological evidence of concurrent involvement of the gall bladder in a cat. Journal of Small Animal Practice 51(5), 280-287.

Peters, L.M., Glanemann, B., Garden, O.A. and Szladovits, B. (2016) Cytological findings of 140 bile samples from dogs and cats and associated clinical pathological data. *Journal of Veterinary Internal Medicine* 30, 123–131.

Verwey, E., Gal, A., Kettner, F., Botha, W.J. and Pazzi, P. (2021) Prevalence of subclinical bactibilia in apparently healthy shelter dogs. *Journal of Small Animal Practice* 62(11), 948–958.

8 Urogenital Fluids

8.1 Anatomy and Physiology

Urine is a liquid solution containing metabolic wastes and certain other substances that excretory organs withdraw from the circulatory fluid and expel from the body. In dogs and cats, the formation of urine begins in the nephron by filtration of blood plasma. As the fluid passes along the nephron tube, water and other useful plasma components such as amino acids, glucose, and electrolytes are reabsorbed into the bloodstream, leaving a concentrated solution of waste material.

Composition

Urine consists of water, urea, creatinine, inorganic salts, uric acid and pigmented products of blood metabolism, one of which (urobilin or urochrome) gives urine its typical yellow/straw colour. Protein is only found in traces. Other substances that are not reabsorbed into the blood remain in the urine.

8.2 Urinalysis

Urinalysis is commonly performed as part of:

- General health screen.
- Workup of clinical signs related to the urogenital tract.
- Screening for breed-related urinary tract disorders.
- Assessment of patients with systemic illness.
- Monitor the response to treatment in established diseases.
- Monitor possible side effects of specific medications (e.g. cyclophosphamide, tyrosine kinase inhibitors).

Specific indications for performing urinalysis include:

- Azotaemia.
- Dysuria/stranguria.
- Haematuria/pigmenturia.
- Pollakiuria.
- Polyuria/polydipsia.
- Urinary incontinence.

Urinalysis consists of three components:

- Physical examination: volume, colour, clarity/turbidity, urinary specific gravity (USG).
- Chemical examination: assessed via dipstick colorimetric test or Pyrogallol red molybdate and Coomassie brilliant blue (e.g. urine protein:creatinine ratio).
- Microscopic examination: assessed via microscopic examination of unstained and/or stained urine sediment.

DOI: 10.1079/9781789247787.0008

This section will focus on the microscopic examination of the wet sediment analysis and urine cytology.

8.3 Sampling Collection and Techniques

- For the evaluation of kidney function, first-morning pre-prandial urine samples are preferred, they are most likely to be concentrated and having the highest USG.
- For sediment examination and urine culture, a randomly timed urine sample may be preferred. Cytomorphology and viability of fastidious microorganisms may be better preserved since urine is stored within the bladder for relatively less time than a morning sample.

Different methods of collection are available, and they may influence the interpretation of the results. They include:

- Cystocentesis.
- Transurethral catheterization.
- Free catch.

Materials

Cystocentesis

- Clippers, disinfectant, and sterile gloves.
- Needles:
  - 22–23 G.
  - 1.0 to 1.5 inches for small dogs and cats. 3.0 inches might be required in large and obese dogs.
- Syringes: from 3 ml to 12 ml; 5 ml syringe usually provides adequate volume for most urinalysis evaluation.

Catheterization

- Sterile urinary catheter. Catheters vary from 3 Fr to 10 Fr in diameter and 13 cm to 50 cm of length. Flexible catheters (e.g. silicone, nylon, latex and rubber) with stylets may be preferred, as they are less traumatic.
- Otoscope/sterile speculum (for female patients).

Free catch

- Kidney dish or similar container.

Materials common to all procedures

- Tubes/containers:
  - Capped sterile container: routine urinalysis.
  - Preservative tubes (e.g. boric sample): urine culture.
  - EDTA tube: cytology.

Patient preparation

- Use of chemical restraint is common for obtaining a sample via catheterization and occasionally for cystocentesis, with the aim of reducing excessive movement of the patient during the procedure. However, this is under the clinician discretion and largely depends on the temperament of the animal and tolerance for discomfort.

Techniques

Cystocentesis:

- This procedure allows to obtain a urine sample from the urinary bladder via transabdominal needle puncture.
- It requires specialized personnel and is the preferred technique when urine culture is required.
- Patient can be placed in a in a standing position or in lateral or dorsal recumbency position.
- Surgical preparation of the abdominal skin site is usually not required; however, the area must be clean and may be clipped.
- The bladder can be identified by palpation or via ultrasound guidance.
  - Palpation:
    - immobilize the bladder with one hand, pushing it dorsally and posteriorly. With the other hand, insert the needle with a syringe attached through the ventral abdominal wall at a 45° angle to the long axis of the patient.
  - Ultrasound guidance:
    - Locate the bladder with the transducer and insert the needle taking care to keep its tip within the plane of the ultrasound beam.
  - Blind method:
    - With the patient in dorsal recumbency, identify the insertion point on the abdominal midline halfway between the umbilicus and the pelvic brim and prepare the area. Insert the needle, generally perpendicular to the long axis of the patient.
  - Apply negative pressure to the syringe and continue the aspiration until at least 5 ml of urine are collected.
    Stop applying negative pressure and withdraw needle from the abdomen.

Catheterization

- There are multiple techniques to obtain a urine sample via catheterization, in particular in female patients. This depends on patient factors and preferences of the operator.
- This technique does not require the bladder to be distended and the patient being willing to urinate. It is a useful collection method when a urinary catheter is already present for another reason.
- Although not ideal due to the risk of contamination, the samples obtained by catheterization may be used for urine culture, as long as a quantitative urine culture is performed.
- Select a suitable urinary catheter. The appropriate length should be checked by holding the catheter lateral to the patient's body and approximating the course of the urethra from the cranial part of the prepuce or vulva to the neck of the bladder.
- Male dogs and cats:
  - Position the patient in lateral recumbence, expose the distal part of the penis to visualize the urethral orifice and clean the area. Large dogs may be catheterized in standing position.
  - Lubricate the insertion tip of the catheter, place it into the urethral orifice and gently advance the catheter. Resistance may be felt and can be overcome by gentle rotation of the catheter. This should be advanced until urine starts dripping.

  - If possible, obtain at least 5–10 ml of urine for analysis.
  - Gently remove the catheter by steady withdrawal in a sterile manner.
- Female dogs and cats:
  - Position the patient in standing or ventrally recumbent position.
  - Clean the vulva and adjacent skin, clip any long hair.
  - Apply sterile lubricant to the insertion of the sterile cone that is attached to the otoscope and insert it through the vulva towards the vagina in order to identify the urethral orifice in the urethra papilla.
  - Alternatively, a digital palpation method (dogs) or a blind technique (dogs, cats) can be used to facilitate the slipping of the catheter into the urethral orifice.
  - Insert the catheter through the otoscope cone and the into the urethra until reaching the bladder. At that point, the otoscope is detached urethra into the bladder lumen and then detach the otoscope.
  - Obtain at least 5–10 ml of urine for analysis, if possible.
  - Gently remove the catheter by steady withdrawal.
- Traumatic catheterization: this technique is adopted to obtain a cytology sample during the investigation of low urinary tract masses (urethra and bladder). A sterile catheter is used to disrupt tissue fragments from the mass. The catheter is placed at the level of the tissue to be sampled and its position is monitored via the ultrasound during its manipulation. Biopsies are obtained by applying suction with a syringe when the side of the catheter tip is in contact with the lesion.

Void sampling

- Samples can be collected during normal voiding or by manual external compression of the urinary bladder. Collection of a urine sample from a surface (e.g. floor and litter tray) is also possible, but risk of sample contamination is very high.
- Sample contamination from the distal urethra and external skin is a common disadvantage but can be minimized by collecting a midstream urine sample. A freshly voided sample may be used for urine culture, as long as a quantitative urine culture is performed.
- Free catch:
  - Clean the back area of the animal and pat dry.
  - Wear latex gloves and, as soon as the micturition posture is assumed, place the collection box underneath the animal, directly in the urine stream. Specific commercial collection devices are preferred to jam jars or similar non-sterile containers.
  - Obtain at least 5–10 ml of urine for analysis.
- Manual expression:
  - This technique should be avoided in post-operative cystotomy or laparotomy patients.
  - Place the patient in lateral recumbency or standing position and identify the bladder by palpation.
  - Perform a gentle bladder expression and place the container underneath the animal, directly in the urine stream.
  - If a urine stream has not been produced within a few seconds of pressure, reposition the hands anteriorly or posteriorly from the original site and reapply the pressure. The procedure may also induce the animal to void naturally.

Complications and contraindications

- Manual compression may traumatize the bladder and may force urine into ureters, kidneys and prostate. It may also cause spurious/traumatic haematuria and haemoabdomen/uroabdomen. This technique is not possible if there is urethral obstruction.
- Transurethral catheterization may increase the risk of urinary tract infections, as bacteria can be introduced into the urinary tract. This is particularly concerning in patients predisposed to urinary tract infections (e.g. lower urinary tract disease, renal failure, diabetes mellitus and hyperadrenocorticism). There is also a potential risk of urinary tract trauma or perforation. The technique is not possible if there is urethral obstruction.
- Cystocentesis may result in inadvertent intestinal or blood vessel sampling, urinary bladder laceration, induction of a vagal response, seeding of neoplastic cells along the needle (urothelial carcinoma) and leakage of urine into the abdomen. It is contraindicated in animals with coagulopathy, receiving anticoagulant therapy and in patients that have had recent cystotomy.

Pearls and Pitfalls

- Dipstick results may be artefactually altered by chemicals present in the disinfectants used to clean the floor or table surfaces from which a voided urine sample can be collected (e.g. bleach).
- Owners should be discouraged from using containers from home, which may contain contaminants (e.g. detergent, food and medications) that may alter results.
- Contamination of urine sample with ultrasound gel and lubricant material should be avoided when cytology is required. Gel stains deeply purple with traditional stain products and may affect overall quality of cytology samples (it may obscure cells or cause cell undertstaining).
- Percutaneous FNA of urethral, bladder or prostatic masses is controversial. This is due to several, albeit infrequent, reports of urothelial carcinoma (transitional cell carcinoma) seeding along the FNA needle tract. Although the true incidence of needle tract metastasis secondary to this procedure is unknown and the exact factors that contribute to its development are poorly understood, many clinicians prefer and recommend traumatic catheterization as method of choice for bladder, prostatic and urethral masses.

Table 8.1. Advantages and disadvantages of different urine sampling techniques.

Free catch	
Advantages	– Normal voiding: no risk and pet owners can obtain sample – Manual compression: distended urinary bladder compressed at more convenient time
Disadvantages	– Samples are often contaminated – Manual compression: (1) urinary bladder may be traumatized, (2) technique cannot be used immediately post cystotomy, and may be uncomfortable in other post-operative patients
Catheterization	
Advantages	– Bladder does not have to be distended
Disadvantages	– Can only be performed by trained personnel – Risk for iatrogenic infection, haemorrhage and contamination – Risk for trauma or perforation of the urethra or urinary bladder – Not possible if there is urethral obstruction
Cystocentesis	
Advantages	– Better tolerated than catheterization – Less risk for iatrogenic infection and contaminants – Ideal sample for urine culture
Disadvantages	– Can only be performed by trained personnel – A sufficient amount of urine in the bladder is required – Risk for microscopic haematuria – Inadvertent intestinal sampling – Urinary bladder tear, leakage of urine into abdomen – Contraindicated in the presence of a coagulopathy or anticoagulant therapy

8.4 Sample Handling, Analysis and Slide Preparation

8.4.1 Sample handling

- Urine should be collected and aliquoted in the following tubes:
  - Sterile plain container: used for routine urinalysis. This should be capped to avoid leakage and evaporation. This sample may also be used for cytologic evaluation and for culture.
  - EDTA tube: preferred sample for cytologic evaluation. It can also be used for cell evaluation in wet sediments. The anticoagulant delays cell deterioration, prevents overgrowth of bacteria and avoids clotting in case of severe haematuria.
  - Boric acid or other preservative tubes: used for storage and culture testing. The sample should ideally be placed into a preservative tube immediately after collection.
    - Boric acid at a concentration of 0.1–0.2% holds the bacterial population steady for up to 48 h, and other cellular components remain intact.
    - Boric acid tube is a consideration for free-catch urine samples as it prevent overgrowth of contaminants. For an aseptically collected cystocentesis sample, it is generally not required.
    - Underfilling of the boric acid tube may lead to false-negative results.
- Urine should be analysed as soon as possible, ideally within 1 h from collection. If not possible, it should be refrigerated and protected from light to prevent overgrowth of microorganisms and photodegradation of bilirubin, respectively. The sample should be brought to room temperature prior to analysis.

8.4.2 Urinalysis

- Macroscopic evaluation: the fluid is evaluated for volume, colour, clarity/turbidity and odour. Urine is normally pale yellow, yellow or amber, clear to slightly turbid.
- USG: it is a measure of the concentration of the urine and reflects the kidney function. Values encountered typically for normally hydrated individuals are often closer to 1.015 to 1.045 in dogs and 1.035 to 1.060 in cats.
- Urine chemistry (pH, protein, glucose, ketones, blood and bilirubin): urine from dogs and cats typically has a pH in the range of 6.0–7.5, contains little to no protein, glucose, blood and bilirubin (dog); urine does not contain ketones.
- Urine sediment examination: urine sediment samples from healthy animals may contain rare erythrocytes, leucocytes, scattered epithelial cells, granular/hyaline casts (in concentrated samples only) and selected crystals, in particular struvite and calcium oxalate dihydrate. These are particularly common if urine sample has been stored and refrigerated.
- Urine culture should be processed ahead of remaining urinalysis components or from a separate aliquot.

Unstained urine sediment preparation

- Place a standard volume of urine (typically 5–10 ml) in a clean centrifuge conical tube.
- Centrifuge at low speed (~400 g) for 5 min. At the end of the process, the sediment may or may not be visible at the bottom of the tube.
- Remove most of the supernatant (typically 4.5 ml) with a sterile pipette. Leave a few drops (typically 0.5 ml), which are needed to re-suspend the sediment. Gently tap the tube with a finger to mix the sediment and avoid any vigorous shaking.
- Transfer with a pipette a drop of the resuspended sediment to a clean microscope slide, and place a coverslip on top to allow the sediment to distribute over the slide.
- Put the slide on to the microscope tray being sure the microscope substage condenser is lowered (or the diaphragm partially closed) and reduce the light power.
- Examine the sediment at low power (10×) and then at higher magnification (40×).

Stained urine sediment preparation

- Transfer a drop of resuspended urine sediment on a clean slide, and smear the fluid by using the pull and push or squash technique.
- Alternatively, a cytospin preparation may be prepared.
- Allow the slide to air dry and stain with any type of Romanowsky stain.

Pearls and Pitfalls

- If the sample is shipped to an external laboratory, submission of an air-dried smear of a fresh urine sediment is also encouraged, as cells in urine deteriorate rapidly. The slide may be prepared by blood smear, line or squash preparation technique.
- Urine submitted in EDTA is not appropriate for culture testing as EDTA has a bacteriostatic activity.
- For result interpretation and sample result comparisons, laboratories should use a standardized technique for urine sediment preparation and evaluation.
- Bacterial quantification, in conjunction with knowledge of the urine collection technique, can help in discriminating genuine urinary tract infection versus contamination when bacteria are seen but inflammatory cells are not present. No laboratory test can accurately differentiate between subclinical bacteriuria and urine tract infection (UTI); therefore, results need to be interpreted alongside clinical history.
- Regardless of the urine collection technique adopted, the diagnosis of urinary tract infection through urinalysis and culture is best determined when the patient has not received antibiotics for at least 3–5 days prior to sample collection.
- Examination of urine sediment may also be achieved with the use of supravital stain applied directly to the drop of urine sediment on the slide. This procedure may facilitate the identification of cells. However, it will dilute the sample, affecting the semi-quantitative evaluation of some results, and it is a potential source of contamination (stain precipitate, bacteria). For these reasons, it is not recommended by the authors.

8.5 Urinary Sediment Findings

- Examination of urine sediment is usually the final part of urinalysis; nontheless, it is very important, as it allows the identification of several pathologies of the urinary tract (e.g. urinary tract inflammation and infection, haematuria, urinary tract neoplasms).
- In this chapter, 'urine sediment' refers to both unstained and stained sediments. The latter may also be reffered to as 'urine cytology' by some sources.
- The majority of microscopic findings are reported semi-quantitatively as numbers on low (10×) or high (40×) power field from a standard amount of urine wet sediment (1–2 drops). Each element is counted by averaging the numbers counted in 10 consecutive microscopic fields. The result is reported as the average number per field (low- or high-power field).
- Small numbers of epithelial cells, erythrocytes, leucocytes, granular and hyaline casts, and various types of crystals may be found in the urine of healthy dogs and cats.
- Bacteria and squamous epithelial cells derived from external genital surfaces may be present in voided and catheterized urine.
- Delayed examination and refrigeration may lead to cast dissolution and spurious crystalluria (e.g. struvite and calcium oxalate).
- The biochemical characteristics of the urine may influence some of the sediment findings, e.g.:
  - Erythrocytes may lyse in urines with a low specific gravity.
  - Different types of crystals may form *in vitro* depending on the pH of the urine.

8.5.1 Casts

- Cylindrical structures mainly composed of precipitated proteins (Tamm-Horsfall mucoproteins) produced by the renal tubular cells of the distal nephron. They can be admixed with cells or other components.
- They usually take the shape of the tubules in which they form. They are elongated cylindrical structures with variable diameter and parallel sides. Narrower casts are thought to originate from proximal or distal tubules, while wide casts are thought to originate from the collecting tubules or ducts. The end of the cast may be rounded, tapered or straight.
- Casts tend to degenerate quickly, in particular in alkaline urine. Therefore, evaluation for casts should be performed within 30 min to 1 h of urine collection for accuracy.
- Casts are quantified as the number seen per low-power field. Rare hyaline or granular casts (<2/lpf) may be seen in urine from normal dogs and cats.
- Increased cast formation and excretion in the urine (also known as cylindruria) can occur with diseases in any area of the kidney (glomeruli tubules, interstitium). The number of casts present does not predict the severity or reversibility of the disease. At the same time, the absence of casts in the urine sediment cannot be used to exclude the possibility of renal disease.
- Mucous threads or fibres should not be mistaken for casts. Mucous threads are distinguished by their variable width, curvilinear shape and tapered ends.
- Casts are classified based on whether or not anything is incorporated into the mucoprotein.

Casts	Cytological features	Clinical relevance
Hyaline casts Composed of Tamm–Horsfall mucoproteins only.	• Pale, colourless, elongated structures. They frequently have rounded ends. • Reduced lighting is essential to see hyaline casts in urine sediment preparations.	• Rare hyaline casts (<2/lpf) can be found in concentrated urine samples from normal dogs and cats. • Increased numbers may be associated with various conditions (fever, strenuous exercise, diuretics, protein-losing glomerular disease).
Cellular casts Composed of Tamm–Horsfall mucoproteins admixed with different types of cells.	• Elongated structures containing different cell types: epithelial cells, leucocytes, and/or red blood cells. • Sometimes, the cell type present within the casts cannot be identified, in which case they are defined as mixed.	• Cellular casts are not seen in urine from normal dogs and cats. • Epithelial cells casts are commonly seen in active renal tubular necrosis or damage (e.g. renal toxins, infarcts, ischemia, and acute nephritis). • Severe dehydration may result in decreased renal perfusion and the ischemic injury may cause degeneration of tubular cells; rehydration with fluid therapy may result in flushing of numerous epithelial casts out of the tubuli. • White cells casts are caused by intrarenal inflammation, such as acute bacterial pyelonephritis and interstitial pyelonephritis. • Red blood cells casts form during intrarenal haemorrhage e.g. renal trauma or haemorrhagic nephritis/ glomerulonephritis.
Granular casts Composed of Tamm–Horsfall mucoproteins and fragments of renal tubular cells.	Elongated structures with an internal granular texture. Granules may vary in size, shape and colour within the same cast. They often have broken ends.	• Rare granular casts (<2/lpf) may be found in urine from healthy dogs and cats. • Increased numbers are commonly associated with renal tubular pathology (generally acute), causing necrosis or degeneration of renal tubular cells and incorporation within the cast.

Casts	Cytological features	Clinical relevance
Waxy casts End stage of the granular casts.	Cylindrical colourless structures with homogenous appearance. They are often large due to urine stasis and their formation in dilated renal tubules. Ends may be straight, blunt or ruptured.	They represent the end stage of granular casts degeneration; therefore, they are seen in the presence of long-standing renal disease, often associate with a reduced urine flow.
Fatty casts Composed of Tamm–Horsfall mucoproteins and lipid material.	Granular or hyaline casts containing variable numbers of fat droplets. These appears as refractile round structures, clear to yellow in colour. They are often seen in urine samples in which free lipid droplets are present as well.	Mainly observed in cats but reported also in dogs in particular in association with disorders of lipid metabolism, such as diabetes mellitus.
Haemoglobin casts Composed of Tamm–Horsfall mucoproteins and haemoglobin.	Elongated structures with yellow to golden brown colour and granular texture.	Commonly associated with intravascular haemolysis and rarely renal haemorrhage from the breakdown of red blood cells casts.

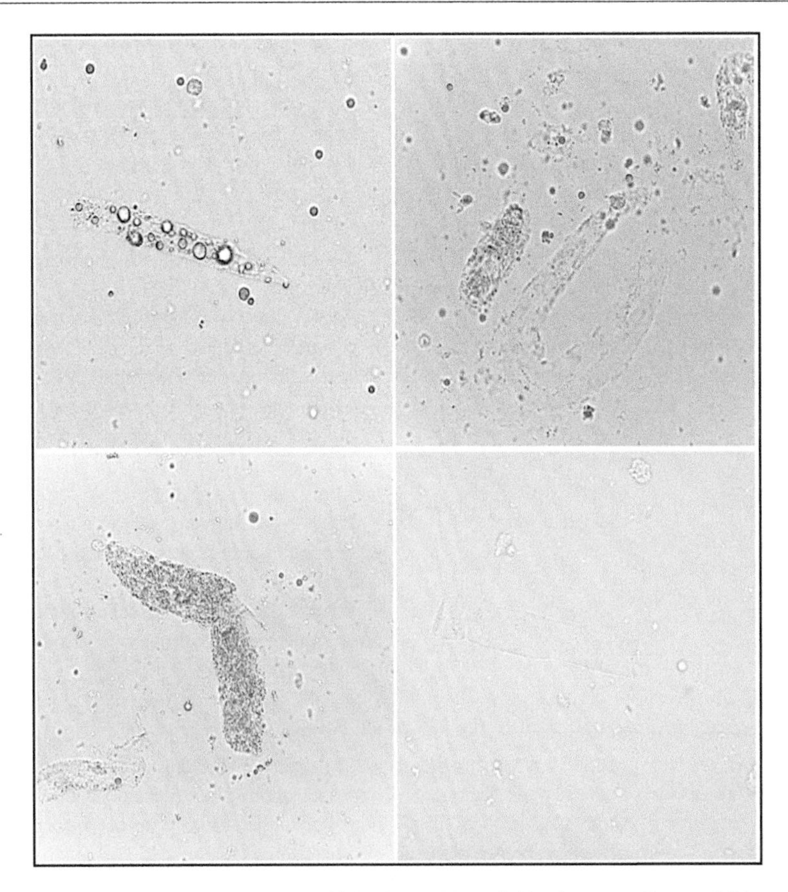

Fig. 8.1. Urine. Unstained wet sediment. (Top left) lipid cast; (Top right) hyaline cast; (Bottom left) granular cast; (Bottom right): waxy casts. (*Courtesy of* Giuseppe Menga *and Rachel Whitman.*)

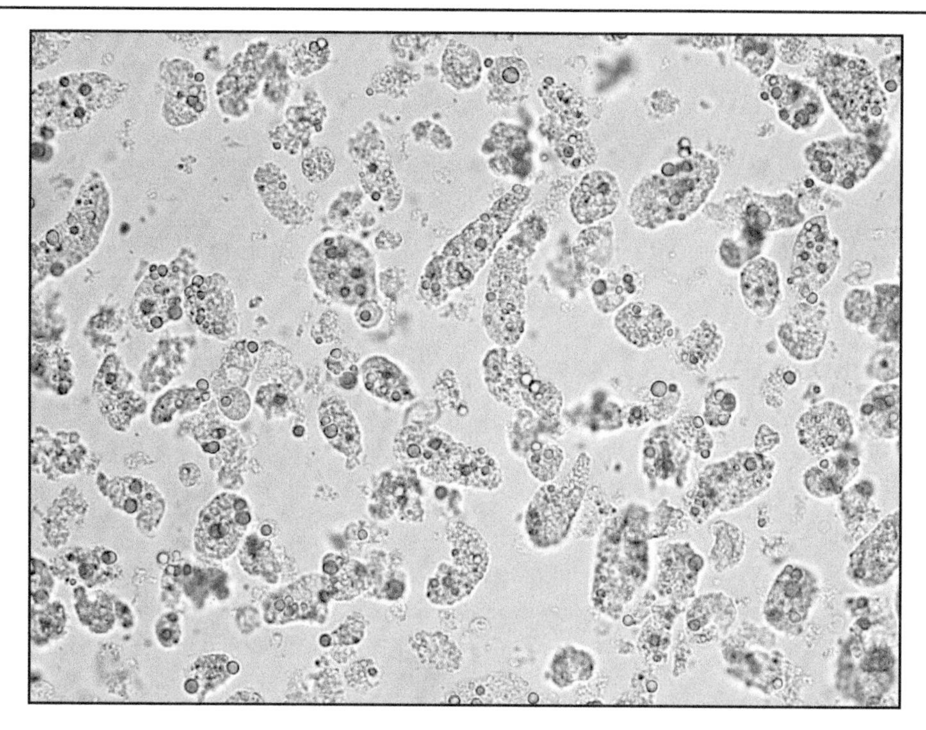

Fig. 8.2. Cat. Unstained urine sediment. Lily toxicity, high numbers of granular casts seen.

8.5.2 Crystals

- Crystalluria occurs secondary to saturation of urine by dissolved minerals or other substances that may precipitate. They can form *in vitro* or *in vivo* secondary to either pathological or non-pathological conditions.
- Crystals are quantified as the number seen per low-power field (10×). Selected crystals (e.g. struvite, calcium oxalate dihydrate and amorphous crystals) may be seen in urine sediment from normal dogs and cats.
- For accuracy, evaluation for crystalluria should be performed within 30 min to 1 h of urine collection.
- Crystalluria may spuriously occur in urine samples that are not fresh, as the result of refrigeration, prolonged storage, post-collection alterations of urine pH or evaporation of water from the sample. Any crystals detected in urine that have been stored for longer than 1 h should be re-evaluated in a freshly collected urine sample.
- The finding of crystalluria does not necessarily indicate the presence of uroliths or even a predisposition to form uroliths. Similarly, absence of crystals does not rule out underlying urolithiasis.
- The pH of the urine favours the precipitation of specific types of crystals:
  - Neutral or acidic pH: amorphous urates, sodium urate, uric acid, calcium oxalate, bilirubin, cystine, xanthine, calcium hydrogen phosphate, sulfa and tyrosine crystals.
  - Neutral or alkaline pH: struvite, amorphous phosphate, calcium phosphate, ammonium biurate and calcium carbonate crystals.

Crystals	Cytological features	Clinical relevance
Struvite/triple phosphate crystals (magnesium, ammonium and calcium phosphate)	• Variably sized, colourless, refractile prismatic structures, often with an internal X ('coffin lid' shaped).	• They can be seen in urine from normal dogs and cats, in urine samples that underwent refrigeration and/or had delayed examination (in vitro/spurious formation). • When found in high numbers in fresh specimens, they are often associated with bacterial infection caused by urease-producing bacteria (e.g. Staphylococcus spp. and Proteus spp.), which increase urine pH. In this case, they are typically accompanied by pyuria, haematuria and bacteriuria. • Struvite crystals can also be seen in patients with alkaline urine secondary to other reasons (e.g. diet) or in patients with mixed crystalluria.
Calcium oxalate crystals (monohydrate and dihydrate)	• Monohydrate calcium oxalates have variable sizes and morphologies: picket-fence-like, spindle-shaped, oval, barrel or dumbbell. • Dihydrate calcium oxalate: colourless, octahedral structures with typical envelope appearance or 'Maltese cross' in the middle. They may also have a cube-like form and vary significantly in size.	• Dihydrate calcium oxalate crystals may be seen in urine from normal dogs and cats. • Their presence may also be spurious in samples that have been stored or that became acidic after it (overgrowth of lactic acid producing bacteria). • Increased numbers of these crystals may be seen in animals that ingested oxalate containing plants (e.g. Brassica), in case of ethylene glycol toxicity (in particular monohydrate forms), and conditions causing increased calciuresis, as seen with hypercalcaemia and/or hypercortisolaemia. • Their presence may result in urolith formation and consequent pyuria and haematuria.
Calcium phosphate crystals	Colourless plate or needle-shaped structures.	They may be seen in association with conditions promoting hypercalciuria and/or hyperphosphaturia (e.g. hyperparathyroidism, idiopathic hypercalciuria and distal renal tubular acidosis)

Crystals	Cytological features	Clinical relevance
Ammonium urate crystals (or biurate)	Brown or yellow-brown spherical structures often with long and irregular protrusions. Smooth surface may also occur.	• They may be seen in healthy Dalmatians, English bulldogs, Schnauzer and a few other breeds. These lack the uricase enzyme that converts uric acid to allantoin, resulting in hyperuricosuria and consequent predisposition to ammonium urate and uric acid crystalluria. • In other canine breeds and in cats, ammonium urate crystalluria is associated with congenital portosystemic vascular anomalies (shunts) and liver insufficiency secondary to reduced hepatocellular mass (e.g. cirrhosis).
Cystine crystals	Colourless, flat and hexagonal structures of variable sizes.	• Their presence is indicator of a defect in cystine metabolism and may lead to development of cystine uroliths. This may be congenital (detect of proximal renal tubular transport of amino acids) or acquired (proximal renal tubular disease). • Selected canine breeds may be predisposed (e.g. Australian Cattle Dog, Bassett Hound and Bulldog). In cats, they have been recognized in Siamese and American Domestic Shorthair cats.
Uric acid crystals	Brown or yellow-brown diamond or rhomboidal structures sometimes containing concentric rings. Smooth surface may also occur.	Same as per ammonium urate/ biurate crystals.
Xanthine crystals	• Brown or yellow-brown spherical structures. • They may resemble ammonium urate crystals.	• Secondary to allopurinol administration in dogs. • They may also be observed in dogs (in particular Cavalier King Charles Spaniels, Dachshunds, Toy Manchester Terrier, Chihuahua and English Cocker Spaniel) and cats with congenital defects (hereditary xanthinuria).

Crystals	Cytological features	Clinical relevance
Amorphous crystals (phosphates, urates, xanthine, silicate)	• Small granular crystals with no distinctive features. In alkaline urine, they are primarily phosphate crystals; in acid urine, they are mainly urate crystals. • They can sometimes be mistaken for degenerate cells or bacteria (less pleomorphic and not as refractile).	• Amorphous phosphate crystals are usually not diagnostically significant, although they may contribute to urolith formation in dogs and cats. • Amorphous urate may be seen in animals with hepatic disorders. They have also been reported in a dog after L-asparaginase treatment for lymphoma related to tumour lysis syndrome and purine metabolism.
Thyrosine crystals	Refractile and needle-shaped structures	They may be associated with hepatic insufficiency resulting in impaired amino acids metabolism.
Bilirubin crystals	Golden to golden-brown, needle-like structures that often form small bundles.	• Rarely seen in sediment from healthy male dogs with well concentrated urine. • Increased numbers may be secondary to hepatic/post-hepatic biliary disease or haemolytic disease. Raised serum hyperbilirubinaemia is expected in those cases.
Cholesterol crystals	Large, clear, rectangular, flat plates, sometimes with a notch on the corner.	• They may be seen in healthy animals. • They can also be observed in association with excessive cellular degeneration, in patients with protein-losing nephropathy (PLN) or previous haemorrhage.
Drug induced crystals	Sulfonamide crystals appear as brown needle-like crystals in sheaves or rosettes. They may also occur as round globules with radial striations.	None.

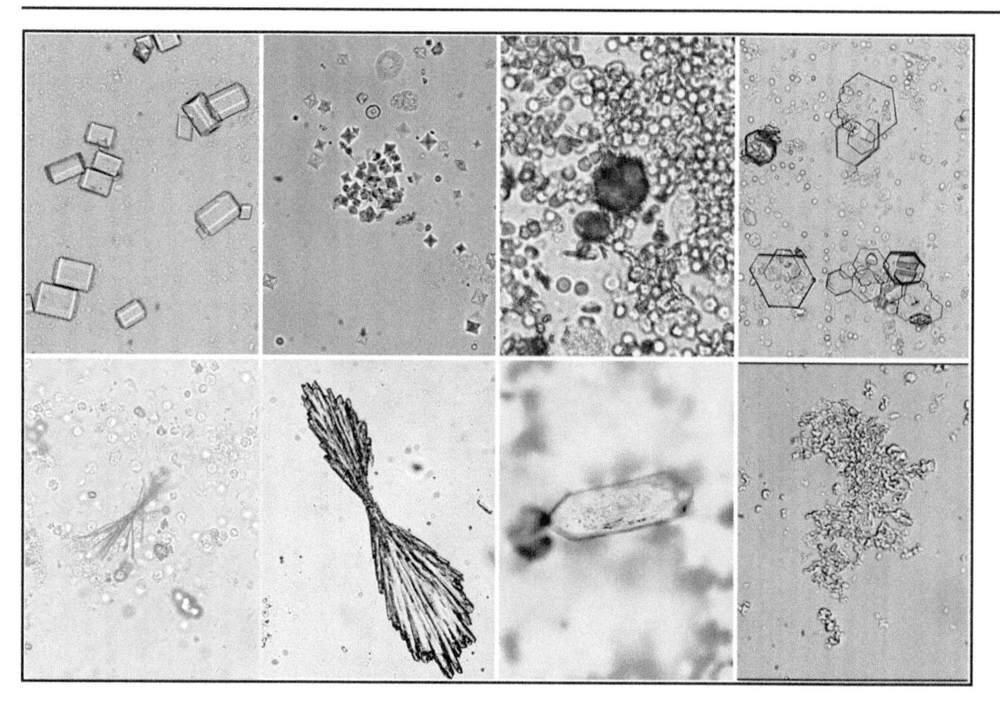

Fig. 8.3. Urine sediment. Top left to right: struvite, calcium oxalate dihydrate, ammonium urate, cystine, bilirubin crystals (*courtesy of Giulia Mangiagalli*), calcium phosphate (*courtesy of Giuseppe Menga*), calcium oxalate monohydrate, amorphous crystals.

8.5.3 Erythrocytes/Red blood cells (RBCs)

- Rare erythrocytes (<5/hpf) may be seen in urine samples of healthy dogs and cats.
- This number may slightly vary depending on the sampling technique.
- No iatrogenic haematuria is expected in free catch urine samples.

Cytological features

- In unstained urine sediment, erythrocytes appear as small, round and pale biconcave disks. They are generally the smallest cell component seen in a urine sediment. In concentrated urine, they may look even smaller and show a variable degree of crenation.
- In hypotonic and/or alkaline urine, erythrocytes swell and may lyse.
- They should not be confused with leucocytes, which are larger and with a granular texture, or lipid droplets, which are usually variable in size and often on a different plane of focus.
- In stained urine sediment, erythrocytes appear as small, round, often crenated, lightly pink/orange structures with smooth surface, and resemble the red blood cells seen in the peripheral blood.

Clinical relevance

- Increased numbers of erythrocytes (>5/hpf) are supportive of haematuria.
- Genuine haematuria may be seen with infection, inflammation, necrosis, neoplasia, haemorrhagic diathesis, toxicity (e.g. cyclophosphamide), trauma and glomerular disease. Voided urine samples from dogs in oestrus might also be haematuric due to genital tract haemorrhage.

- Haematuria may be spurious and secondary to blood contamination at the time of sampling. Iatrogenic haematuria may occur with samples collected by cystocentesis and catheterization, but not with free-catch samples.
- Positive dipstick for blood and presence of red blood cells in the urine sediment confirms haematuria. Positive dipstick in the absence of red blood cells on the sediment may suggest haemoglobinuria. Alternatively, red blood cells may have lysed due to urine low specific gravity.

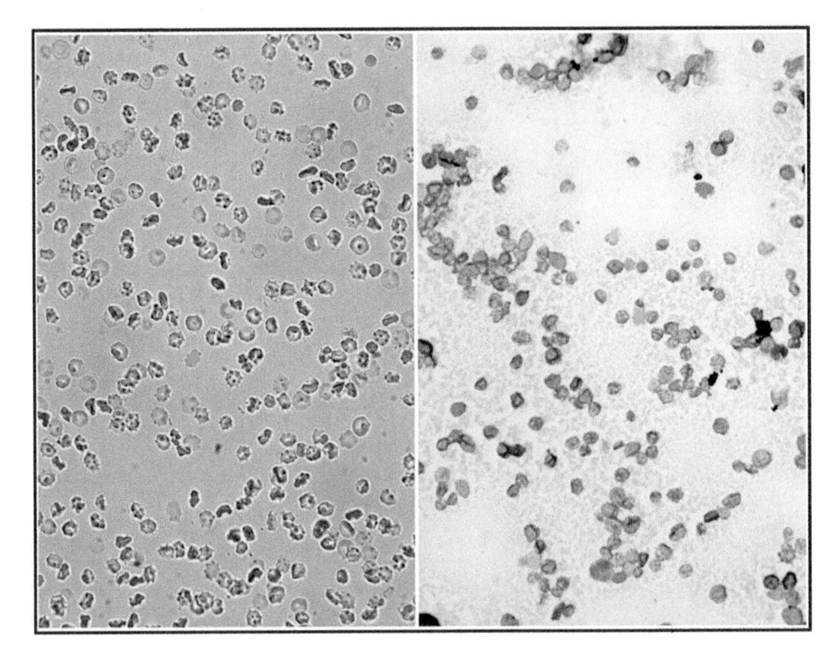

Fig. 8.4. Dog. Urine sediment. Haematuria unstained (left) and stained (right) urine sediment.

8.5.4 Leucocytes/White blood cells (WBCs)

- Rare leucocytes (<5/hpf) may be seen in urine samples of healthy dogs and cats.
- This number may slightly vary depending on the sampling technique (<3/hpf for cystocentesis samples, <8/hpf for samples obtained by catheterization or midstream voiding).

Cytological features

- In unstained urine sediment, leucocytes appear as round, colourless structures with grainy and sometimes slightly refractile appearance; rarely, the lobulation of the nucleus can be appreciated. They are generally larger than red blood cells and smaller than most epithelial cells.
- Urine sediment should be stained if there is any doubt. In particular, leucocytes may shrink in hypertonic urine, and lyse in hypotonic or alkaline urine, making their identification difficult and sometimes impossible.
- In stained urine sediment, leucocytes are most frequently neutrophils and present with a typical U shaped and lobulated nucleus and clear cytoplasm. Other cell types, in particular macrophages and lymphocytes, may be seen in chronic processes. In patients with eosinophilic cystitic, the urine sediment may contain eosinophils.

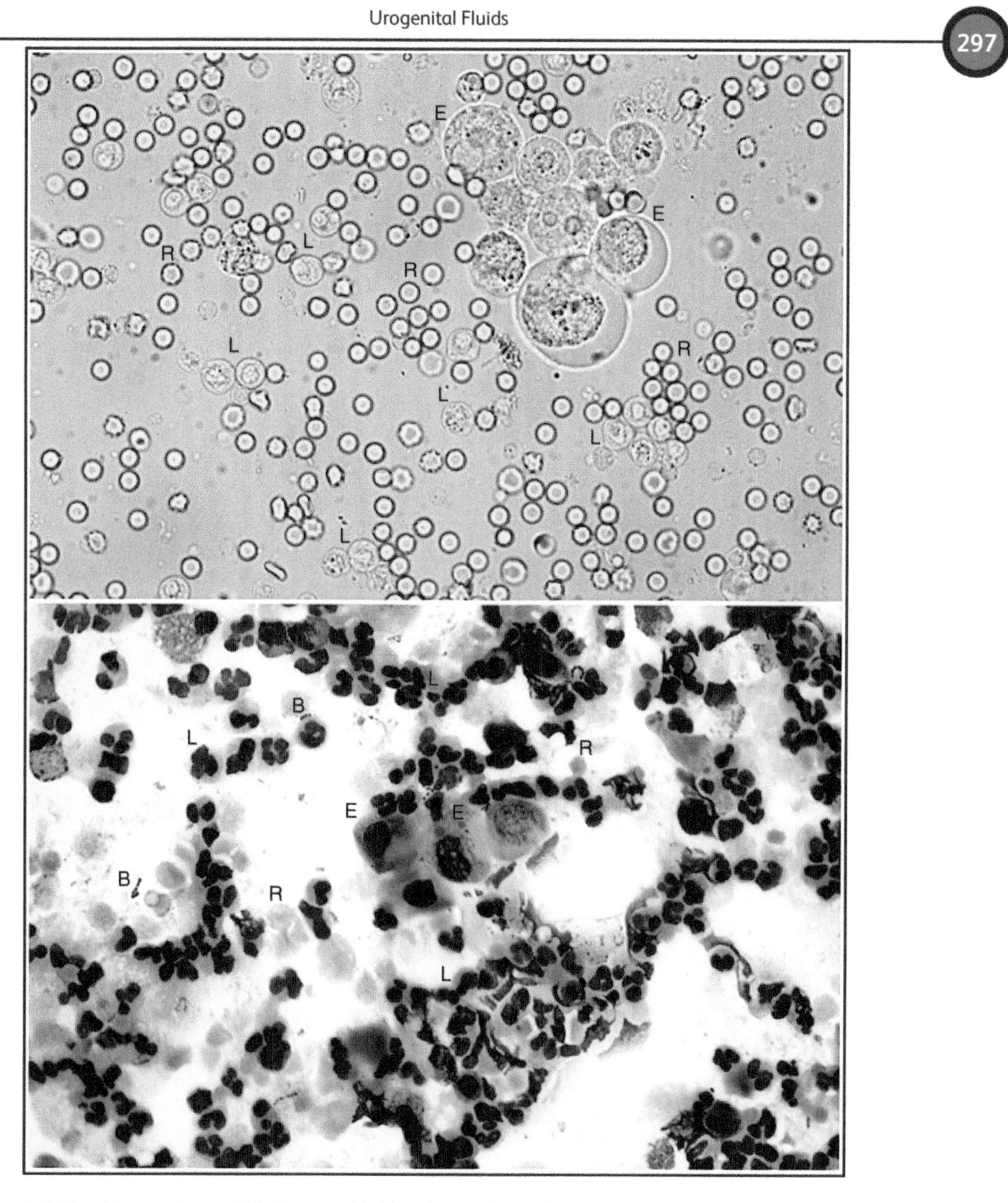

Fig. 8.5. Dog. Urine sediment. UTI. Unstained (left) and stained (right) urine sediment. L: leucocytes; R: red blood cells; E: epithelial cells.

Clinical relevance

- Increased numbers of leucocytes (>5/hpf) support inflammation (pyuria) affecting any segment of the urogenital tract.
- Knowing the collection technique may help localizing the origin of the inflammation. For example, increased leucocytes in a sample obtained by cystocentesis indicate the inflammation involves kidneys, ureters, bladder and/or proximal urethra.
- The absence of pyuria does not exclude urinary tract infection as immunosuppressed animals may develop infection without detectable leucocytes (silent urinary infection in patients with hypercortisolaemia, diabetes mellitus or other immunosuppressive conditions). In patients with polyuria, leucocytes (and bacteria) may also be diluted below the detection limit of microscopy.
- Inflammation may be septic or sterile. The presence of intracellular bacteria (recognizable only in stained sediment samples) from a fresh urine sample is proof of infection. Absence of bacteria does not exclude infection and requires culture to further confirm this.
- Most dipsticks for leucocytes have been developed using human leucocytes and should not be used for animals. In dogs, this test is poorly sensitive (many false-negatives), while in cats it is poorly specific, leading to many false-positives results. Therefore, the diagnosis of inflammation should rely on sediment examination only.

8.5.5 Epithelial cells

- Evaluation of their morphology and differentiation between different subtypes requires cytological examination of the stained urine sediment. This is of paramount importance when urinary tract neoplasia is suspected.
- They are usually present in low numbers. However, their degree of exfoliation greatly depends on the collection technique and may be particularly high in catheterized samples.

Squamous epithelial cells

Cytological features

- Large polygonal cells with abundant basophilic cytoplasm and distinctive angular borders (keratinized). Nuclei, when present, are small, round, centrally located. These cells are often seen individually but can occur in sheets.
- Non-keratinized forms are indistinguishable from transitional epithelial cells.

Clinical relevance

- Squamous cells are often the result of contamination from the distal tract of the urogenital tract or from the external skin; they are more common in catheterized and voided urine samples. Their diagnostic significance is minimal.
- Rarely, their presence may suggest squamous metaplasia of the prostate (secondary to hormonal imbalance), metaplasia of the bladder (secondary to inflammation/trauma) or presence of squamous cell carcinoma of the bladder.

Transitional (urothelial) epithelial cells

Cytological features

- Most common type of epithelial cells seen in urine samples.
- Size and shape are very variable. Most cells are medium-sized (two to four times a leucocyte), round, oval to polygonal with moderate amounts of variably basophilic cytoplasm and a round-to-oval nucleus often centrally located. These cells may exfoliate individually or form variably sized clusters.

Clinical relevance

- Normal lining cells of the urinary tract from the renal pelvis to the proximal urethra (including part of the prostate).
- The presence of a few cells with no signs of atypia is considered of no diagnostic significance.
- Causes of high numbers of transitional cells include catheterized urine samples, uroliths, inflammation (septic and sterile), neoplasia (often associated with variable degree of atypia) or chemical irritation.

Caudate epithelial cells

Cytological features

- Transitional epithelial cells with characteristic caudate, tail-like shape, exfoliating as individual elements or forming small clusters.

Clinical relevance

- Caudate cells originate from the renal pelvis.
- Low numbers may be seen in urine samples from healthy animals.
- Marked increase of this cell type may be associated with pyelonephritis.

Renal tubular (cuboidal epithelial cells)

Cytological features

- Small, round cuboidal cells with eccentric nucleus. They may contain small to a few large clear (fatty) vacuoles, in particular in cats.

Clinical relevance

- Renal tubular cells originate from renal tubuli.
- Low numbers may be seen in urine samples from healthy animals.
- Increased numbers may be associated with acute renal tubular injury.

Prostatic epithelial cells

Cytological features

- Small cuboidal to columnar cells. They have a small to moderate amount of lightly basophilic to amphophilic cytoplasm, often with a grainy texture and occasionally vacuolated. Nuclei are small, round, with granular chromatin and basally placed. Cells are often arranged in clusters with a typical honeycomb arrangement.

Clinical relevance

- Prostatic cells are observed in prostatic wash samples.
- Prostatic wash amples from healthy animals and patients with benign prostatic hyperplasia (BPH) often contain morphologically unremarkable, well differentiated prostatic epithelial cells.
- The presence of atypia supports a diagnosis of prostatic neoplasm, especially with compatible clinical presentation and absence of inflammation and infection.

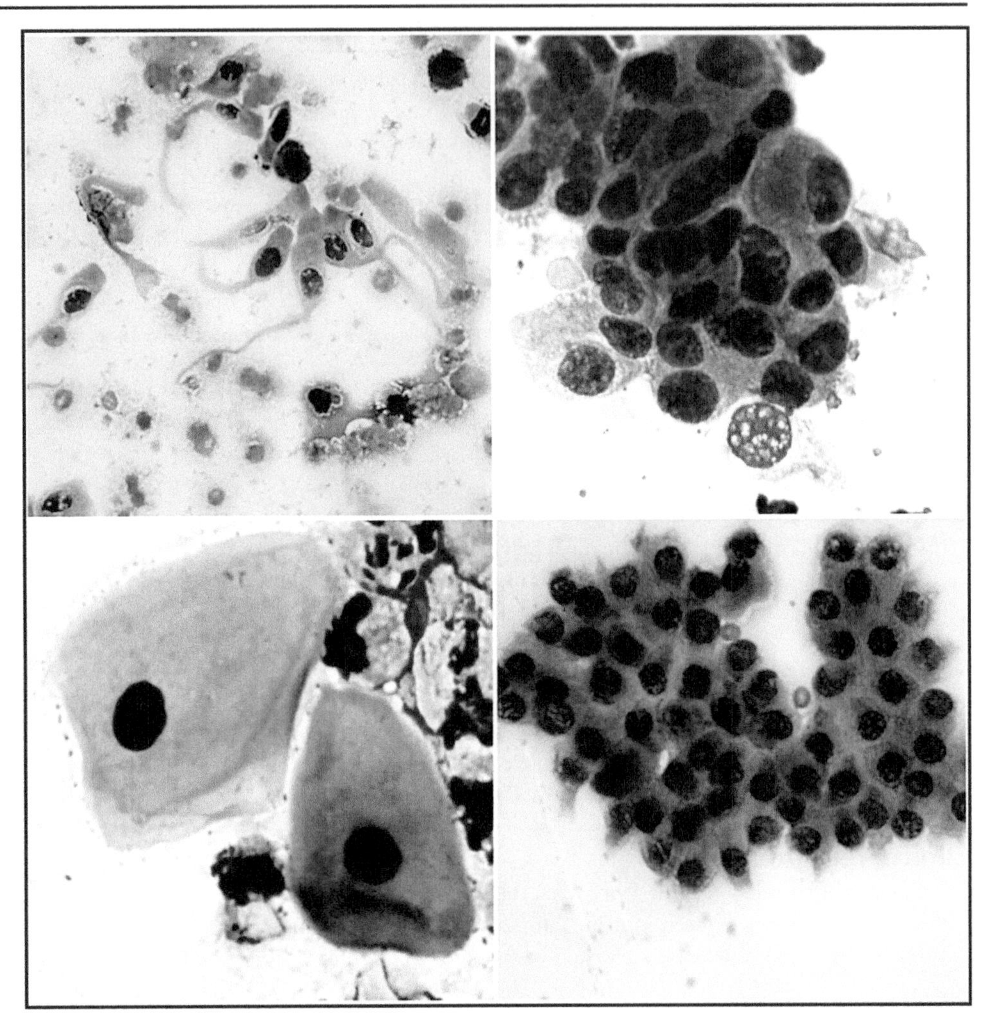

Fig. 8.6. Urine sediment. (top left) caudate epithelial cells; (top right) transitional (urothelial) epithelial cells; (bottom left) squamous epithelial cells; (bottom right) prostatic glandular epithelial cells.

8.5.6 Infectious agents

Bacteria

Cytological features

- Round (cocci) or elongated (rods) small structures; rarely filamentous or spores forming. They may form groups/colonies.
- They may be confused for amorphous debris. If doubt exists, stained urine sediment preparation is beneficial.
- Their presence is often expressed in a semiquantitative manner (e.g. small/moderate/high numbers).

Clinical relevance

- Evidence of bacteria, in particular when intracellular and associated with increased leucocytes (pyuria), is supportive of infection.
- Presence of numerous bacteria, mainly extracellular, not associated with increased numbers of leucocytes, suggest bacterial contamination or bacteria overgrowth. This is particularly common in samples obtained by catheterization or free-catch voided samples. However, silent infection (presence of bacteria not associated with increased leucocytes) may occur in selected patients (e.g. immunocompromised or diabetic animals).
- The absence of bacteria on cytology does not rule out infection, in particular when leucocytes are increased. This is because cytology has lower Se and Sp than culture testing in identification of bacteria.

Table 8.2. Significance of urine culture results.

	Evidence of bacteria on sediment	Absence of bacteria on sediment
Negative bacterial culture	Non-viable bacteria (exposure to antibiotics, prolonged storage, no urine transport medium) Fastidious bacteria (e.g. anaerobes) Bacteria requiring longer incubation or different medium to grow (>24 h) Misinterpretation of bacteria on sediment (confused for debris)	No evidence of infection or contamination
Positive bacterial culture	Urinary tract infection or contamination	Urinary tract infection or contamination (culture has higher sensitivity and specificity than cytology for identification of bacteria)

Fungal spores and hyphae

Cytological features

- Fungal spores: round-to-oval small structures, often brown in colour and with internal septae (also called macroconidia).
- Fungal hyphae: long-branched structures with parallel walls and perpendicular septae.

Clinical relevance

- Often result of contamination, commonly seen in free-catch urine samples. Rarely, they may be part of a genuine fungal infection, in which case concurrent leucoytes are also noted.

Parasites

- *Capillaria plica* and *Capillaria felis cati*: they may be found in urine of dogs and cats, respectively. Animals are often asymptomatic. Eggs are oval, colourless, with a slightly pitted surface and bipolar plugs. They may be associated with haematuria and pyuria. They should be differentiated from *Trichuris vulpis*, which may be seen in voided samples with faecal contamination.

- *Dioctophyma renale*: rare parasites resulting from consumption of infected fish or frogs. Eggs may be found in urine and appear as oval structures with thick, pitted shells except at their poles. They may be associated with haematuria and pyuria.
- *Dirofilaria immitis*: microfilariae may be rarely seen in urine, mainly due to haemorrhage into the urinary tract. They appear as elongated structures (~300 µm) with straight posterior end and tapering anterior end. Their presence indicates heartworm infection and requires treatment.

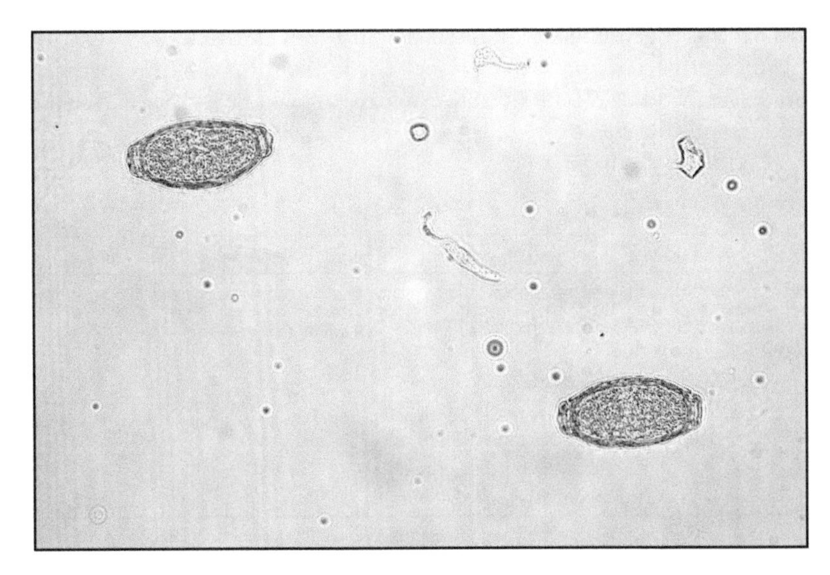

Fig. 8.7. Dog, urine wet sediment. Eggs of *Capillaria plica*. (*Courtesy of Giuseppe Menga.*)

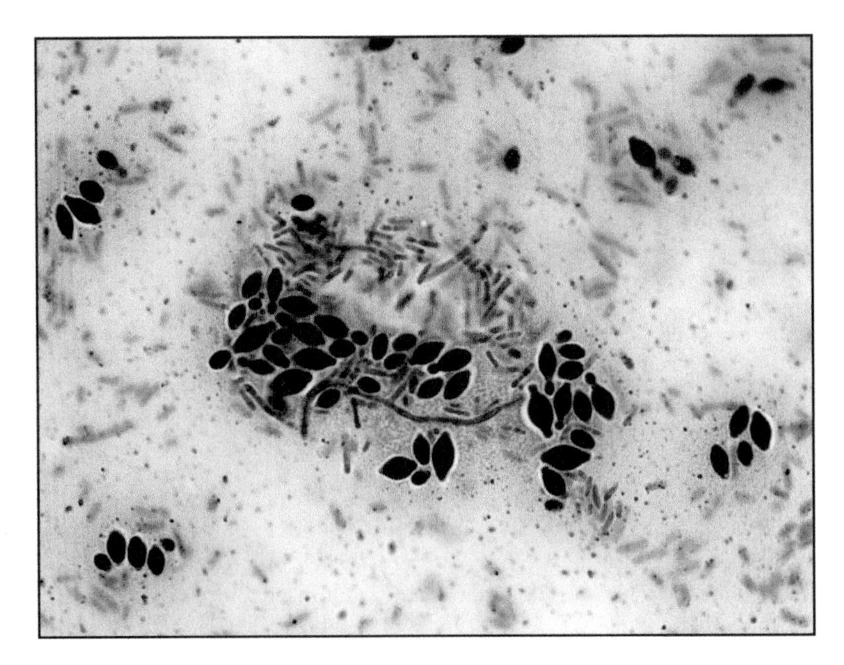

Fig. 8.8. Urine sediment. Mixed bacteria and budding yeasts in the absence of leukocytes, likely due to external contamination. Wright-Giemsa.

8.5.7 Other elements

Other elements	Cytological features	Clinical relevance
Spermatozoa	Oval heads and long, thin tails.	• Incidental finding in urine from intact males. • May be found in free-catch urine samples from females post breeding.
Pollens	Round-to-oval structures, often with yellow-to-brown tint. They may have little stem.	• Result of contamination; may be observed in free-catch urine samples. • Attention must be paid to differentiate them from parasite eggs.
Lipid droplets	• Variably sized (often very small), perfectly spherical structures with defined borders. • They have high refractive index and may appear floating on a different plane of focus.	• Increased numbers may be seen in patients with diabetes mellitus and may be the reflection of the lipid content of renal tubular cells. • They may also result from contaminating lubricants.
Air bubbles	Variably sized, perfectly spherical structures with defined borders, often appearing on a different plane of focus. Unlike fat, they appear flat.	None. They are the result of air trapped between the coverslip and the smear.
Starch granules	Clear hexagonal granules with central fissure.	Incidental finding, resulting from contamination with glove powder used in urine collection.
(Cotton) Fibres	Linear structures of variable length. Internal structure may vary.	Incidental finding, resulting from contamination.
Lubricant/ ultrasound gel	Amorphous deeply eosinophilic/pink material.	Incidental finding, resulting from contamination with lubricant (in catheterized samples) or ultrasound gel (in cystocentesis samples).

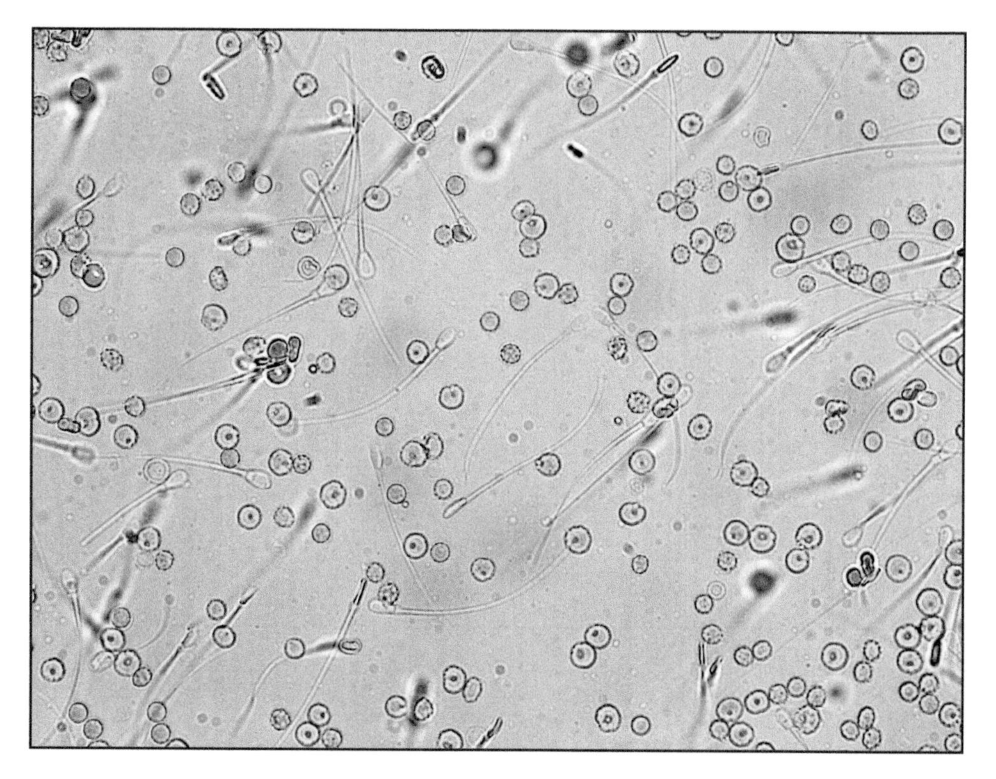

Fig. 8.9. Dog. Urine wet sediment. Spermatozoa admixed with red blood cells.

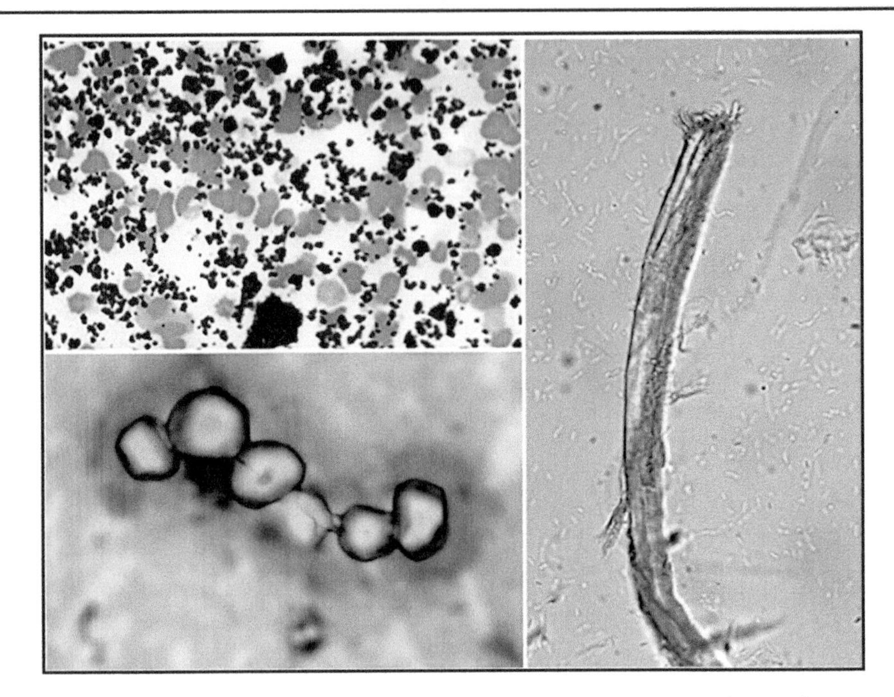

Fig. 8.10. Urine wet sediment. (top left) lubricant gel; (bottom left) starch granules; (right) cotton fibre.

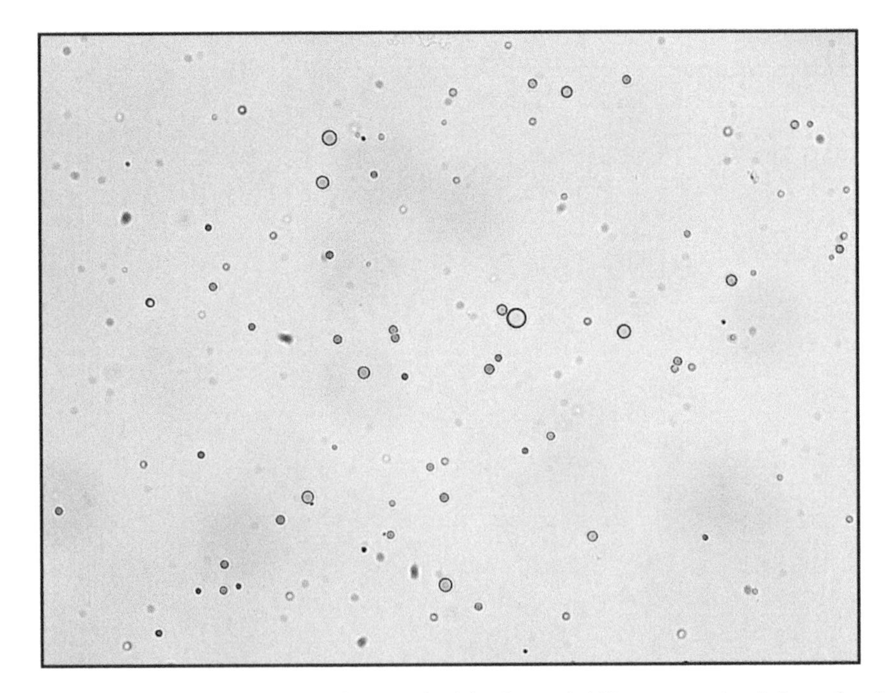

Fig. 8.11. Urine wet sediment. Air bubbles. Similar to lipid droplets, air bubbles can occasionally be confused with red blood cells due to their spherical shape and smooth appearance. However, they occupy a distinct focal plane and exhibit varying sizes, in contrast to the consistent nature of red blood cells.

8.6 Urinary Tract Inflammation

Inflammation of the urinary tract could be septic (e.g. UTI) or sterile.

Urinary tract infection (UTI)

Urinary tract infection, often abbreviated to UTI, is a bacterial infection of the urinary tract (most commonly bladder), associated with compatible urinary tract signs.

Clinical features

- UTI is a common diagnosis in dogs and cats and most frequently involve the bladder (cystitis). In cats, UTI is less common as most cases of cystitis are sterile and idiopathic.
- Typical clinical signs include dysuria/stranguria, haematuria and pollakiuria. When there is involvement of the renal parenchyma (pyelonephritis), systemic signs may also occur (e.g. fever, lethargy) and may be accompanied by kidney injury.
- Bacteria causing UTI are most commonly ascending from the external genitalia and urethra. Less frequently, UTI can be caused by haematogenous bacterial spread and secondary urinary tract colonization.
- Most of the UTIs (~75–90%) involve a single agent, with *Escherichia coli* being responsible for up to half of the infections in dogs and cats.
- In 2019, the International Society for Companion Animal Infectious Diseases revised the classifications of the infections of the lower urinary tract and identified the following categories:
  - Sporadic bacterial cystitis: this term refers to sporadic bacterial infections affecting dogs that are otherwise healthy, with no known urinary tract anatomical and functional abnormalities or relevant comorbidities. To fall into this category, patients must have had fewer than three episodes of known or suspected bacterial cystitis in the preceding 12 months. This condition was previously referred as *simple uncomplicated* UTI.
  - Recurrent bacterial cystitis: this term is used when the patients experience three or more infections within 12 months or two or more episodes in the previous 3–6 months. Recurrent UTI may result from relapsing or persistent infection or reinfection. Causes/predisposing factors include:
    - Incomplete bladder emptying: e.g. lower motor neuron disease or dysautonomia.
    - Anatomical abnormalities of the genitourinary tract.
    - Altered immune function: e.g. diabetes mellitus, hyperadrenocorticism. In diabetic patients, bacterial growth is also promoted by the glucosuria.
    - Urolithiasis.
    - Neoplasia.
    - Ineffective antibiotic therapy.
    - Prostatic disease.
  - Subclinical bacteriuria (SB): this term indicates the presence of bacteria in urine as determined by positive bacterial culture from a properly collected urine specimen, in the absence of clinical signs referrable to UTI. It was formerly referred to as *occult* UTI.
- Bacterial cystitis has a higher incidence in females, probably due to the shorter urethra.
- Diagnosis of UTI should be made in patients with lower urinary tract signs, with supporting laboratory findings (haematuria, pyuria, cytologically evident bacteriuria), and based on quantitative urine culture. Samples for culture should be collected by cystocentesis if no contraindications for this procedure are present.

Cytological features

- Cellularity: variably increased.
- Background: variably haemodiluted.
- On wet preparation, high numbers of leucocytes are seen per high-power field. These are recognized as neutrophils in stained samples. Neutrophils can be variably degenerate, and they may contain phagocytosed bacteria. Bacteria are also frequently found free in the background.
- Depending on the aetiologic agent involved, bacteria could be cocci, bacilli (rods) or coccobacilli. However, cytological appearance alone is not always accurate in predicting the type of bacteria involved, as the morphology can be affected by the fluid environment and overlaps between different organisms of relevance for the site.
- Poor agreement between cytological bacteriuria and positive urine culture has been reported in dogs.
- The presence of inflammatory cells has a positive correlation with positive cultures, but inflammation can occur with sterile cystitis and other causes (e.g. urolithiasis and crystalluria).
- Absence of inflammation does not exclude UTI (e.g. immunocompromised patients). In subclinical forms or in immunocompromised patients, bacteria may be seen without a concurrent inflammatory response.

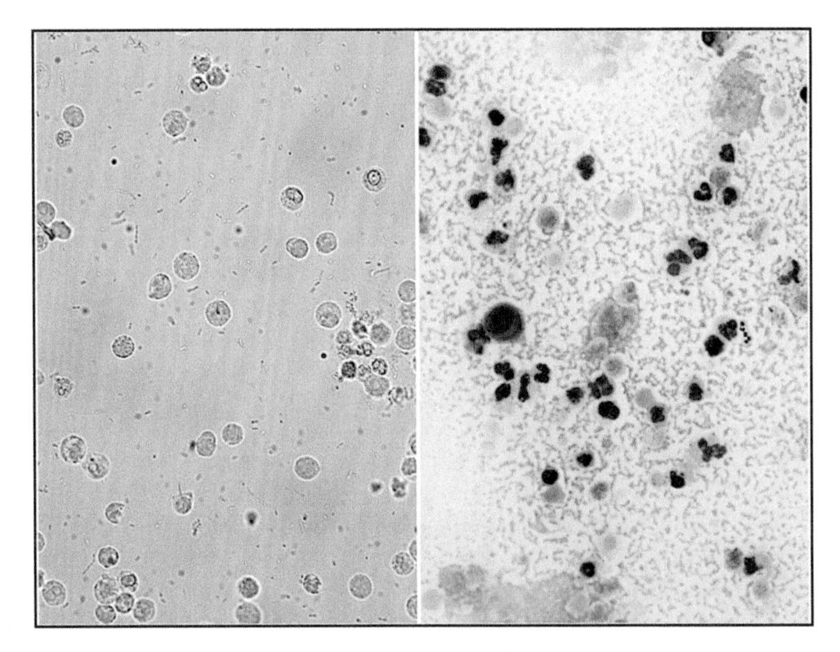

Fig. 8.12. Dog. Urine sediment. UTI. Unstained (top) and stained (bottom) urine sediment.

Feline idiopathic cystitis

Also known as interstitial cystitis.

Clinical features

- Most common clinical signs are dysuria, haematuria, pollakiuria and/or inappropriate urination.
- Age: 4–10 years old.
- The pathogenesis of the disease is not fully understood and may implicate several body systems. Proposed contributing factors include decreased urinary excretion of glycosaminoglycans, increased bladder permeability and neurogenic inflammation. Stress and diet can also increase the risk of feline idiopathic cystitis (FIC).
- FIC is a diagnosis of exclusion.

Cytological features

- Urine sediment analysis (wet and stained) is often negative.
- In some cases, haematuria with or without inflammatory cells may be present, but no recognizable cause is found.
- Microbiology is negative.

Eosinophilic cystitis

This is not very common and is usually described in older dogs with history of chronic urolithiasis. Occasionally, low numbers of eosinophils may be seen in the stained urine sediments.

Sterile haemorrhagic cystitis

Causes

- Cyclophosphamide: the activated metabolites of the drug cause ulceration, oedema and haemorrhage of the urinary bladder mucosa.
- Idiopathic cystitis in cats.
- Urolithiasis.
- Coagulopathy.
- Trauma.

Cytological features

- The urine sediment contains numerous erythrocytes.
- Inflammatory cells may or may not be present.

Differential diagnosis

Idiopathic renal haematuria.

Further reading

Marques, C., Gama, L.T., Belas, A., Bergström, K., Beurlet, S. *et al.* (2016) European multicenter study on antimicrobial resistance in bacteria isolated from companion animal urinary tract infections. *BMC Veterinary Research* 12(1), 213.

Weese, J.S., Blondeau, J., Boothe, D., Guardabassi, L.G., Gumley, N. *et al.* (2019) International Society for Companion Animal Infectious Diseases (ISCAID) guidelines for the diagnosis and management of bacterial urinary tract infections in dogs and cats. *Veterinary Journal* 247, 8–25.

8.7 Prostatic Wash

- Prostatic disease is relatively frequent in dogs, especially older intact male dogs; it is very rare in cats.
- Clinical signs are variable and often non-specific. They may include tenesmus, stranguria, haematuria, pyuria, preputial/urethral discharge and locomotor difficulties.
- Rectal palpation and imaging studies may also show non-specific findings, such as prostatomegaly, change in echogenicity of glandular parenchyma and presence of cysts.
- Cytological evaluation of the prostatic fluid, aspirates and/or histopathology of the gland are often required to achieve a definitive diagnosis.
- The most common prostatic disorders include benign prostatic hyperplasia (BPH), prostatitis, prostatic abscesses, prostatic/paraprostatic cysts and neoplasia.

8.7.1 Sampling techniques, handling, slide preparation and staining

Techniques

The most common ways to collect prostatic samples are:

- Prostatic massage and wash.
- Ejaculation.
- Perirectal and rectal aspiration (FNA).
- Transabdominal ultrasound-guided aspiration (FNA).

FNA techniques will not be described in this textbook.

Materials

- Sterile urinary catheter.
- Syringes: from 3 ml to 12 ml.
- 5–10 ml of sterile saline.
- Tubes:
  - Capped sterile tube (for bacterial culture).
  - EDTA tube (for cytological evaluation).
- Glass slides:

Patient preparation

- Use of chemical restraint is common for prostatic massage and wash. This is aiming to avoid excessive movement of the animal during the procedure.

Techniques

- Prostatic massage and wash:
  - Aseptically catheterize the bladder, remove the urine and rinse it several times with sterile saline. Last rinse should be kept as a pre-massage sample.
  - Using transrectal guidance, retract the catheter to the prostatic urethra and vigorously massage the prostate for 1–2 min.
  - Slowly inject 5–10 ml of sample and aspirate it back, as the catheter is slowly advanced into the bladder (post-massage sample).
  - Both pre and post-massage samples should be kept and analysed.
- Collection and fractionation of the ejaculate:
  - This procedure allows to obtain a more voluminous sample with greater concentration of potentially diagnostic material.
  - The third fraction of the ejaculate is preferred, as it usually derives from the prostate and is more abundant.

    - Ejaculation can be achieved via manual stimulation into either an artificial vagina or into funnels.
    - At the moment of the ejaculation, the prostatic portion of the ejaculate may be separated from the sperm rich fraction.
- Ultrasound-guided aspirates:
    - For culture purposes, ultrasound-guided aspirates or prostatic tissue biopsies can be more specific than ejaculate fluid or fluid collected by prostatic lavage, as contamination is less likely to occur. However, the procedure is more invasive and may not be required.
    - If there are pockets of fluid within the prostatic tissue, sampling of these for culture may also be more fruitful (e.g. prostatic abscesses).
    - A positive urine culture (sampled via cystocentesis) may indicate prostatic infection; however, discrepancies between culture of cystocentesis samples and prostatic washes have been reported.

Prostatic wash cytology preparation

- Centrifuge at low speed (~400 g) for 5 min using a clean conical tube. At the end of the process, the sediment may or may not be visible at the bottom of the tube.
- Remove most of the supernatant with a sterile pipette. Leave a few drops and re-suspend the sediment. Gently tap the tube with a finger to mix the sediment and avoid any vigorous shaking.
- Transfer with a pipette a drop of the resuspended sediment onto a clean microscope slide, prepare some smears, dry rapidly and stain with any type of Romanowsky stain.

Complications and contraindications

- Urinary tract infections following improper procedure for prostatic wash and massage are possible, and priapism following manual ejaculation has been reported.

Pearls and Pitfalls

- In rare cases, fine-needle aspirates and incisional biopsies of the prostatic gland in course of urothelial carcinoma have been associated with tumour seeding along the needle tract. The use of this technique is controversial and discouraged by some oncologists. Urethral catheterization may be preferred.
- Similarly, aspiration from prostatic abscessation or bacteria prostatitis can cause peritonitis.

8.7.2 Cell types

- Prostatic wash cytology findings from healthy animals include a few erythrocytes, rare leucocytes, spermatozoa (in entire males), normal urothelial cells, glandular prostatic epithelial cells and often squamous cells.
- Prostatic epithelial cells: cuboidal to columnar epithelial cells. They are arranged in clusters with a typical honeycomb appearance. Nuclei are small, round and basal. They have granular chromatin and sometimes a single small nucleolus can be seen. The cytoplasm is scant to moderate, pale amphophilic and microvesciculated. It can occasionally contain small clear vacuoles.
- Spermatozoa: composed of oval-shaped heads and long, thin tails.
- Urothelial (transitional) epithelial cells: round, oval to polygonal cells with a moderate amount of variably basophilic cytoplasm and a round-to-oval nucleus often, centrally located. These cells may exfoliate individually or form variably sized clusters. Size and shape of these cells may vary.
- Squamous epithelial cells: large polygonal cells with abundant basophilic cytoplasm and distinctive angular borders (keratinized). Nuclei, when present, are small, round, centrally located. These cells are often seen individually but can occur in sheets. They originate from distal urethra or the external genitalia (contaminants) and may be associated with bacteria. They may derive from the prostate in case of squamous metaplasia.

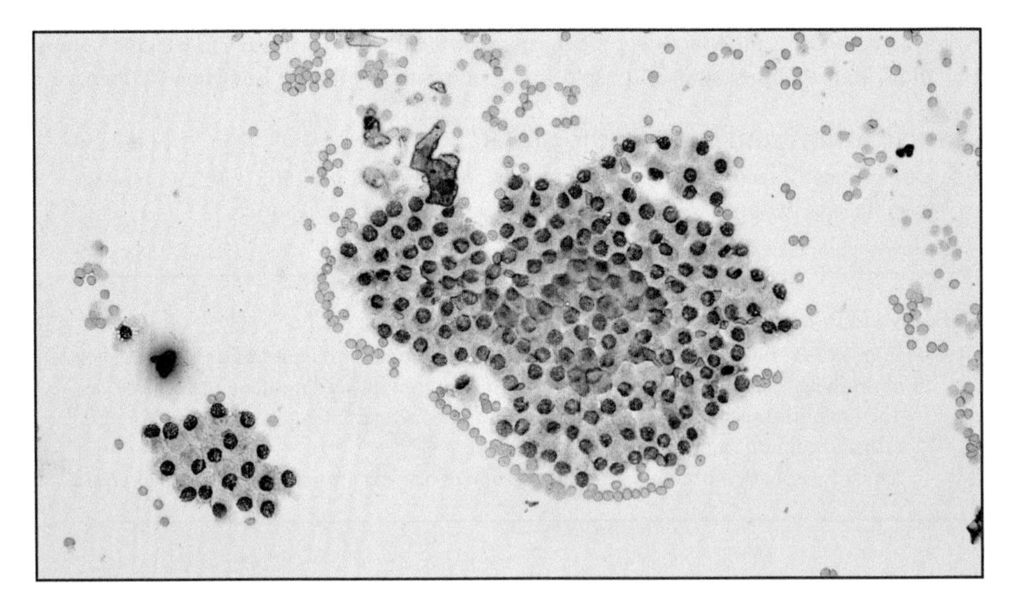

Fig. 8.13. Dog. Well differentiated prostatic epithelial cells arranged in a cluster with honeycomb appearance. Wright-Giemsa.

8.7.3 Prostatitis

Inflammation of the prostatic gland.

Clinical features

- Common disease seen in entire dogs, especially when older. Reports in castrated dogs are rare and mainly occur in patients with recent castration.
- In cats, prostatitis is very rare and is mainly secondary to bacterial colonization from the urinary tract.
- It can be acute or chronic, infectious and non-infectious (sterile).
- In acute forms, the prostate is usually enlarged and painful. Clinical signs include fever, anorexia, depression, straining to urinate or defecate, caudal abdominal pain, haematuria, pain on rectal palpation, and occasionally oedema of the scrotum, prepuce and hindlimb.
- Inflammatory leucogram and non-regenerative anaemia are often present.
- Asymptomatic forms of prostatitis may occur, in particular when chronic. Chronic prostatitis is usually associated with signs of recurrent urinary tract infections, poor semen quality, infertility, decreased libido, and intermittent urethral discharge. Chronic prostatitis may also be associated with gland hyperplasia and cysts formation.
- Infectious agents commonly isolated in prostatitis include:
  - Bacteria: *Escherichia coli*, often ascending from the urethra, is the most common isolate in dogs. Other isolates include *Proteus* spp., *Staphylococcus* spp., *Streptococcus* spp., *Pseudomonas* spp., *Klebsiella* spp., *Enterobacter* spp., *Pasteurella* spp., *Haemophilus* spp., *Mycoplasma* spp. and *Ureaplasma* spp., may also rarely cause of prostatitis; special culture methods may be required. *Brucella canis* is more commonly associated with testicular infections; however, it may also be a cause of prostatitis. Serological testing rather than culture is recommended if *B. canis* infection is favoured because of the laboratory biosafety hazard associated with the isolation of this bacterium and the potential for false-negative cultures.
  - Fungi: *Blastomyces dermatitis*, *Cryptococcus neoformans* and *Coccidioides immitis*. One case of *Pythium* spp. infection has been reported in one dog. Fungal infections at this level are rare and are most commonly associated with systemic infection.
  - Protozoa: *Leishmania* spp.
- Prostatic abscess may be a sequela of chronic prostatitis or can occur in association with acute bacterial prostatitis and cystic hyperplasia. Rarely, it may be secondary to bacteriaemia.

Cytological features

- Cellularity is variable, often high.
- Background: it can be pale basophilic and finely granular (proteinaceous) and variably haemodiluted.
- Acute prostatitis: prevalence of neutrophils with degenerative changes. Small numbers of macrophages with signs of phagocytosis can be observed. In bacterial forms, intracellular and extracellular bacteria are often seen.
- Chronic prostatitis: increased numbers of macrophages, lymphocytes and/or plasma cells, often associated with neutrophils. Squamous metaplasia of prostatic epithelium may be seen, in which case, squamous epithelial cells might be found in the cytology specimens.

- Clusters of well-differentiated prostatic epithelial cells may also be seen. Occasionally, they may exhibit increased cytoplasmic basophilia, mild anisocytosis/anisokaryosis and increased N:C ratio.
- Necrotic material may also be present as aggregates of amorphous blue grey to purple material.

Pearls and Pitfalls

- Because prostatic fluid constantly flows both retrograde into the bladder as well as antegrade out the urethra, cases of prostatitis can be misdiagnosed as urinary tract infections.
- Antimicrobial susceptibility testing should consider soft tissue rather than urinary breakpoints for cases of prostatitis. Furthermore, not all antimicrobials penetrate the blood-prostate barrier and this needs to be considered when selecting an appropriate antimicrobial treatment.

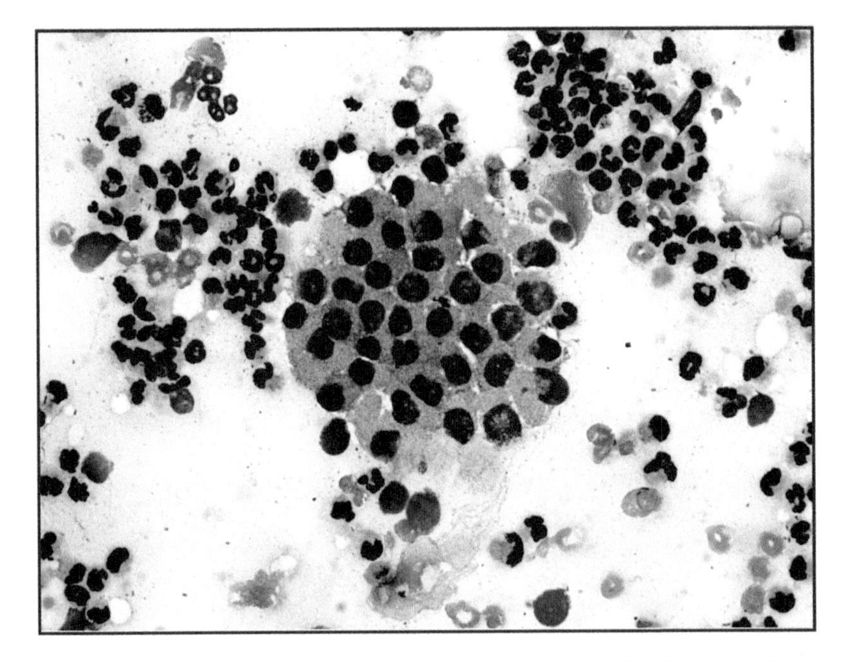

Fig. 8.14. Dog. Septic prostatitis. Prostatic wash. Large numbers of neutrophils, often containing intracellular bacteria (rods), admixed with a cluster of well-differentiated prostatic epithelial cells with typical honeycomb appearance. Wright-Giemsa.

Further reading

Christensen, B.W. (2018) Canine prostatic disease. *Veterinary Clinics of North America: Small Animal Practice* 48, 701–719.

Palmieri, C., Fonseca-Alves, C.E. and Laufer-Amorim, R. (2022) A review on canine and feline prostate pathology. *Frontiers in Veterinary Science* 26(9).

8.7.4 Benign prostatic hyperplasia

Clinical features

- Condition associated with ageing and sex hormone dysregulation.
- Particularly common in older intact male dogs. Reported prevalence is 80% in dogs >6 years and >95% in dogs >9 years old.
- Characterized by diffuse, symmetrical, often non-painful prostatic enlargement growing outward from the urethra. Intraparenchymal variable-sized cysts are often seen.
- Clinical signs are the result of prostatomegaly and include urethral discharge, tenesmus, haematuria, fertility abnormalities and occasionally a stilted gait caused by prostatic pain.
- Presumptive diagnosis is based on the combination of physical examination, ultrasonographic findings, clinical signs and often result of fine-needle aspirates or prostatic washes.
- Prostatic hyperplasia can be associated with other prostatic disorders, including prostatitis and prostatic neoplasia.
- A breed predisposition in Rhodesian Ridgeback dogs has been reported in one study, although this finding should be further investigated and confirmed in a large-scale study.

Cytological features

- Cellularity is variable, often higher than in samples from normal prostate, and may depend on sampling technique.
- Background: variably haemodiluted. Eosinophilic/pink amorphous material may be seen and represents the secretory proteinaceous material produced by the gland.
- Depending on the quality of the wash, prostatic epithelial cells should be the main cellular component.
- Hyperplastic prostatic epithelial cells are morphologically similar to normal prostatic epithelial cells. They are cuboidal to columnar and are often arranged in variably sized clusters with honeycomb appearance. Acinar arrangement may be seen.
- Mononuclear cells (macrophages, lymphocytes) may be seen in some cases of hyperplasia and reflect concurrent chronic inflammation.

Pearls and Pitfalls

Since the term hyperplasia is already defining a benign process, it is preferable to use prostatic hyperplasia (PH) instead of BPH.

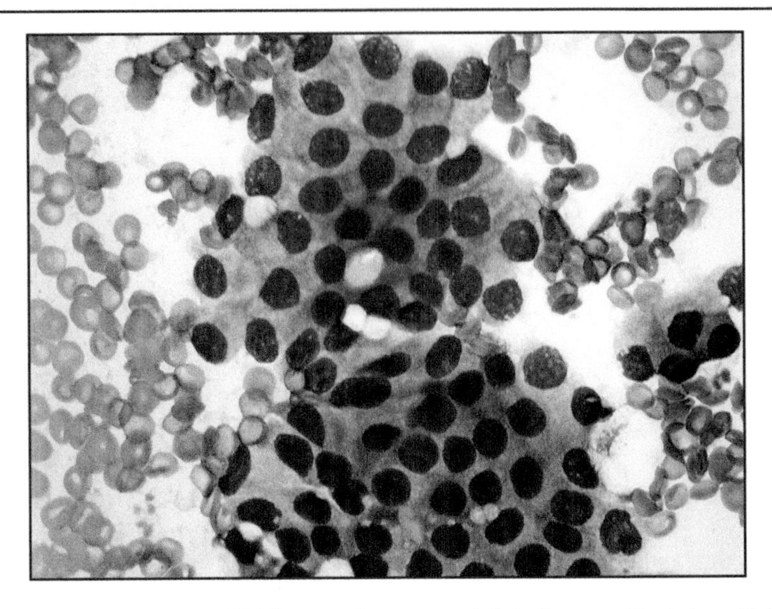

Fig. 8.15. Dog. Prostatic wash. BPH. Well differentiated prostatic epithelial cells arranged in clusters with honeycomb appearance. Wright-Giemsa.

Further reading

Christensen, B.W. (2018) Canine prostatic disease. *Veterinary Clinical of North American: Small Animal Practice* 48, 701–719.
Palmieri, C., Fonseca-Alves, C.E. and Laufer-Amorim, R. (2022) A review on canine and feline prostate pathology. *Frontiers in Veterinary Science* 26(9).

8.7.5 Other non-neoplastic conditions

Squamous metaplasia

Transformation of the prostatic epithelium from columnar glandular to stratified and squamous epithelium.

Clinical features

- Relatively common in dogs; very rare in cats.
- Clinical signs usually relate to hyperoestrogenism and include bilateral symmetrical alopecia, hyperpigmentation, gynecomastia, galactorrhoea, pendulous prepuce, and atrophy of the penis and the contralateral testicle.
- This is not considered a pre-neoplastic condition, but it can lead to formation of cysts and abscesses.

Causes

- Idiopathic.
- Oestrogen producing Sertoli tumour (rarely also interstitial cell tumour).
- Exogenous oestrogen administration.
- Chronic irritation or inflammation (prostatitis).

Cytological features

- Sheets of large, angular and flattened, well-differentiated squamous epithelial cells with abundant pale to light blue cytoplasm with angular borders, and a central, pyknotic or karyorrhectic small dark nucleus are seen.
- Concurrent presence of leucocytes, bacteria or hyperplastic prostatic cells is not uncommon, in particular when this is associated with chronic prostatitis.

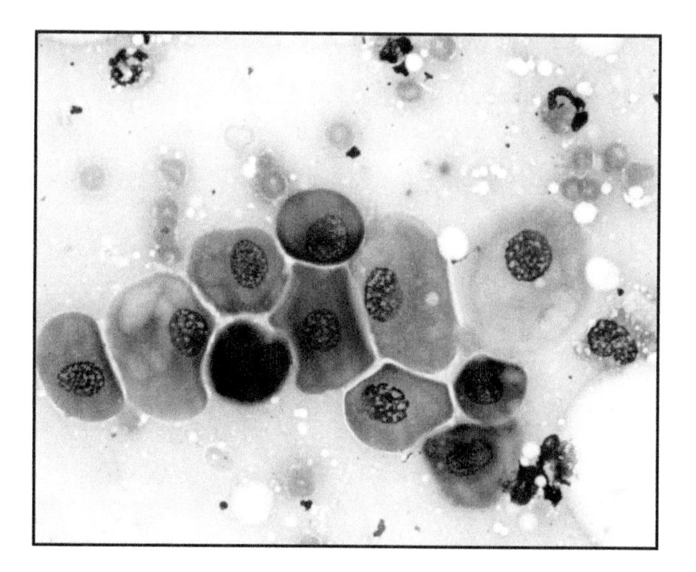

Fig. 8.16. Dog. Prostatic wash. Squamous metaplasia. (*Courtesy of Jim Meinkoth.*)

Prostatic and paraprostatic cysts

Clinical features

- Intraparenchymal (retention) cysts: they are the result of accumulation of fluid due to obstruction of prostatic canaliculi. They can also contain urine and have a connection with the urethra. They are considered an evolution of cystic prostatic hyperplasia but may also occur secondary to squamous metaplasia or prostatitis. They may predispose the animal to abscessation.
- Paraprostastic cysts: they form outside the glandular parenchyma and often arise from a cystic uterus masculinus, a remnant of the paramesonephric duct. They are commonly located in the craniolateral or dorsal aspect of the gland. They are large nodular lesions enclosed by a capsule. They may undergo ossification and mineralization. Only a single case of paraprostatic cyst has been reported in a cat.
- Clinical signs are uncommon unless the size of the cyst becomes large enough to cause dysuria, tenesmus and haematuria.
- Diagnosis is mainly based on transabdominal aspiration more than prostatic wash, unless the cyst is in communication with the gland lumen.

Cytological features

- Samples are acellular or hypocellular similar to a transudate and may contain a few normal prostatic epithelial cells, occasional leucocytes, erythrocytes and cellular debris.

Further reading

Christensen, B.W. (2018) Canine prostatic disease. *Veterinary Clinics of North America: Small Animal Practice* 48, 701–719.

Palmieri, C., Fonseca-Alves, C.E. and Laufer-Amorim, R. (2022) A review on canine and feline prostate pathology. *Frontiers in Veterinary Science* 26(9).

8.8 Neoplasms

- Over 90% of the tumours of the bladder and urethra in dogs and cats are epithelial in origin and malignant (carcinomas).
- The most common are urothelial carcinoma (UC), formerly known as transitional cell carcinoma (TCC), and prostatic adenocarcinoma. These two neoplasms are often indistinguishable from both clinical, imaging, and morphological points of views; therefore, the generic term carcinoma may sometimes be used.
- Squamous cell carcinomas (SCCs) and adenocarcinomas arising from foci of metaplasia of the transitional epithelium have also been rarely reported.
- Benign epithelial neoplasms are rare and include papilloma and adenoma.
- Approximately 10% of the canine urinary bladder neoplasms are mesenchymal and include leiomyoma/ sarcoma, rhabdomyosarcoma, and fibro/sarcoma. Diagnosis of these tumour is achieved via histopathology as they do not exfoliate into urine, and therefore they are not described in this textbook.
- Round cell tumours, in particular lymphoma, may also occur.

8.8.1 Carcinomas

Clinical features

- Urothelial carcinoma
  - Malignant epithelial neoplasia arising from the transitional epithelium lining the urinary tract.
  - Most common type of bladder cancer in dogs and cats. In dogs, it accounts for 2% of all malignant neoplasms and over 70% of bladder tumours. In cats, the incidence is comparatively low.
  - It occurs more frequently in older (average 9–11 years) female neutered dogs. In cats, it is seen in older animals (average 15 years).
  - Urinary bladder, and in particular the trigone area, is the most common anatomical location in dogs; in cats, based on a recent study, only 27% of cases occured there. UC can appear anywhere from the renal pelvis, prostatic urethra, to distal urethra. Lesions are usually solitary, intraluminal, often sessile, with variably echogenicity. Multiple lesions or the involvement of the entire bladder mucosa have been reported.
  - Over 90% of dogs with UC have clinical signs referable to the urinary system (e.g. haematuria, pyuria, pollakiuria and dysuria). Small percentages of dogs present for unrelated signs (e.g. lameness due to bone metastases, dyspnoea due to pulmonary metastases). Similar clinical signs are described in cats.
  - Diagnosis can be achieved via cytology. Occasionally, neoplastic cells can also be noted in urine sediment; however, the submission of urine for cytopathology rarely results in a definitive diagnosis of neoplasia because of poor cellular preservation, low cellularity or concurrent inflammation. Squash preparation from solid biopsy collected via transurethral cystoscopy may also be considered and increases the chances to obtain a cellular sample.

Continued

- Histologically, it can be low or high grade. Carcinoma in situ (CIS) is the most common low-grade form. The vast majority of UC in dogs (>90%) are anaplastic, show signs of invasion (breaching the basement membrane and deeper structures) and are classified as high-grade.
- High-grade UC has a high metastatic potential, with metastasis often found at the time of the diagnosis in more than 20% of dogs. Most common sites include lymph nodes (primarily internal iliac and sublumbar) and lungs. Bones (in particular lumbar and pelvis) are involved relatively frequently. Other internal organs (e.g. liver and spleen) and skin (especially near vulva and prepuce) may also be involved in a smaller percentage of cases. Metastatic disease occurs also in cats and involved 12.7% of cases according to the study mentioned above.
- Prognosis for dogs with high-grade UC is grave, with less than 20% of treated dogs surviving for 1 year or more. In cats, estimated 1-year survival varies from 6% to 28% in untreated cats and patients undergoing cystectomy, respectively.
- Over-represented canine breeds: Scottish Terriers (18- to 20-fold higher risk of UC than other dogs), Airedales, Shetland sheepdogs, West Highland White Terriers, Fox Terriers, and Beagles.

- Prostatic (adeno) carcinoma
  - Malignant epithelial neoplasia arising from the prostatic acinar epithelium.
  - It is the second most common prostatic neoplasia observed in dogs after urothelial carcinoma, from which it is often difficult to be distinguished both cytologically and histologically. Therefore, when a carcinoma is noted in the prostatic gland, the generic term prostatic carcinoma is often used instead.
  - Clinical signs, prognosis and treatment are very similar to urothelial carcinoma, and the distinction is often considered not clinically important.
  - Histologically, prostatic adenocarcinoma may display a high degree of morphological heterogeneity with multiple subtypes described from tubular to solid, cribriform, micropapillary and cribriform patterns. The tubular pattern is more common and is characterized by the formation of small acini and tubules. This form is usually cytologically distinguishable from urothelial carcinoma.

Cytological features

- Given the significant morphological overlap between prostatic adenocarcinoma and urothelial carcinoma, this section describes these two neoplasms in combination.
- Cellularity may depend on the sampling technique.
- Background: variably haemodiluted and often containing a variable amount of necrotic material.
- Neoplastic cells often exfoliate in variably sized, often disorganized clusters; individualized elements are also common. Cells shape varies from round, polygonal, angular and spindleoid.
- In the presence of glandular or acinar-like structures from a sample from the prostatic gland, a diagnosis of adenocarcinoma is favoured.
- Nuclei are round to oval, often large, with coarse, granular, or clumped chromatin. They are variably located within the cells. Multiple prominent and irregularly shaped nucleoli are frequently seen.
- The cytoplasm is variably basophilic, and moderate to abundant. It may contain Melamed-Wolinska bodies, which can displace the nucleus to the periphery giving the cell a signet ring appearance.

- Melamed-Wolinska bodies consist of 2-6 µm vacuoles containing a pink to magenta fine granulation. They are usually single but may be multiple within the same cell. These structures are PAS+. Although they have been more frequently been associated with UC, they are not pathognomonic, as they may also be occasionally observed in normal urothelial cells, in other carcinomas and in mesothelial cells.
- Cytological features of atypia are often prominent. Anisocytosis and anisokaryosis are variable to marked and the N:C ratio is variable. Binucleation, multinucleation, mitotic figures and nuclear molding are often seen. A recent study has shown that the absence of neutrophilic infiltration, the presence of multinucleated cells, and nuclear molding are associated with malignancy.
- In some cases, the pleomorphism is less prominent.
- Concurrent increase in leucocytes, in particular neutrophils, may be present, as concurrent pyuria (with or without infection) is common. Variable amounts of necrotic material may be observed in fine-needle aspirates.

Pears and Pitfalls

- Seeding of neoplastic cells via aspirational cytology of the bladder tumour has been reported but is uncommon to rare. This event is mainly observed after surgical celiotomy for mass biopsy/excision and usually occur within the first few months post-surgery. For this reason, traumatic urethral/bladder catheterization may be preferred for diagnostic purposes.
- Definitive diagnosis via cytology may be challenging in well-differentiated forms (e.g. UC *vs* polypoid cystitis) or in the presence of concurrent inflammation (neoplasia *vs* dysplasia). In those cases, further tests should be considered:
  - Histopathology: diagnosis is often straightforward and also allows to establish tumour grade. Problematic diagnosis may occur when (a) the biopsy sample is too small (cystoscopy), (b) the tumour is low-grade and very well-differentiated, resembling normal transitional epithelium, (c) sample is from the prostate and it is difficult to differentiate urothelial origin vs prostatic origin, and (d) sample is from a tissue other than urogenital tract, for example in the evaluation of a possible metastatic lesions to other organs.
  - Immunohistochemistry: Uroplakin III (UPIII) can be used to rule in/out urothelial carcinoma cells (a) in a biopsy from a metastatic lesion of unknown origin, (b) in small bioptic samples from the bladder in which the tumour origin is not certain, and (c) in samples from the prostate where it is difficult to differentiate between UC and prostatic adenocarcinoma. UPIII expression can be lost in some high-grade forms.
  - BRAF mutation detection assay: PCR-based test that searches for a single mutation in the BRAF gene within the transitional epithelial cells. This mutation has been identified in up to 85% of UC cases and, to date, it has never been recorded in urine specimens neither from healthy dogs nor in patients with inflammatory or dysplastic processes affecting the genitourinary tract. The presence of BRAF mutation is considered confirmatory for UC (or prostatic carcinoma). However, the absence of mutation does not entirely rule it out, since false-negative results may occur. The great advantage test is that it can be performed on almost any diagnostic sample that contains transitional epithelial cells, including pre-stained cytology smears with equivocal diagnosis, meaning that no additional samples are required. Based on recent publications, BRAF mutation status does not seem to have a prognostic significance on survival.

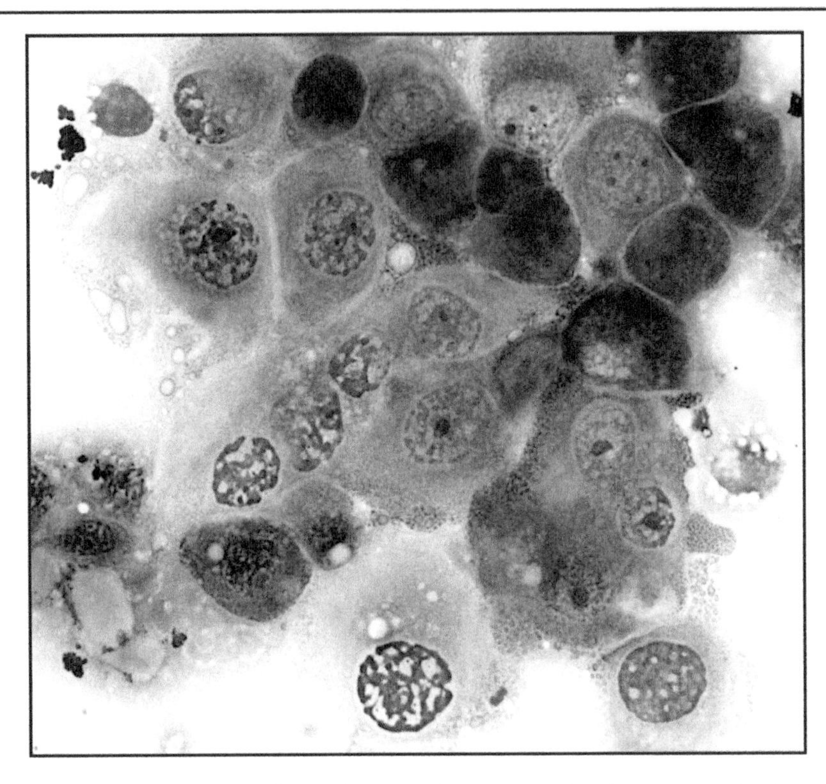

Fig. 8.17. Dog. Urothelial carcinoma. Cluster of polygonal transitional cells with coarse granular chromatin and prominent nucleoli. Wright-Giemsa.

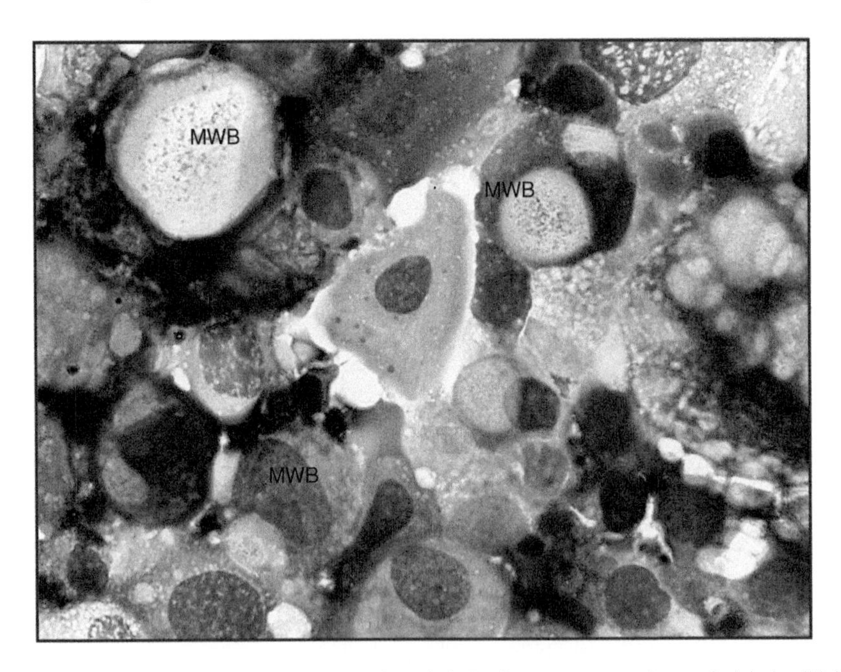

Fig. 8.18. Dog. Urothelial carcinoma. Transitional epithelial cells containing pink-round globules (Melamed-Wolinska bodies) displacing the nucleus to the periphery. Wright-Giemsa.

Further reading

Christensen, B.W. (2018) Canine prostatic disease. *Veterinary Clinics of North America: Small Animal Practice* 48, 701–719.
Gedon, J., Kehl, A., Aupperle-Lellbach, H.A., Bomhard, W. and Schmidt, J.M. (2022) BRAF mutation status and its prognostic significance in 79 canine urothelial carcinomas: a retrospective study (2006–2019). *Veterinary and Comparative Oncology* 20(2), 449–457.
Griffin, M.A., Cump, W.T.N., Giuffrida, M.A. et al. (2020) Lower urinary tract transitional cell carcinoma in cats: Clinical findings, treatments, and outcomes in 118 cases. *Journal of Veterinary Internal Medicine* 34(1), 274–282.
McAloney, C.A., Evans, S.J.M., Hokamp, J.A., Wellman, M.L. and White, M.E. (2021) Comparison of pathologist review protocols for cytologic detection of prostatic and urothelial carcinomas in canines: a bi-institutional retrospective study of 298 cases. *Veterinary and Comparative Oncology* 19(2), 374–380.
Palmieri, C., Fonseca-Alves, C.E. and Laufer-Amorim, R. (2022) A review on canine and feline prostate pathology. *Frontiers in Veterinary Science* 26(9).
Pierini, A., Criscuolo, M.C., Bonfanti, U., Benvenuti, E., Marchetti, V. *et al.* (2022) Usefulness of squash preparation cytology in the diagnosis of canine urinary bladder carcinomas. *Veterinary Clinical Pathology* 51(4), 498–506.
Wycislo, K.L. and Piech, T.L. (2018) Urinary tract cytology. *Veterinary Clinics of North America: Small Animal Practice* 49(2), 247–260.

8.8.2 Lymphoma

Lymphoma may involve the urinary tract with variable frequency, and the diagnosis can rarely be achieved by urinalysis.

Renal lymphoma

Clinical features

- It may occur in both dogs and cats, but it is mainly observed in the feline species.
- It may be confined to the kidneys, or it may be associated with alimentary or multicentric lymphoma. In cats, it is most frequently B-cell in origin.
- To the authors' knowledge, there is only one reported case in the literature of renal lymphoma diagnosed by cytology of the urine. This was a T-cell lymphoma in an adult Brittany Spaniel dog that underwent further confirmatory tests (flow cytometry, PARR).
- Clinical signs associated with renal lymphoma are largely consistent with renal insufficiency and include hyporexia, weight loss and polyuria/polydipsia. Renomegaly is common and often bilateral. In cats, extension of renal lymphoma into the CNS is more commonly reported than with other lymphomas.
- Eryhrocytosis secondary to paraneoplastic increased erythropoietin (EPO) production may occur.

Bladder lymphoma

Clinical features

- Very rare extra-nodal lymphoma described in both species. To the authors' knowledge, diagnosis of bladder lymphoma by urine cytology has been reported in three dogs and one cat. Both T- and B-cell forms have been described. One of the B-cell cases in a dog was associated with IgG monoclonal gammopathy and Bence-Jones proteinuria.
- Clinical signs vary and are not always present. They include haematuria.
- On diagnostic imaging, bladder lymphoma may present as mural mass or diffuse infiltration. Imaging findings may be similar to other urinary tract neoplasms, requiring cyto/histopathology for a definitive diagnosis.

Cytological features

- Cellularity is variable.
- Background: clear and often haemodiluted.
- Neoplastic lymphoid cells are mainly intermediate to large. Only one case of small-cell lymphoma in a dog has been described.
- Nuclei are round, intermediate to large, sometimes indented, paracentral to eccentric, with coarse, stippled chromatin and often visible nucleoli.
- The cytoplasm is scant to moderate, blue/basophilic, with defined borders. Clear intracytoplasmic vacuoles may be observed.
- Mitotic figures are often seen and may be numerous and atypical.
- Because neoplastic lymphocytes are often fragile and prone to disruption during sample collection, the samples may contain numerous bare nuclei from ruptured cells (smudge cells).
- Low numbers of transitional epithelial cells are often seen and may show some signs of atypia.
- A concurrent septic or sterile inflammation may be present, in which case degenerate and non-degenerate neutrophils are seen, respectively.

Pearls and Pitfalls

- Examination of wet urine sediment only may lead to false-negative results because intermediate to large lymphoid cells may resemble other leucocytes or small epithelial cells in unstained sediment preparations.

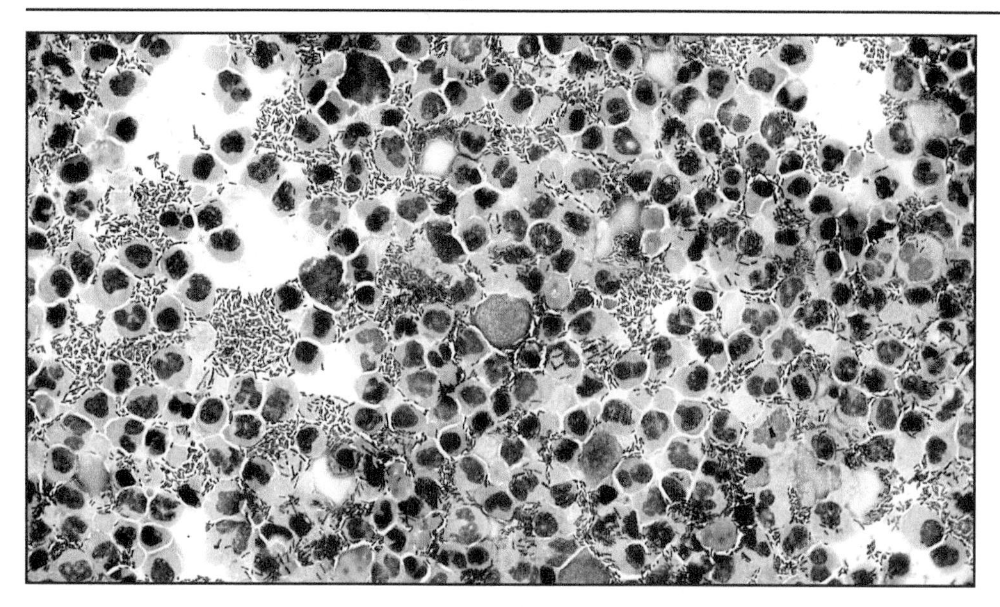

Fig. 8.19. Dog. Urine sediment. Bladder lymphoma. Occasional large lymphoid cells admixed with numerous degenerate neutrophils and large numbers of bacteria (rods). Wright-Giemsa.

Further reading

Benigni, L., Lamb, C.R., Corzo-Menendez, N.C., Holloway, A., Eastwood, J.M. *et al.* (2006) Lymphoma affecting the urinary bladder in three dogs and a cat. *Veterinary Radiology and Ultrasound* 47(6), 592–596.

Capasso A., Monti P., Morey-Matamalas A. *et al.* (2022) Lymphoma of the urinary bladder with concomitant septic peritonitis in a dog. Vet Record Case Reports. Early view.

Geigy, C.A., Dandrieux, J., Miclard, J., Kircher, P. and Howard, J. (2010) Extranodal B-cell lymphoma in the urinary bladder with cytological evidence of concurrent involvement of the gall bladder in a cat. *Journal of Small Animal Practice* 51, 280–287.

Jeffries, C., Russell Moore, A. and Schlemmer, S.N. (2022) Urinary bladder wall mass with neoplastic lymphoid cells in the urine: diagnosis of an IgG secretory B-cell lymphoma with Bence-Jones proteinuria in a dog. *Veterinary Clinical Pathology* 51(3), 426–431.

Taylor, A., Finotello, R., Vilar-Saavedra, P., Couto, C.G., Benigni, L. *et al.* (2019) Clinical characteristics and outcome of dogs with presumed primary renal lymphoma. *Journal of Small Animal Practice* 60(11), 663–670.

Witschen, P.M., Sharkey, L.C., Seelig, D.M., Granick, J.L., Dykstra, J.A. *et al.* (2019) Diagnosis of canine renal lymphoma by cytology and flow cytometry of the urine. *Veterinary Clinical Pathology* 49(1), 137–142.

Additional Techniques to Refine the Cytologic Diagnosis in Fluid Samples

Martina Piviani

The aim of this chapter is to provide a practical guide to the choice of the most suitable additional techniques to complement the cytological examination of fluids and to reach the most specific and accurate diagnosis. These techniques may be even more relevant when evaluating bodily fluids, where histopathology is not an option.

9.1 Cytochemistry

Also called 'special stains' to distinguish these techniques from stains routinely used in cytology in different settings (e.g. quick panoptic stains, Wright-Giemsa, May-Grunwald Giemsa and Papanicolau stain), cytochemistry uses different chemicals to highlight special characteristics of cells or extracellular matrix.

These stains can be applied to unstained slides but also to previously stained slides. Prestained slides can be destained with different methods. In a recent paper, a method using 5% alcohol acid solution (ethanol 70% with 5 ml of concentrated HCl), applied for 1–15 min, depending on the thickness of the smear, was reported to give fast and acceptable results. For some stains, destaining is not necessary.

9.1.1 Cytochemistry to highlight the presence of infectious organisms

Special stains are most often used in cytology to detect microorganisms that may stain poorly with routine stains.

- Acid-fast (also called Ziehl-Neelsen)
  - To detect *Mycobacterium* spp. and *Crypstosporidium* spp. Both organisms uniformly stain fuchsia.
  - To identify *Nocardia* spp., which stains inconsistently and partially fuchsia.
- Fontana-Masson
  - To detect phaeohyphomycosis. The hyphae stain light green even when apparently non-pigmented on routine stains.
- Grocott-Gomori methenamine silver (GMS)
  - To detect fungal hyphae, yeasts and algae, which stain black.
  - Aberrant staining of non fungal organisms (e.g. *Nocardia* spp.) may occasionally be observed.
- Gram
  - To distinguish Gram-positive bacteria, which stain blue, from Gram-negative bacteria, which stain red.
- India ink
  - To identify *Cryptococcus* spp. The capsule remains colourless above a black background. This is not often used, as cryptococcosis does not typically represent a diagnostic challenge.

DOI: 10.1079/9781789247787.0009

- Mucicarmine
    - To identify *Cryptococcus* spp. The capsule stains deep red. As already indicated above, this stain is not typically necessary for diagnosis.

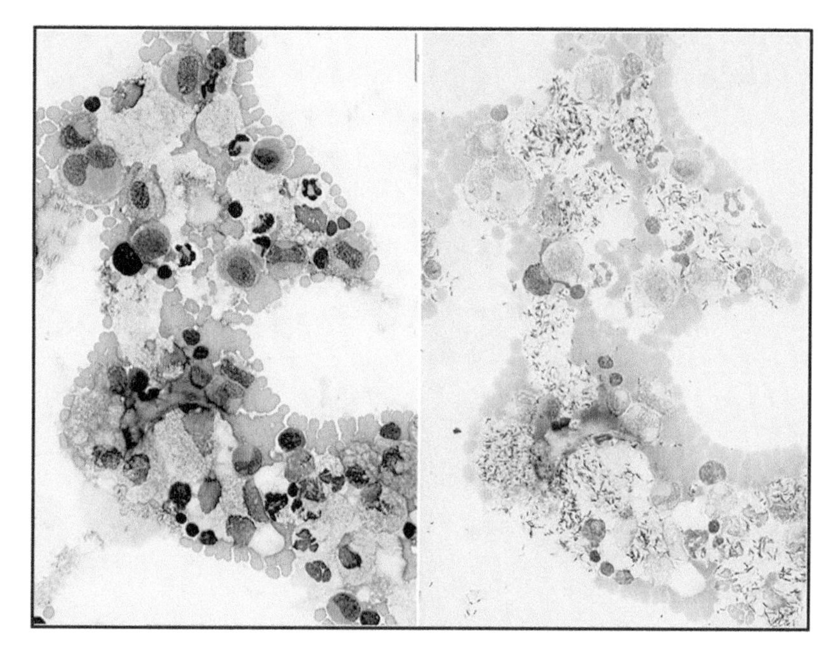

Fig. 9.1. Cat. Peritoneal fluid. Cytospin. Mycobacterosis. (Left) pyogranulomatous inflammation with presence of many negatively staining bacilli within macrophages and free in the background, Wright-Giemsa. (Right) Bacilli stain fuchsia with acid fast.

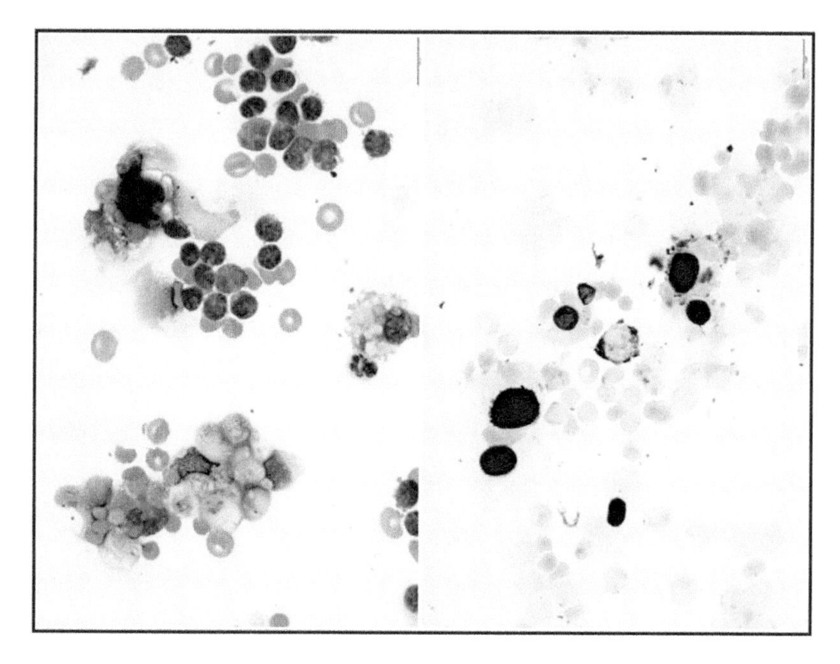

Fig. 9.2. Dog. Cerebrospinal fluid. Cytospin. Protothecosis. (Left) Mixed inflammatory pleocytosis with presence of several round-to-oval structures measuring 5–15 µm in diameter, mostly light blue with vacuolated to clear interior (visible on the left and consistent with empty casings), and rarely with a blue granular interior and a thin colourless wall (right). These algal organisms are seen both intracellularly within macrophages and free in the background. Wright-Giemsa. (Right) The structures stain black with GMS.

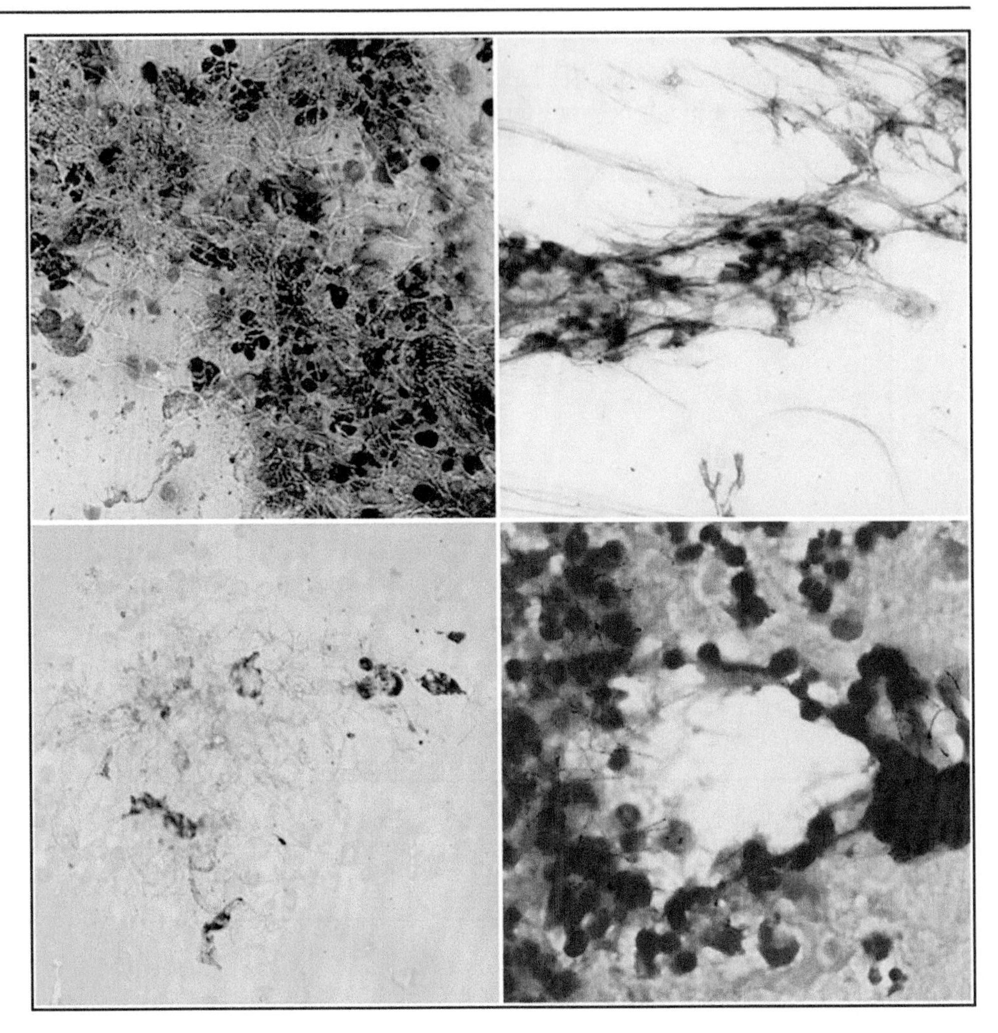

Fig. 9.3. Dog. Pleural fluid, Direct preparation. Septic pyothorax due to *Nocardia* spp. confirmed by culture. (Top left) Neutrophilic inflammatory exudate with presence of many negatively staining filamentous bacteria free in the background. Quick panoptic stain. (Top right) Filamentous bacteria occasionally stain fuchsia. Acid fast. (Bottom left) Filamentous bacteria stain black. GMS. (Bottom right) Filamentous bacteria stain blue. Gram.

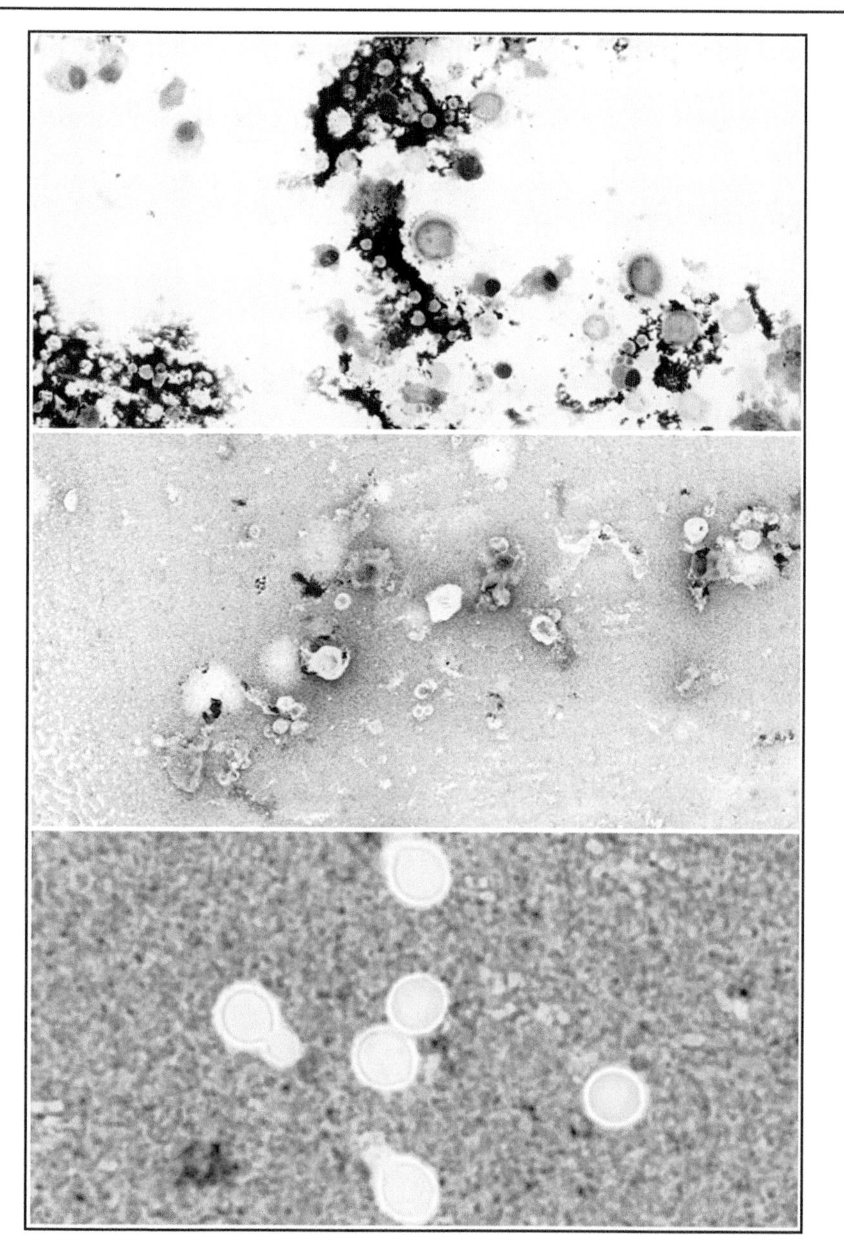

Fig. 9.4. Dog. Cerebrospinal fluid. Cytospin preparation. Cryptococcosis. (Top) Numerous yeast organisms admixed with macrophages and fewer small lymphocytes. Yeasts include larger forms (15–30 μm in diameter) with 2–4 μm thick clear capsule and a light pink interior, and smaller (2–5 μm in diameter) round to oval forms with a thinner (1 μm) clear capsule. Wright-Giemsa. (Middle) India ink stain on prestained slide highlights the thick capsule, which is colourless above the brown-black background. (Bottom) India ink on unstained slide. (*Courtesy of Stephen Cole.*)

9.1.2 Special stains to identify pigment or extracellular substances

- Alcian blue and periodic acid-Schiff
  - To identify mucin and mucin-like substances, e.g. in biliary effusions containing 'white bile'.
  - Variable stain reaction depending on the type of mucins. Positive reaction is blue for Alcian blue and pink/magenta for periodic acid-Schiff.
- Congo red
  - To differentiate amyloid from fibrin, collagen and other extracellular substances.
  - Amyloid can be (rarely) seen in peritoneal effusions of patients with amyloidosis and secondary liver rupture.
  - Positive reaction is peach-pink with an apple green birefringence under polarized light.
- Fontana-Masson
  - To differentiate melanin from haemosiderin. The presence of melanocytes and melanophages in cavitary effusions is very rare.
  - Positive reaction is black.
- Hall's stain
  - To identify bile in effusions caused by biliary peritonitis, although this is typically not challenging in routinely stained slides.
  - Positive reaction is green to blue-green.
- Luxol fast blue
  - To identify myelin in cerebrospinal fluid, either within macrophages (myelomalacia) or free in the background (accidental puncture of spinal cord), although this is typically not challenging in routinely stained slides.
  - Positive reaction is blue.
- Mucicarmine
  - To specifically identify epithelial mucins, but insensitive so rarely useful.
  - Positive reaction is red.
- Prussian blue (Pearl's stain)
  - To highlight the presence of haemosiderin and differentiate it from melanin. Routinely performed in equine bronchoalveolar washes to support a suspicion of exercise-induced intrapulmonary haemorrhage (EIPH).
  - Positive reaction is bright blue to black.

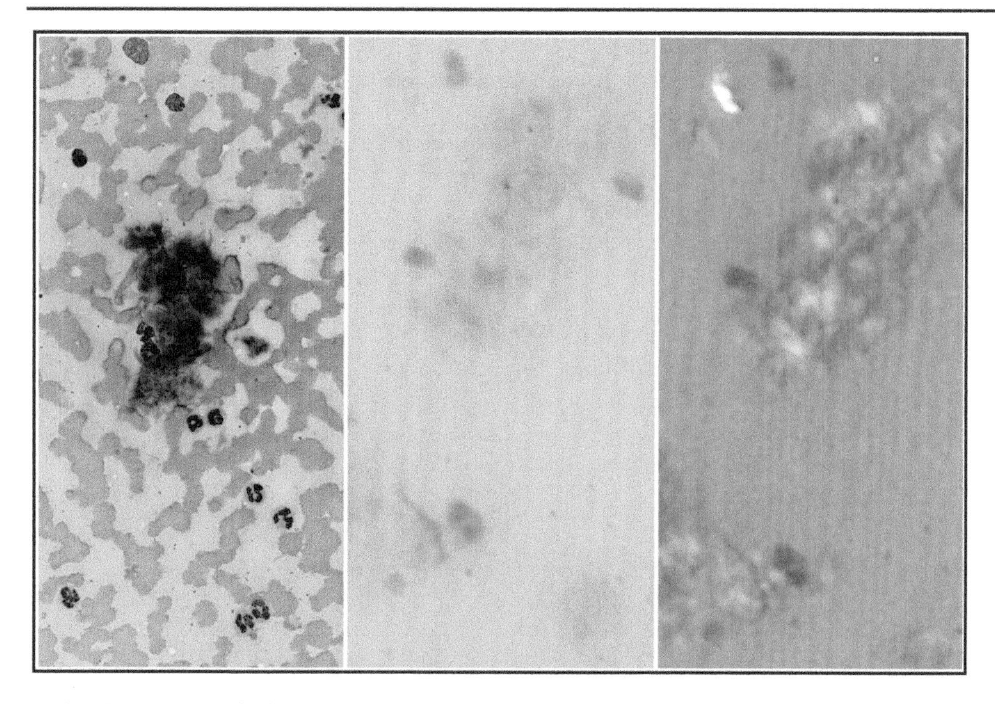

Fig. 9.5. Dog. Peritoneal fluid, direct smear. Haemorrhagic effusion with amyloid. From left to right. (Left) Erythrocytes, few leucocytes and small lakes of pink fibrillar material, Wright-Giemsa. (Middle) The extracellular material stains peach pink with Congo red. (Right) The material has an apple green birefringence under polarized light.

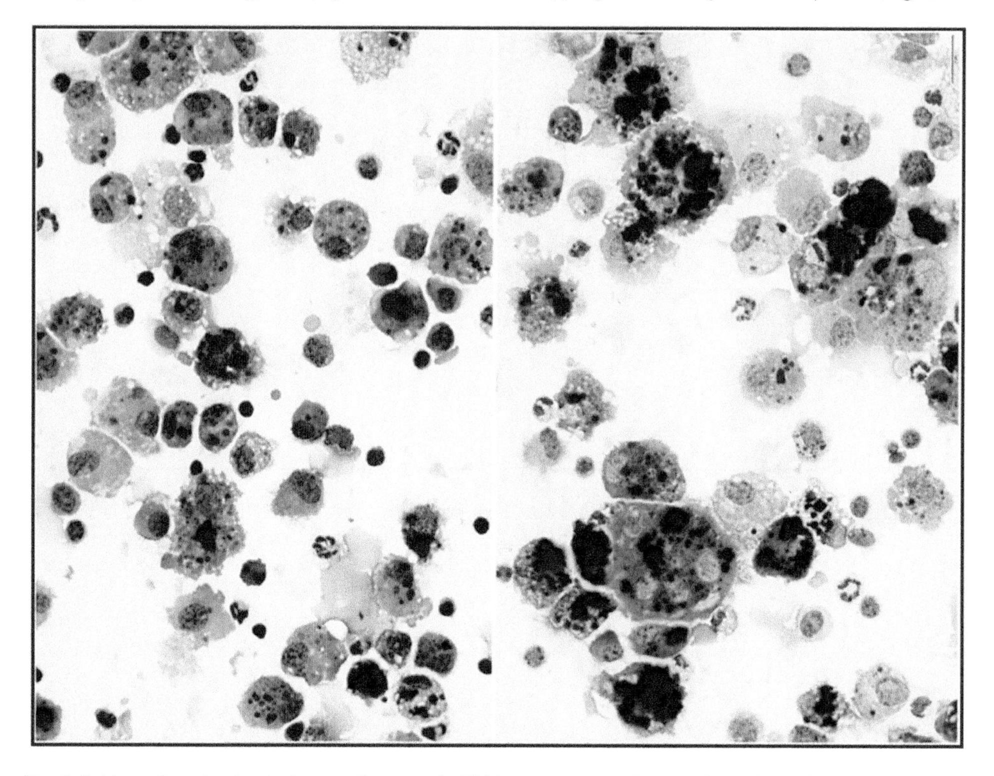

Fig. 9.6. Horse. Bronchoalveolar lavage. Cytospin. (Left) Numerous macrophages admixed with fewer small lymphocytes, occasional neutrophils and eosinophils, and rare erythrocytes. Most macrophages contain scant to abundant blue/green to black pigment. (Right) The pigment appears bright blue to black in the slide stained with Prussian blue.

9.1.3 Special stains helpful to identify specific cell types

- Alkaline phosphatase (nitro blue tetrazolium chloride/5-bromo-4-chloro-3-indolyl phosphate [NBT/BCIP])
  - Easy, cheap and rapid technique using a substrate for the endogenous enzyme alkaline phosphatase combined with a chromogen.
  - Cannot be used on formalin-fixed tissue.
  - Positive reaction is brown/black (blue by some methods).
  - Mesothelial cells, macrophages and leucocytes are negative for alkaline phosphatase in dogs and cats.
  - Cells with atypia seen in effusions and positive for alkaline phosphatase are typically neoplastic and can include osteoblasts, carcinoma cells from primary pulmonary carcinomas and possibly carcinomas of other origin, chrondroblasts and melanocytes.
  - Slides prestained with Romanowski stains can be used but staining intensity may be weaker than when unstained slides are used.
- Toluidine blue
  - Useful to differentiate mast cells from granular lymphocytes in dubious cases. It stains granules in mast cells and basophils, not in granular (LGL) lymphocytes.
  - Positive reaction is red-purple.

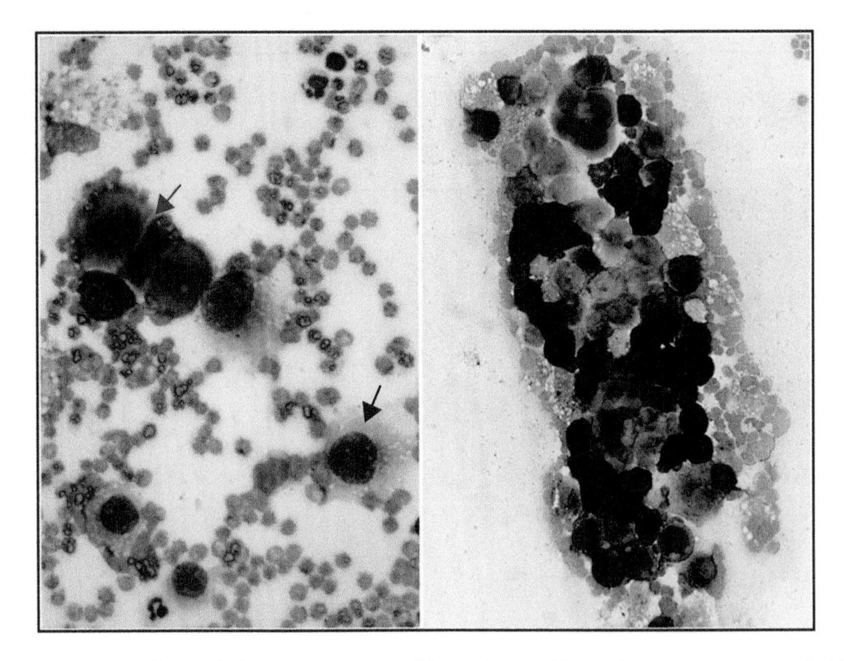

Fig. 9.7. Dog. Pleural effusion. Sediment preparation. Effusion due to effusion due to osteosarcoma. (Left) Vacuolated macrophages mesothelial cells with the typical peripheral pink fringe (red arrow) and individualized atypical cells with large nuclei and prominent nucleoli (black arrow), Wright-Giemsa. (Right) The atypical cells stain brown/black with NBT/BCIP.

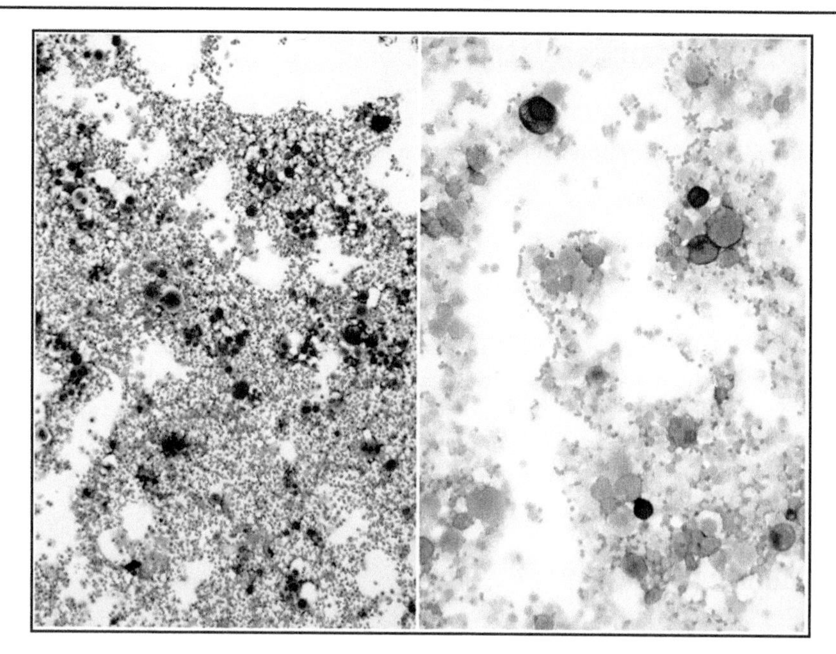

Fig. 9.8. Cat. Pleural effusion. Cytospin. Neoplastic effusion due to carcinoma. (Left) Atypical large cells with multinucleation and karyomegaly, seen individualized or in groups, Wright-Giemsa. (Right) The atypical cells stain brown/black with NBT/BCIP.

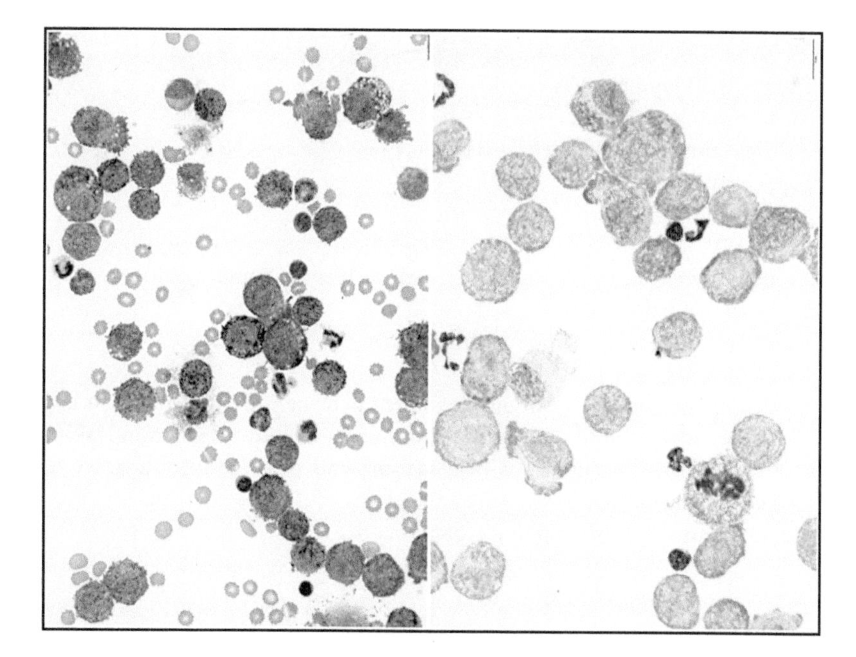

Fig. 9.9. Dog. Peritoneal effusion. Cytospin. Neoplastic effusion due to mast cell tumour. (Left) Many neoplastic round cells admixed with fewer neutrophils and eosinophils. Neoplastic cells contain few to moderate numbers of magenta granules, Wright-Giemsa. (Right) Granules stain pink with Toluidine blue.

9.2 Immunocytochemistry

It is sometimes impossible, even on histopathology, to define the specific cell origin of a cell population based only on morphology and arrangement. In those cases, where special stains (cytochemistry) are unhelpful, immunocytochemistry can be considered. However, this technique is not widely available, and results may be very variable, depending on the specific methods used and laboratory.

The use of precharged slides is ideal to minimize tissue loss during the procedure. The signal is typically stronger on slides not previously stained. However, unstained slides are not always available and need to be fixed or frozen, if not used immediately. Therefore, the technique has also been successfully optimized by some laboratories to be performed using Romanowsky-stained slides. This also allows to check representativeness and quality of the slides prior to ICC. Selected markers from a laboratory performing ICC on prestained slides are listed below. For the selection of the markers, it is recommended to always obtain the advice of the specific laboratory used.

9.2.1 Round cell markers

- CD3
  - To identify T lymphocytes.
  - Membranous and cytoplasmic staining pattern.
- CD20
  - To identify B lymphocytes. Positive in B-cell lymphomas but not in B acute lymphoblastic leukaemia.
  - Membranous and cytoplasmic staining pattern.
- Pax5
  - To identify B lymphocytes.
  - Nuclear staining pattern.
- Multiple myeloma oncogene-1 (MUM1)
  - To identify plasma cells.
  - Nuclear staining pattern.
- c-Kit (CD117)
  - To identify mast cells. Also used in panels to identify spindle cell tumours as gastro-intestinal stromal tumours.
  - Membranous or cytoplasmic staining pattern.
- CD204
  - To identify macrophages. Although expected to be negative in dendritic cells DCs and histiocytes, it was found to be positive in most histiocytic sarcomas in IHC validation studies. Negative in cutaneous histiocytoma and other proliferations composed of Langerhans histiocytes.
  - Membranous cytoplasmic staining pattern.

9.2.2 Epithelial, mesothelial and synovial cell markers

- Cytokeratin and vimentin
  - Neoplastic epithelial cells are positive for pancytokeratin and typically negative for vimentin (except during epithelial-mesenchymal transition). Down-expression below the limit of detection is possible depending on cytokeratin used and type of carcinoma.
  - Neoplastic mesothelial cells are positive for cytokeratin and typically positive for vimentin (may rarely be negative).
  - Synovial cell sarcomas are positive for vimentin, with a small proportion of cells coexpressing cytokeratin.
  - Cytoplasmic and sometimes membranous staining pattern.

9.2.3 Mesenchymal markers

- Vimentin
  - To identify atypical cells as mesenchymal (sarcoma). Macrophages, mesothelial cells and synovial cells are also typically positive.
  - Cytoplasmic staining pattern.
- Factor VIII
  - To identify sarcomas as haemangiosarcomas; platelets and megakaryocytes are also positive.
  - Labile.

9.2.4 Melanocytic markers

- Melan A
  - To identify melanocytes, most relevant in amelanotic or poorly melanotic melanomas.
  - Cytoplasmic staining pattern.
- Melanosome
  - To identify melanocytes.
  - Cytoplasmic staining pattern.

9.2.5 Infectious agents

- Feline coronavirus
  - To support the suspicion of feline infectious peritonitis when there is a significant macrophagic component.
  - Granular cytoplasmic staining pattern within macrophages. A proteinaceous background may complicate interpretation due to background unspecific staining.
  - Suboptimal specificity in one study.
  - Vulnerable epitope, variable results depending on method used.

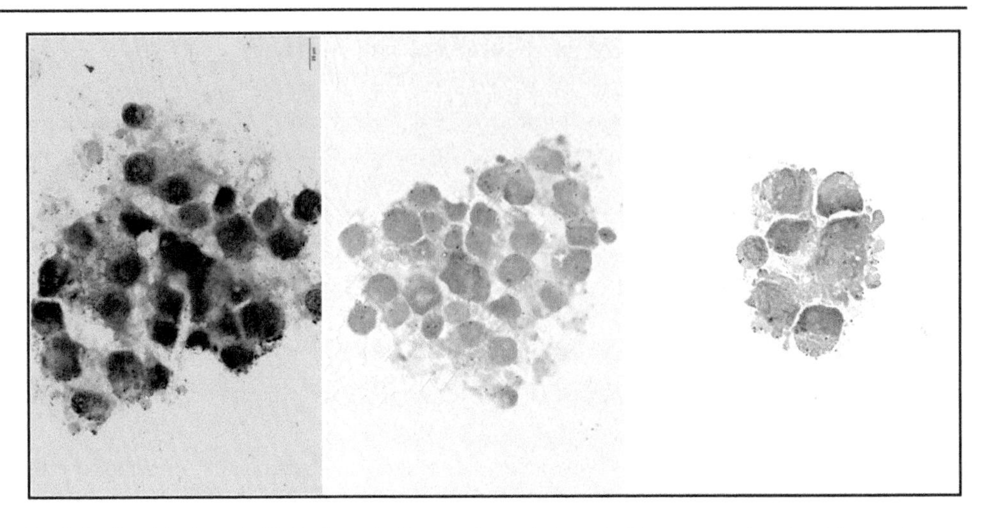

Fig. 9.10. Dog. Cerebrospinal fluid. Cytospin. Malignant neoplasia, probable ependymal or choroid plexus tumour. From left to right. (Left) Atypical oval to spindleoid to vaguely polygonal cells with tendency to cohesion. (Centre) Atypical cells have weak to moderate membranous or cytoplasmic staining for pancytokeratin. (Right) Atypical cells have moderate membranous or cytoplasmic staining for vimentin. (*Courtesy Laura Black.*)

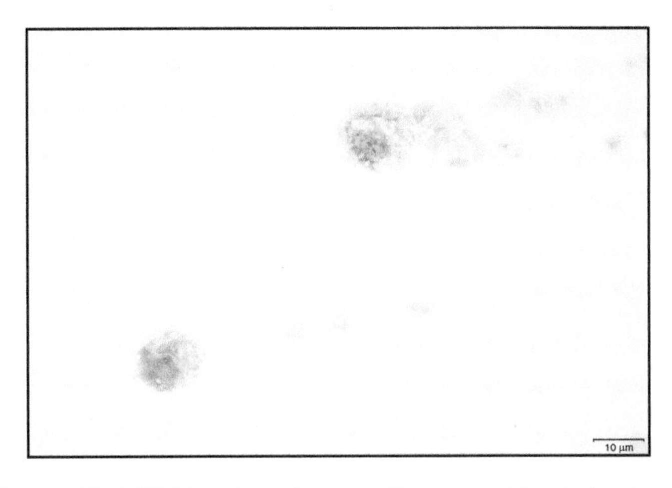

Fig. 9.11. Cat. Peritoneal fluid. FIP. Macrophages have a positive granular intracytoplasmic reaction for FeCoV. (*Courtesy Laura Black.*)

9.3 Cell Pellet Immunohistochemistry

Fluid samples can be transformed into cell pellets using different methods. The simplest method is by centrifugation of the fluid in a plastic tube (Eppendorf) and replacement of the supernatant with formalin solution. After 24 h, the pellet is removed from the bottom of the plastic tube and processed as a routine tissue biopsy sample.

The microhaematocrit tube technique can be useful for markedly haemorrhagic fluids. The great advantage over immunocytochemistry is that the wide library of immunohistochemical markers, and the same methods validated for routine histology samples can be directly applied to cell pellet histology sections. In addition, multiple sections can be easily obtained by a single-cell pellet, allowing for larger panels of markers.

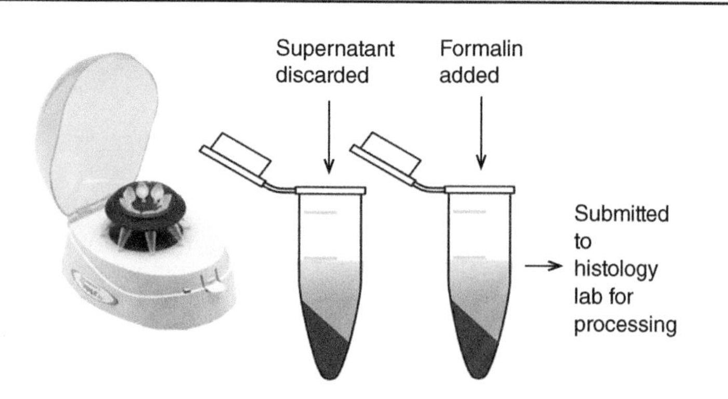

Fig. 9.12. Preparation of cell pellets from fluid samples.

Mesothelial hyperplasia versus neoplasia (mesothelioma and carcinoma)

- Cytokeratin and vimentin
  - Mesothelial cells are positive for cytokeratin and typically positive for vimentin (rarely negative).
  - Carcinoma cells are positive for cytokeratin and typically negative for vimentin (occasionally positive).
  - Cytoplasmic staining in both.
- Wilms tumour 1 (WT1)
  - Positive in mesothelial cells (rarely negative).
  - It does not differentiate between neoplastic and normal or hyperplastic mesothelial cells.
  - Carcinoma cells are negative.
  - Nuclear staining. Faint diffuse cytoplasmic staining is considered unspecific.
- Desmin
  - Often positive in mesothelial cells (both neoplastic and hyperplastic), rarely in carcinoma cells.
  - Cytoplasmic and membranous staining.
- IMP3
  - Potentially helpful in the panel but not fully discriminatory.
  - Mostly positive in mesothelial cells (with both higher intensity and percentage of cells positive in mesothelioma than in hyperplasia).
  - Mostly negative in carcinoma cells.
  - Cytoplasmic staining.

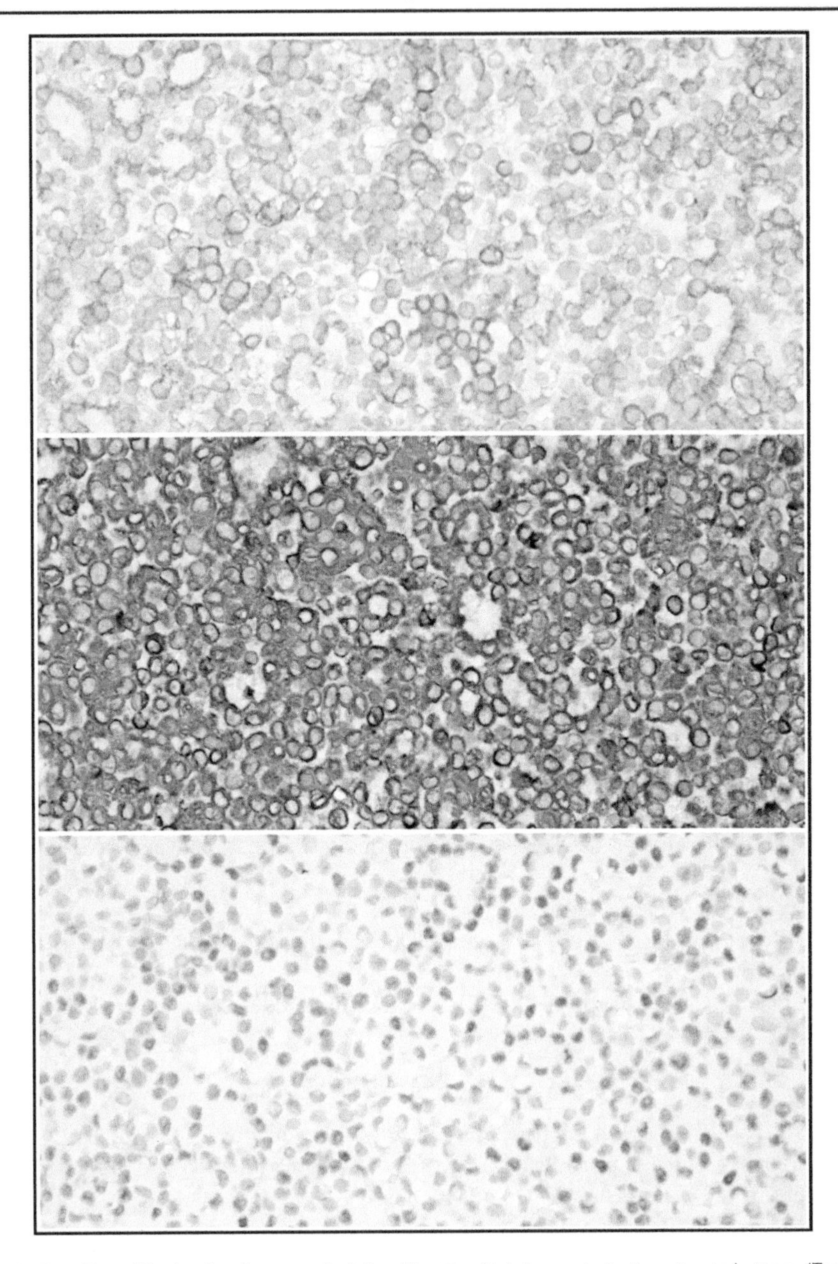

Fig. 9.13. Dog. Pleural fluid, cell pellet, mesothelial proliferation likely hyperplasia. From top to bottom. (Top) Most cohesive cells have positive membranous/cytoplasmic staining for pancytokeratin. (Middle) All cells have positive cytoplasmic staining for vimentin. (Bottom) Most cohesive cells have positive nuclear staining for WT1.

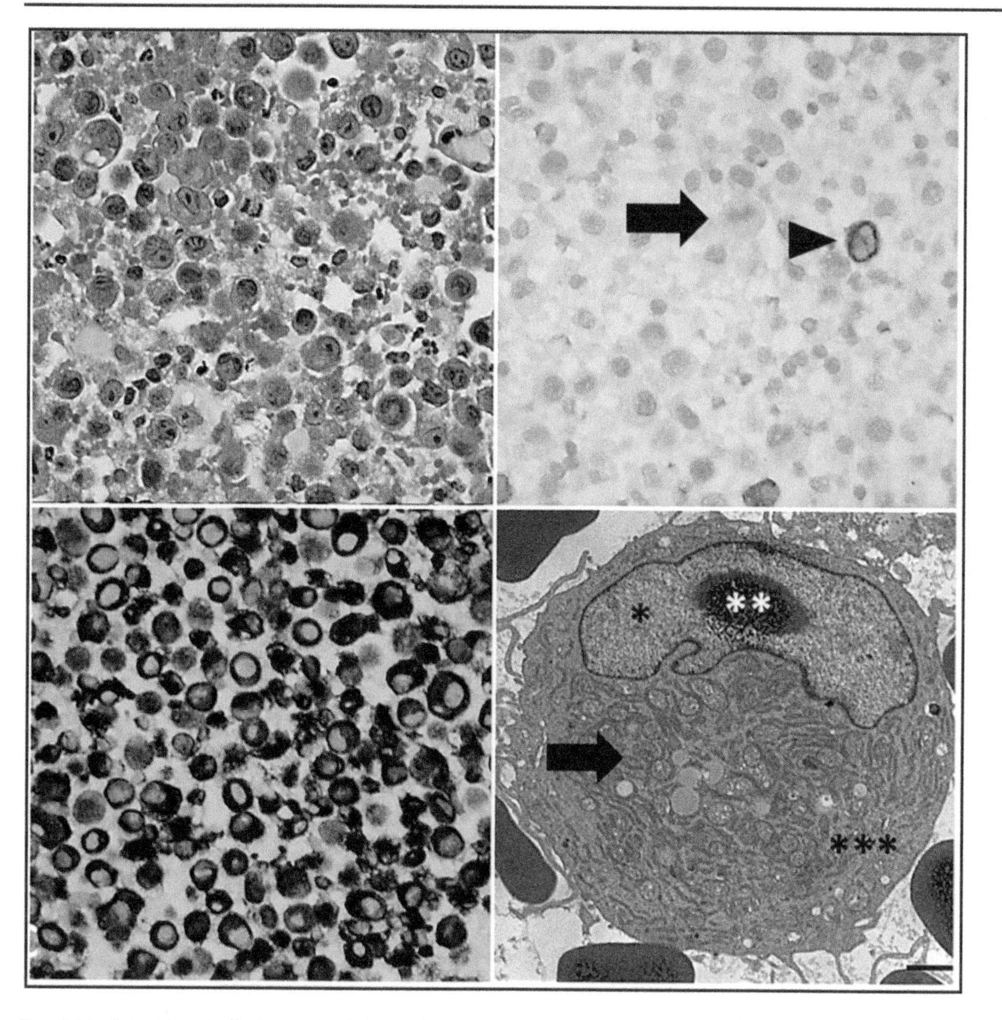

Fig. 9.14. Dog. Pleural effusion, cell pellet, neoplastic effusion due to osteosarcoma (diagnosed via cytology and ALP cytochemistry, same case as in Fig. 9.7). (Top left) Atypical cells admixed with frequent macrophages, few neutrophils and moderate numbers of erythrocytes. (Top right) Only rare cells are positive for cytokeratin (most likely mesothelial cells). (Bottom left) All cells excluding erythrocytes stain positive for vimentin (including neoplastic and mesothelial cells; histiocytic, plasma cell and melanocytic origin were excluded by negative CD18, MUM1 and S100, respectively). (Bottom right) Transmission electron microscopy of one atypical cell, not compatible with histiocyte, myocyte, epithelial and mesothelial cell. (*Courtesy of Lorenzo Ressel.*)

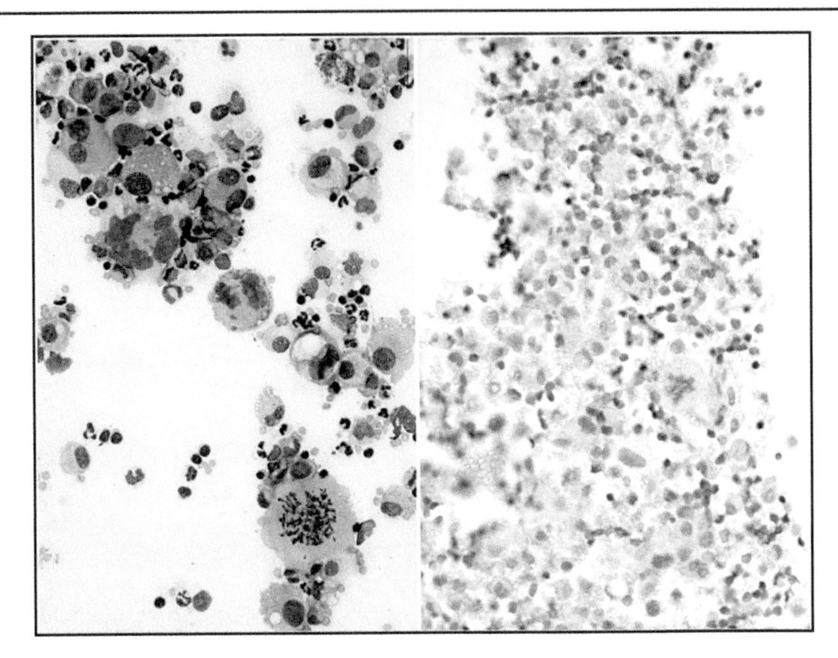

Fig. 9.15. Cat. Peritoneal effusion. Neoplastic effusion due to leiomyosarcoma (confirmed on post-mortem and immunohistochemistry). (Left). Cytospin slides containing several cells with marked atypia. (Right) Cell pellet, with occasional cells positive for alpha-smooth muscle actin (IHC for pancytokeratin, Iba1 and vimentin were negative). *(Courtesy of Guido Rocchigiani and Lorenzo Ressel.)*

NOTE: This is not an all-inclusive list and is based only on markers optimized for prestained slides at Specialty VETPATH, Seattle, WA. Other markers may have been validated at other laboratories.

9.4 Flow Cytometry, Clonality Testing and BRAF

Flow cytometry and clonality testing (PARR) can also be performed on fluids, with the main aim of confirming a cytological suspicion of lymphoma. As for any ancillary test, these techniques are best used in combination, and in light of the cytological findings, and should not be used as first-line test to establish a diagnosis of lymphoma.

CSF is often an unsuitable sample either for flow cytometry or PARR, due to the small sample volume and insufficient DNA material, respectively, even when a pleocytosis is present.

9.4.1 Flow cytometry

- Its basic principle is based on the measurement of light scattered by cells (size and granularity/complexity), and the fluorescence observed when these cells are passed in a stream through a laser beam and are exposed to fluorescent markers (antibodies). These are used to detect the expression of cellular molecules, called clusters of differentiation (CDs), which are specific for each myeloid and lymphoid subpopulations.
- Flow cytometry can be used to:
  - Confirm the cytological suspicion of lymphoma.
  - Immunophenotype the lymphoma and provide prognostic information.
- It requires fresh fluid. A cytofixative is not required for fluid with high protein content.

9.4.2 PARR

- Stands for PCR for antigen receptor rearrangements. It is a clonality assay that identifies and amplifies specific sequences of lymphocyte DNA. A clonal result for immunoglobulin or T-cell receptor supports a diagnosis of lymphoid neoplasia.
- The result should not be used to determine the phenotype of the neoplastic cells, due to the phenomenon of lineage infidelity.
- Before considering PARR, myeloid neoplasms and histiocytic sarcoma should first be excluded by other means, as they can occasionally give clonal results.
- Any type of cellular sample is suitable, including fresh fluid in EDTA, prestained and unstained slides and, if no other samples are available, cell pellet. Prestained slides are ideal, to confirm that the cells of interest are present in sufficient numbers.

9.4.3 BRAF

- Recent studies have identified BRAF V595E mutation in up to 85% of dogs with urothelial carcinoma (UC), both bladder and prostatic forms. A PCR-based molecular test that searches for a single mutation in the BRAF gene within transitional cells has been recently made available on the market for diagnostic use.
- Specificity appears to be 100% as to date this mutation has never been recorded in urine specimens neither from healthy dogs nor in patients with inflammatory or dysplastic processes affecting the genitourinary tract. This means that finding the BRAF mutation is confirmatory for UC, but the lack of it does not entirely rule it out, since false-negative results may occur. Rarely, cells from other types of tumours may bear a BRAF mutation, but they are typically not present in urine.
- BRAF mutation status does not appear to be an independent prognostic factor for overall survival in dogs with urothelial carcinoma.
- Sample requirements may vary depending on the laboratory offering the test and include fresh urine, prestained and unstained slides and formalin-fixed paraffin-embedded tissue specimens. Prestained slides are ideal to confirm a cytological suspicion of UC assuming that the cells of interest are present in sufficient numbers.

Further reading

Akiyoshi, M., Hisasue, M., Asakawa, M.G., Neo, S. and Akiyoshi, M. (2022) Hepatosplenic lymphoma and visceral mast cell tumor in the liver of a dog with synchronous and multiple primary tumors. *Veterinary Clinical Pathology* 51(3), 414–421.

Bauer, N.B., Bassett, H., O'Neill, E.J. and Acke, E. (2006) Cerebrospinal fluid from a 6-year-old dog with severe neck pain. *Veterinary Clinical Pathology* 35(1), 123–125.

Dehghanpir, S.D. (2023) Cytomorphology of deep mycoses in dogs and cats. *Veterinary Clinics of North America: Small Animal Practice* 53(1), 155–173.

Evans, S.J. (2023) Flow cytometry in veterinary practice. *Veterinary Clinics of North America: Small Animal Practice* 53(1), 89–100.

Gerdon, J., Kehl, A., Aupperle-Lellbach, H., Von Bomhard, W. and Schmidt, J.M. (2022) BRAF mutation status and its prognostic significance in 79 canine urothelial carcinomas: a retrospective study (2006–2019). *Veterinary Comparative Oncology* 20(2), 449–457.

Gruendl, S., Matiasek, K., Matiasek, L., Fischer, A., Felten, S. *et al.* (2017) Diagnostic utility of cerebrospinal fluid immunocytochemistry for diagnosis of feline infectious peritonitis manifesting in the central nervous system. *Journal of Feline Medicine and Surgery* 19(6), 576–585.

Ives, E.J., Vanhaesebrouck, A.E. and Cian, F. (2013) Immunocytochemical demonstration of feline infectious peritonitis virus within cerebrospinal fluid macrophages. *Journal of Feline Medicine and Surgery* 15(12), 1149–1153.

Kato, Y., Funato, R., Hirata, A., Murakami, M., Mori, T. *et al.* (2014) Immunocytochemical detection of the class A macrophage scavenger receptor CD 204 using air-dried cytologic smears of canine histiocytic sarcoma. *Veterinary Clinical Pathology* 43(4), 589–593.

Marcos, R., Santos, M., Santos, N., Malhao, F., Ferreira, F. *et al.* (2009) Use of destained cytology slides for the application of routine special stains. *Veterinary Clinical Pathology* 38(1), 94–102.

Mesquita, L., Mortier, J., Ressel, L., Finotello, R., Silvestrini, P. *et al.* (2017) Neoplastic pleural effusion and intrathoracic metastasis of a scapular osteosarcoma in a dog: a multidisciplinary integrated diagnostic approach. *Veterinary Clinical Pathology* 46(2), 337–343.

Milne, E.M., Piviani, M., Hodgkiss-Geere, H.M., Piccinelli, C., Cheeseman, M. *et al.* (2021) Comparison of effusion cell block and biopsy immunohistochemistry in mesothelial hyperplasia, mesothelioma, and carcinoma in dogs. *Veterinary Clinical Pathology* 50(4), 555–567.

Monti, P., Barnes, D., Adrian, A.M. and Rasotto, R. (2018) Synovial cell sarcoma in a dog: a misnomer – cytologic and histologic findings and review of the literature. *Veterinary Clinical Pathology* 47(2), 181–185.

Owens, S.D., Gossett, R., McElhaney, M.R., Christopher, M.M. and Shelly, S.M. (2003) Three cases of canine bile peritonitis with mucinous material in abdominal fluid as the prominent cytologic finding. *Veterinary Clinical Pathology* 32(3), 114–120.

Raskin, R.E., Vickers, J., Ward, J.G., Toland, A. and Torrance, A.G. (2019) Optimized immunocytochemistry using leukocyte and tissue markers on Romanowsky-stained slides from dogs and cats. *Veterinary Clinical Pathology* 48(S1), 88–97.

Ryseff, J.K. and Bohn, A.A. (2012) Detection of alkaline phosphatase in canine cells previously stained with Wright–Giemsa and its utility in differentiating osteosarcoma from other mesenchymal tumors. *Veterinary Clinical Pathology* 41(3), 391–395.

Thongtharb, A., Uchida, K., Chambers, J.K. and Nakayama, H. (2017) Variations in histiocytic differentiation of cell lines from canine cerebral and articular histiocytic sarcomas. *Veterinary Pathology* 54(3), 395–404.

Suggested Further Reading

Greene, C.E. (2012) *Infectious Diseases of the Dog and Cat.* 4th edn. Elsevier, St. Louis, Missouri.
Meuten, D.J. (2016) *Tumours in Domestic Animals.* 5th edn. Wiley Blackwell, Ames, Iowa.
Raskin, R., Meyer, D.M. and Boes, K. (2022) *Canine and Feline Cytopathology: A Colour Atlas and Interpretation.* 4th edn. Elsevier, St. Louis, Missouri.
Rizzi, T.E., Valenciano, A., Bowles, M., Cowell, R., Tyler, R. and DeNicola, D.B. (2017) *Atlas of Canine and Feline Urinalysis.* Wiley Blackwell, Hoboken, New Jersey.
Sharkey, L.C., Radin, M.J. and Seelig, D. (2020) *Veterinary Cytology.* Wiley Blackwell, Hoboken, New Jersey.
Valenciano, A.C. and Cowell, R.L. (2020) *Cowell and Tyler's Diagnostic Cytology and Hematology of the Dog and Cat.* 5th edn. Elsevier, St. Louis, Missouri.
Villiers, E. and Ristic, J. (2016) *BSAVA Manual of Canine and Feline Clinical Pathology.* 3rd edn. BSAVA, Gloucester, UK.

Websources

https://eclinpath.com